DISEASE REVIEWS
IN PRIMARY CARE

Concise guides written and peer-reviewed by doctors

Editors:
Dr Scott Chambers
Dr George Kassianos
Dr Jonathan Morrell
Dr Michael Schachter

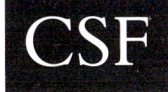

Managing Editor: Dr Scott Chambers
Editorial Controller: Emma Catherall
Operations Manager: Julia Potterton
Designer: Chris Matthews
Typesetter: Julie Smith
Director – Online Business: Peter Llewellyn
Publishing Director: Julian Grover
Publisher: Stephen I'Anson

© 2005 CSF Medical Communications Ltd.

1 Bankside
Lodge Road
Long Hanborough
Oxfordshire
OX29 8LJ, UK

Tel: +44 (0)1993 885370
Fax: +44 (0)1993 881868
Email: *enquiries@csfmedical.com*

www.csfmedical.com

The content of *Disease Reviews in Primary Care* is the work of a number of contributors and has been produced in line with our standard editorial procedures. Whilst every effort has been made to ensure the accuracy of the information at the date of approval for publication, the Authors, the Publisher, the Editors and the Editorial Board accept no responsibility whatsoever for any errors or omissions or for any consequences arising from anything included in or excluded from *Disease Reviews in Primary Care*.

ISBN: 1-905064-83-7

Typeset by Creative, Langbank, Scotland.
Printed and bound in Italy.
Distributed by NBN International, Plymouth, Devon

Contents

Foreword v
Dr Scott Chambers

1. **Allergic rhinitis** 1
   Dr Richard Clark

2. **Alzheimer's dementia** 15
   Dr Richard Clark

3. **Angina** 31
   Dr Richard Clark

4. **Asthma** 49
   Dr Eleanor Bull

5. **Atherothrombosis** 63
   Dr Scott Chambers and Dr Jonathan Morrell

6. **Atopic eczema** 85
   Dr Eleanor Bull and Dr Scott Chambers

7. **Benign prostatic hyperplasia** 101
   Dr Richard Clark

8. **Cholera** 115
   Dr Duncan West

9. **Chronic pain** 129
   Dr Eleanor Bull

10. **COPD** 145
    Dr Susan Chambers and Dr Scott Chambers

11. **Coronary heart disease** 163
    Dr Richard Clark

12. Depression 175
   Dr Richard Clark and Dr Eleanor Bull

13. Diabetes 191
   Dr Richard Clark

14. Erectile dysfunction 203
   Dr Scott Chambers

Foreword

An introduction to *Disease Reviews in Primary Care*

Disease Reviews in Primary Care is a collection of concise, peer-reviewed, disease guides, derived from the medical journal *Drugs in Context*. Published in two volumes, *Disease Reviews in Primary Care* provides a series of structured overviews covering a wide range of diseases that are either directly managed in primary care or are routinely encountered in this setting prior to secondary referral.

Evidence-based peer-reviewed and practice-orientated

Drugs in Context, under the editorship of Dr George Kassianos, Dr Jonathan Morrell and Dr Mike Schachter, was the first medical journal to review the evidence base surrounding various drugs that are used routinely in primary care and to place this evidence in the context of the disease or condition concerned and the practical setting where patients with the condition routinely present. Consequently, *Drugs in Context* is now widely regarded as an invaluable clinical management resource, particularly for healthcare professionals working in the primary-care sector.

The Disease Overview section found in each issue of *Drugs in Context* provides an up-to-date summary of the latest thinking on a specific disease or condition. In response to demand from our readers, we have decided to compile currently published Disease Overviews from *Drugs in Context* into a separate two-volume compendium. We hope that these books will provide you with a readily accessible reference resource for use in your practice, and may prove to be helpful particularly when discussing diagnosis and treatment options with your colleagues and your patients.

Concise and accessible

Each article in *Disease Reviews in Primary Care* focuses on a single condition and highlights key features of the disease in a logical and structured fashion. As such, each review sets out to cover:
- the prevalence and incidence of the condition within the UK, set against the backdrop of its global epidemiology
- the latest thinking on the underlying pathophysiology of the disease
- important risk factors in disease development
- an overview of the aetiology of the condition, including the contribution of genetic and environmental influences

- the clinical presentation of the disease – symptoms and signs
- diagnosis and management, including a discussion of the latest clinical guidelines and management algorithms
- an exploration of the socioeconomic impact of the disease, including quality-of-life issues.

Each disease summary is written by a highly qualified professional writer experienced in medical education and communication, and is peer-reviewed by a clinician with expertise in the clinical field under review. With the inclusion of key references, figures, tables, summaries, key points and call outs, we hope that you find this source of information useful, from both an educational and practical perspective.

Dr Scott Chambers
Managing Editor

1. Allergic rhinitis

Dr Richard Clark
CSF Medical Communications Ltd

Summary

Allergic rhinitis is an extremely common condition which seems to be increasing in prevalence, possibly because of the spread of western lifestyles. However, its prevalence shows a high degree of variability between countries. Allergic rhinitis – whether intermittent (seasonal, for example 'hay fever') or persistent (perennial)[a] – develops after an individual's immune system becomes hypersensitised to an airborne allergen such as pollen or dust mites. The most common symptoms are nasal pruritis, rhinorrhoea, nasal blockage and sneezing. This disease can have a substantial impact on a patient's quality of life. Following a confirmed diagnosis, treatment involves allergen avoidance and pharmacological therapies.

Epidemiology

Allergic rhinitis is an extremely prevalent disease, affecting 10–20% of the UK population and 20–40 million people in the US alone.[1–3] More than 10% of the world's population suffer from allergic rhinitis, though the prevalence shows a high degree of variability between countries, as shown by the International Study of Asthma and Allergies in Childhood (ISAAC).[4,5] The 12-month prevalence of allergic rhinoconjunctivitis in children varies worldwide from 1–40%, with the UK amongst the countries with the highest prevalence (Figure 1).[5,6]

Allergic rhinitis is more common in children than in adults – up to 40% of children are affected compared with 10–30% of adults – and is the most common allergic disease as well as a leading chronic condition in children under 18 years of age.[3] Symptoms generally tend to improve with age, and there is a significant trend for symptom improvement with an earlier onset of the disease.[2]

---

[a]A new subdivision of allergic rhinitis has been established in the *Allergic Rhinitis and its Impact on Asthma (ARIA) guidelines*,[1] with the terms 'intermittent' and 'persistent' replacing 'seasonal' and 'perennial' respectively. These guidelines also classify the severity of the disease as 'mild' or 'moderate–severe'.

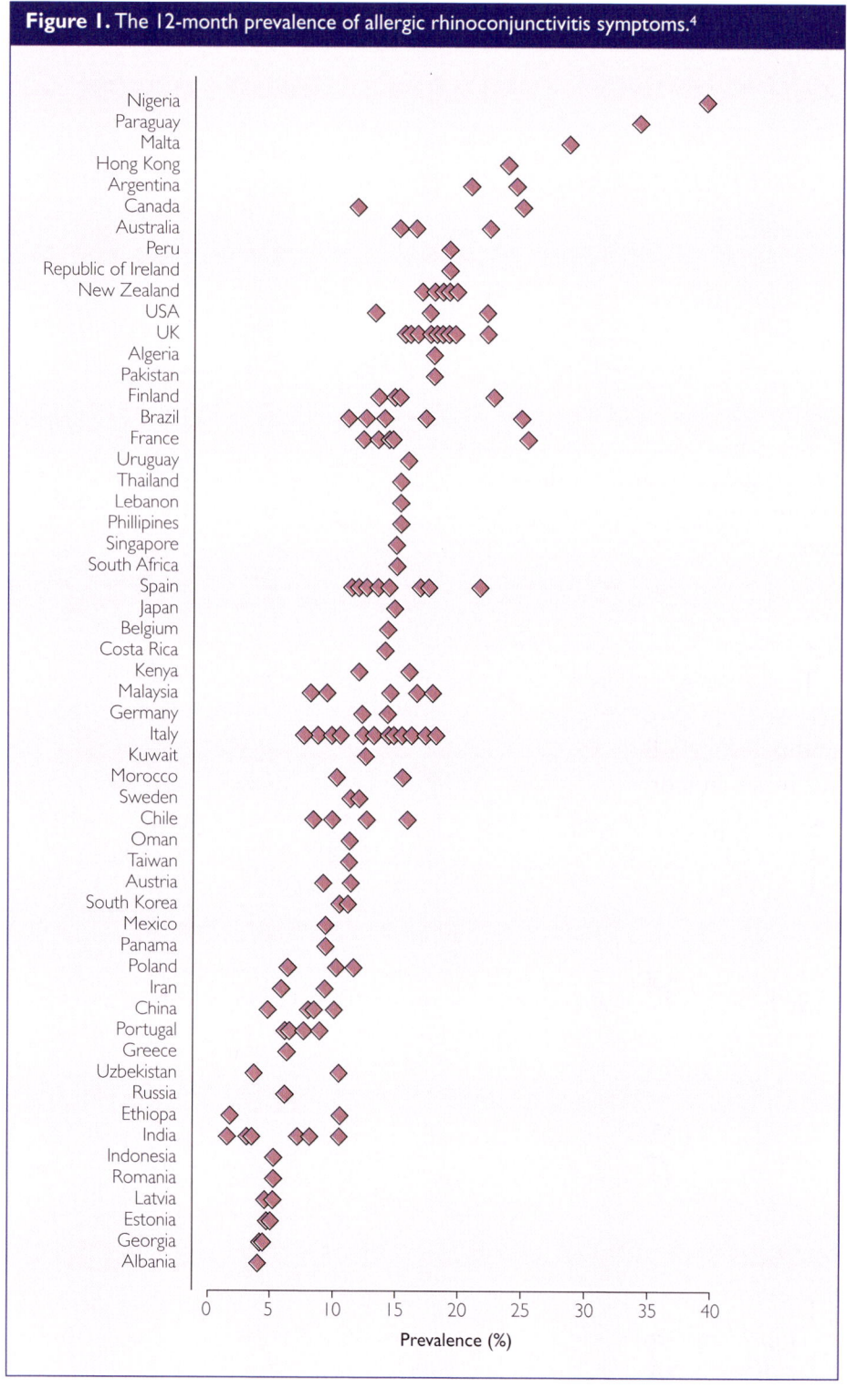

Figure 1. The 12-month prevalence of allergic rhinoconjunctivitis symptoms.[4]

The prevalence of allergic rhinitis is increasing in both adults and children, and is best exemplified by the doubling of the number of children with allergic rhinitis over the past 20 years.[7] Although the cause of this increase is unknown, it is likely to be the result of environmental and lifestyle factors such as higher concentrations of airborne pollution, rising populations of dust mites, poorer ventilation in homes and offices, and dietary factors.[2,7]

Classification

The ARIA guidelines proposed a new classification system for allergic rhinitis.[1] The condition was previously subdivided on the basis of the time of exposure to an allergen into seasonal, perennial and occupational allergic rhinitis. However, the same allergens may be seasonal or irregular in some settings and perennial in others. The new classification system employs symptom and quality-of-life parameters and is based on the duration and severity of the disease. Thus, the condition is subdivided into either 'intermittent' or 'persistent' allergic rhinitis and as either 'mild' or 'moderate–severe' (Table 1). However, the terms seasonal and perennial allergic rhinitis are still commonly used.

The increase in allergens in the home is partly responsible for the increase in the prevalence of allergic rhinitis and other comorbid conditions, including asthma and other allergies. Such allergens include dust mites, indoor moulds, pet-animal dander, cockroaches and other insects.[1,3] Outside the home, common airborne allergens include tree, weed and grass pollen and mould spores.[1,2] Other distinct types of the disease include occupational rhinitis, which is less well documented than

Table 1. Classification of allergic rhinitis.[1]

Intermittent	Persistent
Symptoms are present for: • less than 4 days a week *or* • for less than 4 weeks	Symptoms are present for: • more than 4 days a week *and* • for more than 4 weeks
Mild None of the following is present: • sleep disturbance • impairment of daily activities, leisure and/or sport • impairment of school or work • troublesome symptoms	**Moderate–severe** One or more of the following is present: • sleep disturbance • impairment of daily activities, leisure and/or sport • impairment of school or work • troublesome symptoms

occupational asthma and arises in response to allergens in the workplace (e.g. laboratory animals, wood dust, grains, chemicals, glues, latex and solvents). Drugs such as aspirin and other non-steroidal anti-inflammatory drugs also commonly induce allergic rhinitis. Finally, in rare cases, allergic rhinitis can be triggered through a food allergy.[1]

In addition to airborne allergens, evidence is accumulating that pollutants such as tobacco smoke and urban pollution (e.g. vehicle exhaust fumes, ozone, and nitrogen and sulphur dioxides) may aggravate nasal symptoms in patients with allergic rhinitis.

Pathophysiology

Allergic rhinitis can be defined as an allergen-driven mucosal inflammation resulting from the complex interplay between inflammatory cells, inflammatory mediators and cytokines.[8] It develops after an individual's immune system becomes hypersensitised to an airborne allergen such as pollen or dust mites. Sensitisation occurs when long-term exposure to threshold concentrations of an allergen leads to presentation of the allergen by antigen-presenting cells to T-helper lymphocyte 2 cells.[3,9] These lymphocytes then release the mediators interleukins-3, -4 and -5 and other cytokines,[9] which drive pro-inflammatory processes (e.g. immunoglobulin [IgE] production) against these allergens through the action of mast cells, plasma cells and eosinophils.[3]

Once an individual is sensitised to a particular allergen, subsequent exposure triggers a cascade of events resulting in allergic rhinitis. The allergic symptoms of this disease comprise early and late phases. The early phase can start within minutes of contact with an allergen, and is characterised by sneezing, rhinorrhoea, nasal obstruction and occasionally pruritus.[1] These events are triggered by an interaction between the allergen and mast-cell-bound antibodies, followed by mast cell degranulation, resulting in the liberation of pro-inflammatory molecules such as histamine, leukotrienes, prostaglandins and platelet-activating factor (Figure 2).[10] Histamine in particular has a key role in increasing vasodilation (causing sinusoidal filling, occlusion and congestion of nasal airways), vascular permeability (causing watery rhinorrhoea), mucus secretion and bronchoconstriction.[10]

The late-phase response occurs in approximately 35% of those experiencing the early-phase response and occurs within 4–10 hours of allergen exposure.[1,9] Clinically, this phase is distinct from the early-phase response, as nasal obstruction is the predominant symptom.[3] The late-phase reaction is characterised by an influx of inflammatory cells (eosinophils, T-

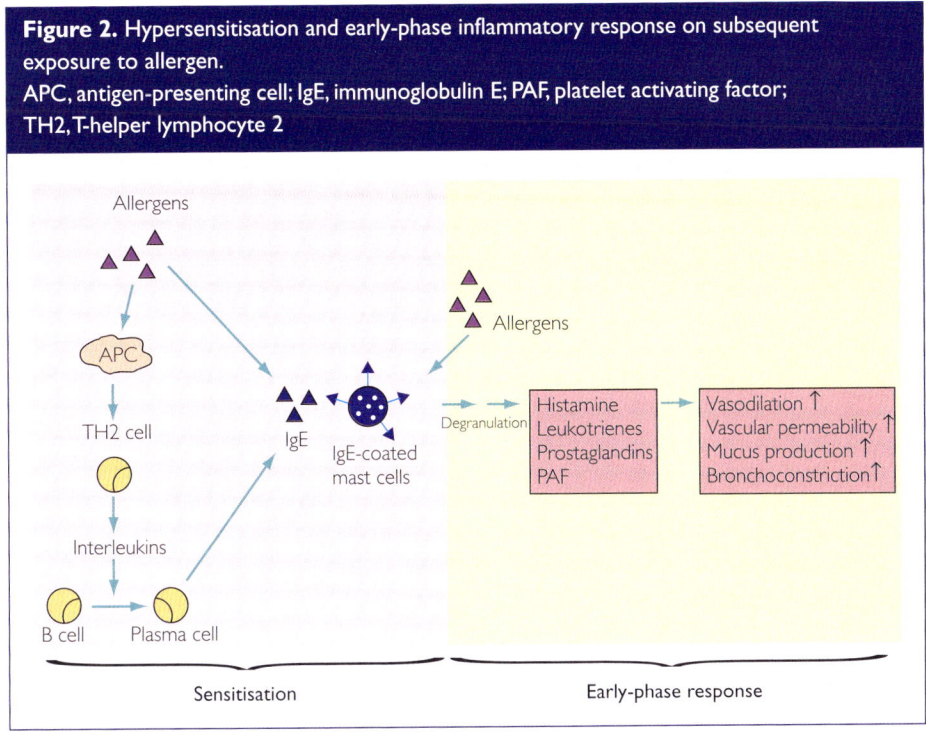

Figure 2. Hypersensitisation and early-phase inflammatory response on subsequent exposure to allergen.
APC, antigen-presenting cell; IgE, immunoglobulin E; PAF, platelet activating factor; TH2, T-helper lymphocyte 2

lymphocytes, basophils and neutrophils) at the site of the allergic reaction, with cytokines and chemokines playing a key role in the recruitment, activation and perpetuation of these cells.[1,10] Chronic inflammation may arise if the allergic response is perpetuated by inflammatory cells following the late-phase response period, and results in airway hyper-reactivity, tissue damage and chronic allergic disease.[3,10]

Risk factors

The prevalence of allergic rhinitis is greatest in:
- higher socioeconomic classes
- non-whites
- polluted areas
- people with a family history of allergy, particularly allergic rhinitis
- people with positive allergy skin tests
- firstborn children
- those born during the pollen season
- those with asthma
- children who are introduced early to foods or formula food, rather than being breast-fed

- those exposed to indoor allergens (e.g. animal dander and dust mites) during childhood
- children with high serum IgE levels (>100 IU/mL) before 6 years of age.[1,3]

Symptoms

The clinical presentation of allergic rhinitis varies depending on the duration of allergen exposure, age and extent of comorbid disease. However, patients with rhinitis can usually be subdivided into 'sneezers and runners' and 'blockers', with those in the 'sneezer and runner' group the most likely to have allergic rhinitis (Table 2).[1] Rhinorrhoea is more common in intermittent than persistent allergic rhinitis, whilst nasal obstruction is associated with the latter form of the disease.[1,11]

The symptoms of allergic rhinitis most easily recognised in adults include nasal pruritis, rhinorrhoea, nasal blockage and sneezing, whereas a wide spectrum of symptoms makes the diagnosis of this disease in children more difficult.[12] Children with allergic rhinitis may suffer from coughing, sneezing, nasal pruritus, nasal congestion, sore throat, halitosis, respiratory distress (in infants), hypernasality and behavioural problems.[12] Although older children with allergic rhinitis may blow their noses frequently, younger children are more likely to sniff, snort and repetitively clear their throats.[3] Nasal pruritis may stimulate grimacing, twitching and picking of the nose, resulting in nose bleeds.[3]

Patients may develop 'shiners' (oedema and darkened tissues under the eyes caused by venous congestion), and whilst being strongly suggestive of allergic rhinitis, this symptom can also be found in patients with chronic non-allergic rhinitis and/or sinusitis.[3,4] Another characteristic of this disease is the 'allergic salute', namely the upward rubbing of the nose with the palm

> The symptoms of allergic rhinitis most easily recognised in adults include nasal pruritis, rhinorrhoea, nasal blockage and sneezing ... a wide spectrum of symptoms makes diagnosis in children more difficult.

Table 2. Clinical symptoms of allergic rhinitis.[1]

'Sneezers and runners'	'Blockers'
Sneezing	Little/no sneezing
Watery mucus (running nose)	Thick nasal mucus (catarrh)
Anterior ± posterior rhinorrhoea	More often posterior rhinorrhoea
Itchy nose	No itching
Nasal blockage (variable)	Nasal blockage often severe
Frequently associated with conjunctivitis	Not associated with conjunctivitis

in an attempt to relieve pruritis, which can result in a permanent line, the *linea nasalis*, in the supratip crease area.[4]

Chronic symptoms of allergic rhinitis include sleep disturbance caused by snoring, itself a consequence of nasal congestion, leading to daytime somnolence and an inability to concentrate.[3,12] Patients' quality of life can be profoundly affected by allergic rhinitis.[13] In fact, this impact on quality of life can be as great as or even greater than that seen in asthma. Adults may experience fatigue, low energy and a decrease in social functioning, whilst children can suffer from learning impairment, an inability to integrate with their peers, anxiety and family dysfunction.[13]

> Impact on quality of life can be as great as or even greater than that seen in asthma.

Diagnostic tests

The diagnosis of allergic rhinitis is normally relatively straightforward, but can be complex in certain cases. The mainstay of diagnosis is an accurate patient history, which should include social, medical and family history, medications used, seasonal variations and any palliating or precipitating factors.[4] The presence of lower respiratory tract disease, skin symptoms and pollen-related food allergies should always be investigated, as they are commonly associated with this disease.[11] A complete head and neck examination is vital and should include visualisation of the anterior nares with a light source and nasal speculum; flexible or rigid nasal endoscopy may also be used.[4] The nasopharynx, oral cavity and hypopharynx should be examined, an otoscope used to evaluate the effects of nasal disease on auditory tube function and the turbinate mucosa checked using a cotton-tipped palpitator to distinguish any swelling from a bony abnormality.[4] Septal deformity in particular should be excluded before a diagnosis of allergic rhinitis is made.[4]

If an allergy is suspected, diagnostic testing is ideally required to confirm the presence or absence of allergic disease. The goal of specific antigen testing is to determine which, if any, antigenic substance is causing the patient's symptoms. These tests usually take the form of a skin-prick test or a laboratory (*in vivo*) test. The skin-prick test involves placing a drop of antigen on the skin then passing a solid needle (lancet) through the droplet to deliver the antigenic substance to the dermal layer.[4] As there are many complexicites to the performance and interpretation of such tests, it is generally recommended that they are performed by appropriately trained healthcare professionals. Laboratory testing generally takes the form of a serum immunoassay (usually of antigen-specific IgE) and is of similar value to skin tests but provides quantitative results. However, laboratory tests may be preferable if:

- patients are uncooperative (e.g. frightened children)
- the patient cannot or did not discontinue antihistamines or other interfering medications
- the patient has a history of severe allergic reactions, with anaphylaxis as a possible risk
- abnormal skin reactivity is a concern.[3,4]

However, in the majority of cases an accurate diagnosis can be made from the skin-prick test in conjunction with a patient's history and a physical examination.[4] Allergens used for skin testing should be selected for each patient on the basis of their prevalence in the patient's geographic area, home and school environment.[3] The most useful allergens for skin-prick testing are shown in Table 3.[3] A further advantage of specific antigen testing is that it can help to convince the patient and their family of the allergy diagnosis and the subsequent need for environmental control and/or treatment.[3] Finally, nasal challenge tests may be helpful to identify occupational rhinitis.

Comorbidity

Allergic rhinitis can result in a chronic state of nasal inflammation and obstruction which is also associated with a number of other conditions affecting the upper and lower respiratory tract. In fact, a number of diseases are highly comorbid with allergic rhinitis and include:
- asthma
- eczema
- otitis media
- sinusitis
- conjunctivitis
- nasal polyps.

Most importantly, there is a particularly high degree of comorbidity between allergic rhinitis and asthma, which has been shown in many

Table 3. Common allergens used for testing intermittent and persistent allergic rhinitis.[3]

Intermittent	Persistent
Weed pollen	House-dust mite (dermatophygoides)
Grass pollen	Animal dander
Tree pollen	Fungi (moulds)

epidemiological studies. Most patients with allergic and non-allergic asthma have rhinitis, whilst many patients with allergic rhinitis have asthma.[14] Asthma is arguably the most serious of the allergic diseases, causing 100,000 hospitalisations per year in England and Wales, and can be fatal.[15] A 23-year follow-up study of people who had allergic rhinitis as college undergraduates showed that only 14% of those with asthma did not have allergic rhinitis and that asthma occurred in 21% of individuals with allergic rhinitis.[14] Amongst individuals with both asthma and allergic rhinitis, improvement in allergic rhinitis was associated with a resolution of asthma symptoms, whereas a worsening of allergic rhinitis was associated with the persistence of asthma symptoms.[16] Furthermore, countries with a low incidence of asthma (<5%, e.g. Albania and Romania) have a low incidence of allergic rhinitis (<6%), whilst countries with the highest incidence of asthma (>30%, e.g. Australia and UK) have some of the highest prevalences of allergic rhinitis (15–20%).[1,5]

Several theories have been proposed to explain these comorbidities, such as the 'one airway, one disease' approach, stating that diseases of both the upper and lower respiratory tract (e.g. allergic rhinitis and asthma) are both clinical manifestations of the same (allergic respiratory) disease.[17] Upper and lower airways are considered to be affected by a common, evolving inflammatory process. Although it is unknown whether aggressive treatment of allergic rhinitis can help prevent asthma, effective treatment may help reduce morbidity associated with other comorbid disorders, including asthma.[17,18] Treatment for allergic rhinitis in patients with comorbid asthma has been associated with up to a 50% risk reduction of asthma-related adverse events.[18] However, the new asthma guidelines developed by the British Thoracic Society/Scottish Intercollegiate Guideline Network did not recognise that treating one condition benefited the other.[19]

Pharmacoeconomics

Pharmacoeconomic data for allergic rhinitis are limited. In the US, direct costs (physician visits, laboratory tests and medication) for intermittent allergic rhinitis were approximately US$1.23 billion in 1994, whilst indirect costs associated with decreased productivity accounted for a further US$1000 per worker per year.[20]

Treatment options

Allergen avoidance

Allergen-avoidance measures should be undertaken in all cases of allergic rhinitis confirmed by specific antigen testing,[1] though evidence demonstrating benefit for appropriate techniques is somewhat limited. Of course, it is not possible to avoid allergens completely, but reducing exposure ('environmental control') can reduce the severity of symptoms and the need for pharmacological treatment.[1,8,11] Protective face masks or eye glasses, closing windows during the day and use of car pollen filters may be helpful for patients suffering from intermittent allergic rhinitis during the summer months.[1] Patients with persistent allergic rhinitis may benefit from using vacuum cleaners with high-efficiency particulate air filtration to reduce the allergen load indoors, together with the destruction of house-dust mites by washing bed linen at temperatures above 55°C.[1] The replacement of carpets with vinyl or polished wood floors may also be of benefit.[1]

Pharmacological treatments

The main pharmacological treatment options and their efficacy in relieving the various symptoms of allergic rhinitis are summarised in Table 4.[21] Second-generation oral antihistamines are considered effective agents in the treatment of mild-to-moderate allergic rhinitis as they relieve symptoms of nasal itching, sneezing and rhinorrhoea, though they are less effective for the treatment of nasal congestion.[11] Thus, combinations of oral antihistamines and decongestants are commonly prescribed in many countries, though such an approach has some associated hazards.[1] First-generation antihistamines should be avoided because of their unfavourable risk–benefit ratio, since they show poor selectivity, and sedative and anticholinergic effects.[1] Intranasal antihistamines may be useful as 'on-demand' medication in addition to oral therapy as they have a rapid onset

> Second-generation oral antihistamines are considered effective agents in the treatment of mild-to-moderate allergic rhinitis.

Table 4. Characteristics of pharmacological treatments for allergic rhinitis.[21]

Characteristic	Oral antihistamine	Nasal antihistamine	Nasal steroid	Nasal decongestant	Ipratropium bromide	Nasal cromone
Rhinorrhoea	++	++	+++	0	++	+
Sneezing	++	++	+++	0	0	+
Itching	++	++	+++	0	0	+
Nasal blockage	+	+	+++	++++	0	+
Eye symptoms	++	0	++	0	0	0
Onset of action	1 hour	15 minutes	12 hours	5–15 minutes	15–30 minutes	Variable
Duration of action (hours)	12–24	6–12	12–48	3–6	4–12	Variable

0, no effect; +, marginal effect; ++++, substantial effect.

of action; however, they have no effect against non-nasal symptoms such as conjunctivitis.[1]

Intranasal corticosteroids are particularly effective for the symptomatic relief of allergic rhinitis and are the treatment of choice for patients with moderate or severe symptoms.[8] However, for patients with intermittent allergic rhinitis, therapy should start before contact with allergens, as there is a delay in the onset of action. Several concerns have been raised about the safety of long-term use of intranasal corticosteroids because of cumulative dosing effects. Effects reported include adrenal suppression and reduced bone density and growth retardation in children.[22] Thus, high doses of corticosteroids for long periods should be avoided, and children's height should be monitored regularly.[23] Oral corticosteroids are not recommended beyond the short-term treatment of severe exacerbations of rhinitis that fail to respond to other treatments.[11] Oral or intramuscular corticosteroids should not be regarded as first-line treatment for allergic rhinitis but as a last resort.[11]

Anticholinergic agents (e.g. ipratropium bromide) may be useful in controlling the symptoms of rhinitis, though little information is available regarding their efficacy in allergic rhinitis.[11] Ipratropium bromide only improves symptoms of nasal hypersecretion in persistent allergic rhinitis, and so other drugs are preferable in the majority of cases.[11]

Mast cell stabilisers such as disodium cromoglycate given intranasally are well tolerated, though are not as effective as corticosteroids or antihistamines, and their usefulness is limited by the need for frequent administration.[8,11] Thus, this category of agents is not considered to be a major therapeutic option in the treatment of allergic rhinitis, though they may be useful in mild childhood rhinitis.[8,11]

Decongestants are very effective in treating symptoms of nasal obstruction resulting from allergic rhinitis. However, prolonged use of topical decongestants (>10 days) should be avoided as this can lead to tachyphylaxis, rebound swelling of the nasal mucosa and 'drug-induced rhinitis'.[11] Immunotherapy may also be considered, particularly for patients in whom allergy avoidance and pharmacological measures provide insufficient control.[11]

An algorithm for the diagnosis and management of allergic rhinitis is shown in Figure 3.[21]

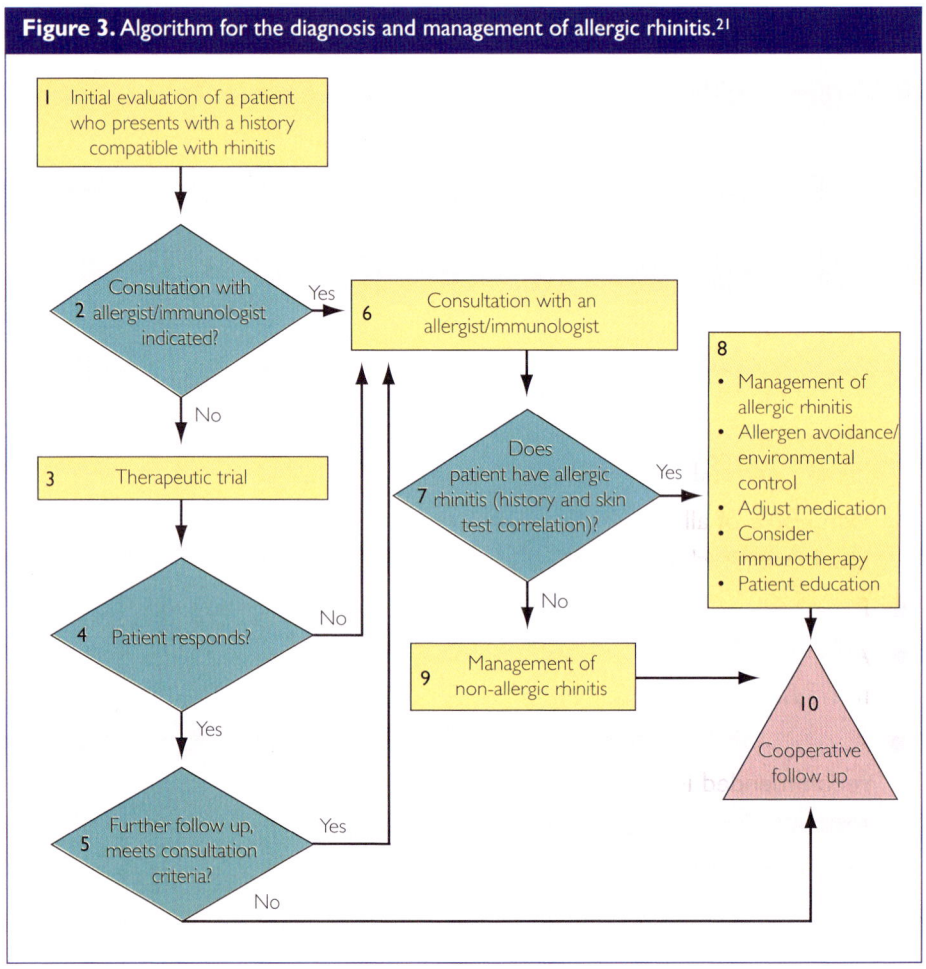

Figure 3. Algorithm for the diagnosis and management of allergic rhinitis.[21]

Key points

- Allergic rhinitis is an extremely prevalent disease, affecting 10–20% of the UK population and over 10% of the world's population.
- The prevalence of allergic rhinitis seems to be increasing, possibly because of the spread of western lifestyles.
- Allergic rhinitis is more common in children and is the most common allergic disease, as well as a leading chronic condition, in children under 18 years of age.
- In general, symptoms of allergic rhinitis tend to improve with age.
- Allergic rhinitis develops after an individual's immune system becomes hypersensitised to an airborne allergen such as pollen or dust mites.
- Symptoms of allergic rhinitis most easily recognised in adults include nasal pruritis, rhinorrhoea, nasal blockage and sneezing.
- Patients' quality of life can be profoundly affected by allergic rhinitis.
- A number of diseases are highly comorbid with allergic rhinitis, most notably asthma.
- Allergen-avoidance measures and pharmacological treatments are recommended in cases of allergic rhinitis confirmed by specific antigen testing.
- Second-generation antihistamines are considered effective agents in mild-to-moderate, intermittent and persistent allergic rhinitis.

References

1. Bousquet J, Van Cauwenberge P, Khaltaev N; ARIA Workshop Group; World Health Organization. Allergic rhinitis and its impact on asthma. *J Allergy Clin Immunol* 2001; **108(5 Suppl)**: S147–334.
2. Schoenwetter WF. Allergic rhinitis: epidemiology and natural history. *Allergy Asthma Proc* 2000; **21**: 1–6.
3. Skoner DP. Allergic rhinitis: definition, epidemiology, pathophysiology, detection and diagnosis. *J Allergy Clin Immunol* 2001; **108**: S2–8.
4. Fornadley JA, Corey JP, Osguthorpe JD *et al*. Allergic rhinitis. Clinical practice guideline. *Otolaryngol Head Neck Surg* 1996; **115**: 115–22.
5. The International Study of Asthma and Allergies in Childhood (ISAAC) Steering Committee. Worldwide variation in prevalence of symptoms of asthma, allergic rhinoconjunctivitis, and atopic eczema. *Lancet* 1998; **351**: 1225–32.
6. Strachan D, Sibbald B, Weiland S *et al*. Worldwide variations in prevalence of symptoms of allergic rhinoconjunctivitis in children: the International Study of Asthma and Allergies in Childhood (ISAAC). *Pediatr Allergy Immunol* 1997; **8**: 161–76.
7. Ceuppens J. Western lifestyle, local defenses and the rising incidence of allergic rhinitis. *Acta Otorhinolaryngol Belg* 2000; **54**: 391–5.
8. Dykewicz MS, Fineman S. Executive summary of joint task force practice parameters on diagnosis and management of rhinitis. *Ann Allergy Asthma Immunol* 1998; **81**: 463–8.
9. Virant FS. Allergic rhinitis. *Immunol Allergy Clin North Am* 2000; **20**: 265–82.
10. Salmun LM. Antihistamines in late-phase clinical development for allergic disease. *Expert Opin Invest Drugs* 2002; **11**: 259–73.
11. van Cauwenberge P, Bachert C, Passalacqua G *et al*. Consensus statement on the treatment of allergic rhinitis. European Academy of Allergology and Clinical Immunology. *Allergy* 2000; **55**: 116–34.
12. Lack G. Pediatric allergic rhinitis and comorbid disorders. *J Allergy Clin Immunol* 2001; **108**: S9–15.
13. Meltzer EO. Quality of life in adults and children with allergic rhinitis. *J Allergy Clin Immunol* 2001; **108**: S45–53.
14. Greisner WA 3rd, Settipane RJ, Settipane GA. Co-existence of asthma and allergic rhinitis: a 23-year follow-up study of college students. *Allergy Asthma Proc* 1998; **19**: 185–8.
15. Jarvis D, Burney P. ABC of allergies. The epidemiology of allergic disease. *BMJ* 1998; **316**: 607–10.
16. Greisner WA 3rd, Settipane RJ, Settipane GA. The course of asthma parallels that of allergic rhinitis: a 23-year follow-up study of college students. *Allergy Asthma Proc* 2000; **21**: 371–5.
17. Corren J. The link between allergic rhinitis and asthma, otitis media, sinusitis and nasal polyps. *Immunol Allergy Clin North Am* 2000; **20**: 445–60.
18. Fuhlbrigge AL, Adams RJ. The effect of treatment of allergic rhinitis on asthma morbidity, including emergency department visits. *Curr Opin Allergy Immunol* 2003; **3**: 29–32.
19. The BTS/SIGN guidelines on the management of asthma. *Thorax* 2003; **58(Suppl 1)**; i1–94.
20. Blaiss MS. Cognitive, social and economic costs of allergic rhinitis. *Allergy Asthma Proc* 2000; **21**: 7–13.
21. Prodigy Guidance – Allergic Rhinitis. April 2002. *http://www.prodigy.nhs.uk/guidance.asp?gt=Allergic%20rhinitis*
22. Committee on the Safety of Medicines. The safety of inhaled and nasal corticosteroids. *Curr Probl Pharmacovigilance* 1998; **24**: 8.
23. Cave A, Arlett P, Lee E. Inhaled and nasal corticosteroids: factors affecting the risks of systemic adverse effects. *Pharmacol Ther* 1999; **83**: 153–79.

Acknowledgements

Figure 1 is adapted from Fornadley *et al.*, 1996.[4]
Figure 3 is adapted from Prodigy Guidance, 2002.[21]

2. Alzheimer's dementia

Dr Richard Clark
CSF Medical Communications Ltd

Summary

Alzheimer's disease is a progressive neurodegenerative disorder, resulting in the syndrome of Alzheimer's dementia. The most common form of dementia, Alzheimer's accounts for about 65% of all dementias and can be either familial or sporadic in nature. Familial Alzheimer's disease is relatively uncommon and predominantly affects patients under the age of 65 years, whereas the sporadic form is rare in people under 60 years of age, yet affects one person in 20 aged over 65 years and one person in five over 80 years of age. Symptoms of Alzheimer's disease are revealed gradually such that a close family member rather than the sufferers themselves are often first to notice a change in personality. In fact, the early symptoms of Alzheimer's disease are frequently mistaken for signs of the normal ageing process or other conditions such as depression. As the disease progresses, patients experience increased memory loss such that they will eventually fail to recognise close family and friends. They also need more and more help to perform normal daily tasks, and eventually become totally dependent on others for nursing care. The economic burden on society is huge as long-term nursing care is costly. Alzheimer's disease is a life-shortening illness, with death usually occurring within 5–10 years of diagnosis. As the disease itself is irreversible, treatments for Alzheimer's dementia address cognitive and behavioural symptoms. Non-pharmacological treatments involve the manipulation of the patient's environment and the introduction of structured behaviours and activities. Most current pharmacological treatments are focused on reducing the cholinergic deficit (i.e. by using cholinesterase inhibitors). Drugs of this class, of which there are three approved treatments currently available for mild or moderate dementia, have shown efficacy in stabilising – and in some patients improving – the decline in cognitive function, delaying the need for placement in a nursing home and improving disruptive behaviours.

The burden and impact of Alzheimer's disease

Alzheimer's disease is a progressive neurodegenerative disorder, causing the syndrome of Alzheimer's dementia (Table 1).[1] Alzheimer's dementia is defined clinically by a gradual decline in memory, plus at least one other area of higher intellectual function.[2] The domains affected are cognition (e.g. memory loss, impaired judgement and disorientation), daily functioning (e.g. difficulty in performing normal day-to-day activities, such as washing/bathing, dressing) and behaviour (e.g. changes in mood, personality and loss of initiative) (Table 2).[2,3] Onset may occur from the age of 45, but usually occurs after 65 years.[4] The early onset of the disease, before 65 years of age, is strongly associated with familial inheritance. It is

Table 1. Definitions of dementia, Alzheimer's dementia and Alzheimer's disease.

Term	Definition
Alzheimer's disease	Progressive neurodegeneration with distinctive histopathology
Alzheimer's dementia	The symptoms of Alzheimer's disease, marked by a gradual decline in memory, plus at least one other area of higher intellectual function
Dementia	Chronic or persistent disorder of the mental processes marked by memory disorders, personality changes, impaired reasoning etc. due to injury or brain disease, the most common form of which is Alzheimer's dementia

Table 2. The domains of function and symptoms of Alzheimer's dementia.

Domains affected	Symptoms
Cognition	Memory loss Language problems Disorientation Impaired judgement Misplacing items
Function	Difficulties in performing day-to-day activities: • instrumental activities of daily living (ADL) • basic activities of daily living Difficulties in performing complex tasks
Behaviour	Changes in mood or behaviour: • aggression, agitation, depression Changes in personality Loss of initiative

important, in terms of treatment approaches, to distinguish Alzheimer's dementia from other common forms of dementia, which include vascular, Lewy body and fronto-temporal dementias, including Pick's disease (Figure 1).[5] Some patients may present with a combination of dementia-related diseases.

Dementia is a common disorder, affecting approximately 18 million people worldwide, with figures predicted to nearly double to 34 million by 2025 in line with shifting population demographics.[6] In the UK, the prevalence of dementia is about 1%, and there are currently over 775,000 cases of dementia.[5,7] By 2010 there will be about 840,000 people with dementia in the UK, a figure that is expected to rise to over 1.5 million cases by 2050.[5]

Dementia is comparatively rare in people under 60 years of age, but its prevalence increases sharply with advancing age amongst those in their 70s and 80s (Figure 2).[8,9] Dementia affects one person in 20 aged over 65 years and one person in five over 80 years of age.[5] Alzheimer's dementia is the most common type of dementia, accounting for over half of all cases. Overall, most studies show that Alzheimer's dementia is as common in men as in women, though some evidence suggests a slightly higher prevalence rate may occur amongst women.[6,9]

The Audit Commission has estimated that dementia costs the UK £6.1 billion annually (1998–99 prices), with £3.3 billion as direct spend by the NHS and social services.[10,11] Patients with dementia are about four-times more likely than those without dementia to require institutionalised care, and institutionalisation is responsible for the largest proportion of costs.[12] The pharmacological treatment of Alzheimer's disease with cholinesterase inhibitors can reduce the economic burden of the disease by delaying

> In the UK, the prevalence of dementia is about 1%, and there are over 775,000 cases of dementia.

> Dementia costs the UK £6.1 billion a year, with £3.3 billion as direct spend by the NHS and social services.

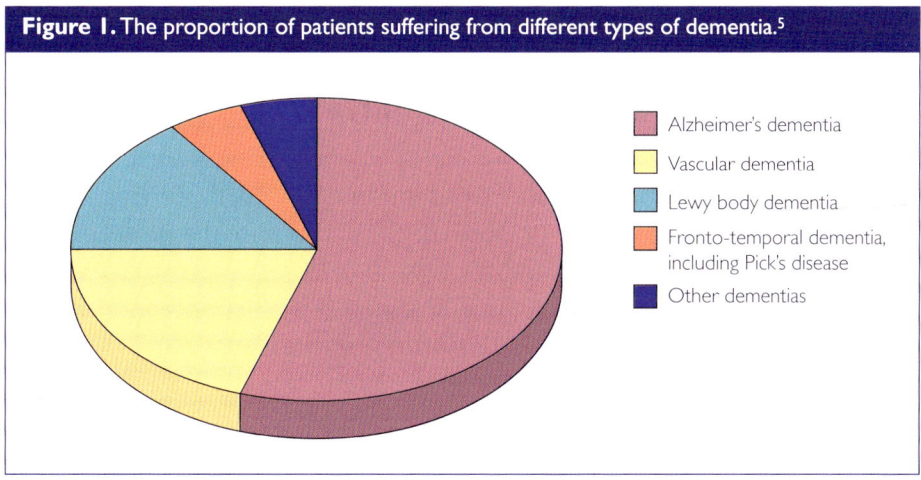

Figure 1. The proportion of patients suffering from different types of dementia.[5]

- Alzheimer's dementia
- Vascular dementia
- Lewy body dementia
- Fronto-temporal dementia, including Pick's disease
- Other dementias

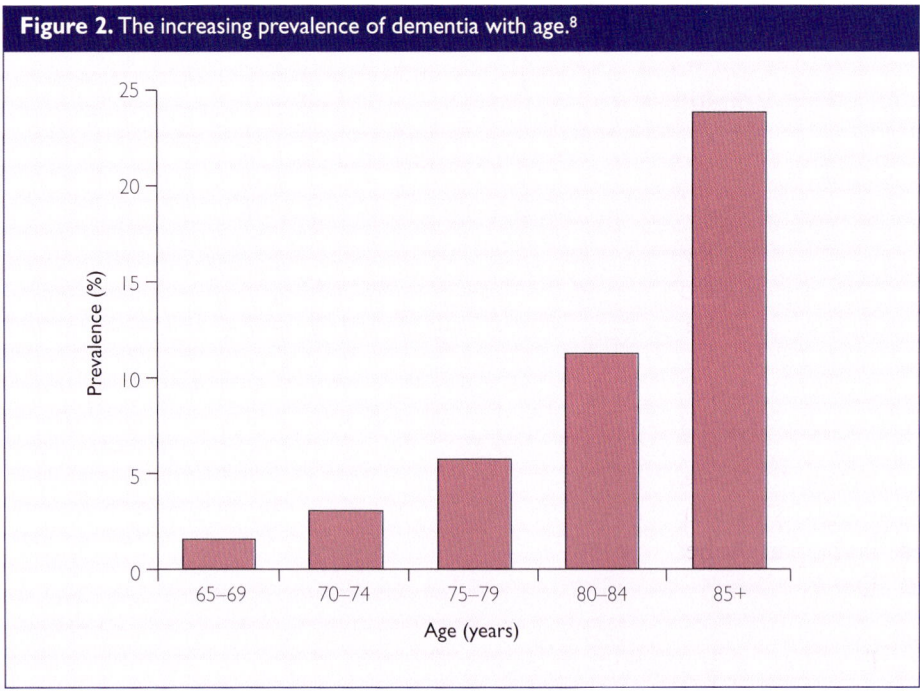

Figure 2. The increasing prevalence of dementia with age.[8]

patients' progression to the nursing home, as reported by a study of tacrine, rivastigmine and in particular, donepezil.[13] Thus, although the annual cost to the NHS of prescribing a cholinesterase inhibitor for Alzheimer's disease is estimated at about £800–1200 per patient, a delay of 12 weeks in nursing home placement would accrue a saving of £4500 per patient.[11,14] The cost of treating Alzheimer's disease increases with the severity of the disease state, as evidenced by the increased costs associated with increments in the Neuropsychiatric Inventory (NPI) scale.[15] Patients with advanced disease are more expensive to treat in terms of their use of hospital resources, the number of physician consultations and the caregiver burden.[16]

Diagnosis and measuring dementia

The symptoms of Alzheimer's disease start gradually and as patients are generally unaware of the gradual deterioration in their memory, it is common for a family member or close friend to recognise the problem.[17] It is important that the emergence of memory and cognitive deficits, as indicators of Alzheimer's disease, are differentiated from other possible causes of cognitive decline, which may include old age, depression, hypercalcaemia and side-effects from concomitant medications. The term mild cognitive impairment (MCI) was proposed to describe the transitional state between normal cognition and Alzheimer's disease. Conventionally defined MCI has reasonable predictive value and specificity for Alzheimer's disease with an estimated 8% of MCI patients converting annually.[18] However, not all patients with MCI and the worsening of episodic memory will convert to Alzheimer's disease.[19]

Since approximately 74% of dementia patients will first present to a doctor in a primary-care setting, GPs, in particular, should be aware of signs that are indicative of Alzheimer's disease.[20] The following points are worthwhile of consideration during a consultation.

- Although a patient may not look ill, has a relative or close friend noticed a change in their personality or memory impairment?
- Does the patient have a tendency to look at an accompanying relative or friend when asked a question?
- Does the patient have difficulty recalling the current date?
- Is the patient hesitant in their use of language?
- Do they have a tendency to minimalise/rationalise symptoms?

Prior to referral to a specialist, patients with suspected Alzheimer's disease should undergo routine blood tests, including:
- a full blood count for macrocytotic anaemia, suggesting vitamin B_{12}/folate deficiency (or an excessive consumption of alcohol)
- thyroid function tests to exclude hypothyroidism
- a fasting blood glucose test
- a serum calcium test.[4]

Importantly, there is an average delay of 4 months from the first onset of noticeable Alzheimer's disease to the first appointment with a doctor, and a 1-year delay from noticing the first symptoms to diagnosis.[20] This emphasizes the importance of the early initiation of treatment for Alzheimer's disease in order to obtain maximum therapeutic benefit (e.g. delaying the progression of Alzheimer's disease and increasing the length of time prior to nursing home placement).[20]

Clinical assessment using rating scales and other assessment tools remains the cornerstone of the diagnostic approach to Alzheimer's disease, although concerns as to the validity and relevance of such scales to the patient population have been voiced. The increased use of positron emission tomography (PET) and magnetic resonance imaging (MRI) to identify changes in glucose metabolism and brain atrophy and the analysis of biomarkers in cerebrospinal fluid and blood serum (e.g. β-amyloid, total and phospho-tau protein) may improve the sensitivity and specificity of diagnosis in the future.

There is an average delay of 1 year from first noticing Alzheimer's disease to its diagnosis.

The International Statistical Classification of Diseases and Related Health Problems, (tenth edition; ICD-10) outlines criteria for a formal diagnosis of Alzheimer's disease.[1]

(1) The presence of dementia:
- disturbance of higher cortical functions including memory, thinking, orientation, comprehension, calculation, learning capacity, language and judgement
- consciousness is not clouded
- impairments of cognitive function are commonly accompanied and occasionally preceded by deterioration in emotional control, social behaviour or motivation
- interference with personal activities of daily living such as washing, dressing, eating, personal hygiene, excretory and toilet activities may occur.

(2) Insidious onset with slow deterioration.

(3) Absence of clinical evidence, or findings from special investigations, that the mental state may be due to other systemic or brain disease which can induce dementia (e.g. hypothyroidism, hypercalcaemia, vitamin B_{12} deficiency, niacin deficiency, neurosyphilis, normal pressure hydrocephalus or subdural haematoma).

(4) Absence of a sudden, apoplectic onset, or of neurological signs of focal damage such as hemiparesis, sensory loss, visual field defects and incoordination occurring early in the illness (although these phenomena may be superimposed later).[1]

A diagnosis of Alzheimer's disease can also be made using criteria set out by the National Institute for Neurological and Communicative Disorders and Stroke – Alzheimer's Disease and Related Disorders Association (NINDS ADRDA), which emphasises memory loss as the main feature to distinguish Alzheimer's dementia from other forms of dementia. The Diagnostic and Statistical Manual of Mental Disorders (fourth edition; DSM-IV) defines Alzheimer's disease by assessing the severity of cognitive and non-cognitive impairment and classifies Alzheimer's disease according to the age of onset of symptoms and the presence or absence of behavioural disturbances.

The most widely used test for screening patients in whom dementia is suspected is the Mini-Mental Status Examination (MMSE).[17] However, the MMSE is relatively insensitive in patients with severe dementia, for whom the Severe Impairment Battery (SIB), which evaluates cognitive aptitudes and other skills, is more appropriate. The MMSE has a maximum (best) score of 30, and can be used to grade Alzheimer's disease:
- mild – MMSE score 21–26
- moderate – MMSE score 12–20

- moderately severe – MMSE score 10–11
- severe – MMSE score of nine or less.[14]

Of the components of the MMSE, the clock-drawing test – used as a cognitive screening instrument – is the most useful and simplistic. Commonly, the fourth quadrant of the clock shows the greatest sensitivity for dementia. Although the MMSE is a good test of cognitive function, it takes up to 10 minutes to complete and so does not fit easily into a standard primary-care consultation. In contrast, the Abbreviated Mental Test Score (AMTS) consists of 10 questions and can be completed during a standard GP consultation (Figure 3).

Figure 3. The Abbreviated Mental Test Score (AMTS).

Each correctly answered question scores one point

1. Age
2. Time to nearest hour
3. An address – for example 42 West Street – to be repeated by the patient at the end of the test
4. Year
5. Name of hospital, residential institution or home address, depending on where the patient is situated
6. Recognition of two persons – for example, doctor, nurse, home help etc.
7. Date of birth
8. Year First World War started
9. Name of present monarch
10. Count backwards from 20 to 1

Total score _____

(A score of less than six is suggestive of dementia.)

Course, symptoms and prognosis

As Alzheimer's disease is progressive, the structure and chemistry of the brain become increasingly altered over time. As a consequence of these changes, Alzheimer's disease is usually considered as three stages – early, middle and late. However, in some individuals certain symptoms may appear earlier, later or not at all, and various stages may overlap.[5] The behavioural and psychological symptoms of dementia (BPSD) can occur and disappear during the course of illness, with different symptoms associated with different stages of the disease. For example, depression and anxiety are more prevalent in early Alzheimer's disease and psychosis, agitation and aggression commonly present later on. Guidelines for the management of BPSD have been published by the Scottish Intercollegiate Guidelines Network (*www.sign.ac.uk*) and the International Psychogeriatric Association.[21]

Early stage

Alzheimer's disease tends to begin gradually, so the early symptoms may go unrecognised, frequently being mistaken as normal signs of ageing. Typical symptoms include:

- loss of short-term memory, forgetting recent conversations or events
- decreased judgement, finding decisions harder to make, inability to manage complex tasks (e.g. financial decisions)
- loss of interest in other people or activities
- lack of initiative and becoming slower to grasp new ideas.[5,17]

Middle stage

Symptoms become more marked as Alzheimer's disease progresses, and as a consequence patients need increased help with their daily tasks, such as eating, washing and dressing. Typical symptoms include:

- increasing decline in short-term memory leading to forgetfulness, with patients being unable to recognise close friends or family, and often repeating the same phrase many times
- becoming easily upset, angry or aggressive, and patients may also become very clinging
- wandering off and becoming lost, and becoming confused about where they are
- difficulty or inability to dress, undress and poor attention to personal hygiene
- behaving in an inappropriate manner, such as going outside in nightclothes
- experiencing paranoid ideas and hallucinations.[5,17]

Specific staging scales can be used to assess the severity of Alzheimer's disease progression and, of these, the Functional Assessment Staging (FAST) system and the Clinical Dementia Rating (CDR) are the most reliable.

Late stage

At this stage, patients require a great deal of help and gradually become totally dependent on others for nursing care. Loss of memory may be close to complete, such that they do not recognise familiar objects or surroundings or closest family members, though flashes of recognition can occur. Other symptoms include:

- increasing frailty, shuffling or unsteady gait, eventually becoming confined to bed and/or a wheelchair
- losing control of bladder and bowel functions
- inability to eat unaided
- considerable weight loss
- progressive loss of speech, though they may cry out occasionally or repeat a few words.[5,17]

Dementia can progress for up to 10 years and is a life-shortening illness, though another condition or illness such as bronchopneumonia, may trigger death and be listed as the cause of fatality on the death certificate.[5] Death usually occurs within 5–10 years of diagnosis.[22] As patients' mobility is affected, this can contribute to a decline in physical health and cardiovascular disease; they can be less likely to cope with infections and more likely to die of a pulmonary embolism or a myocardial infarction.[5] However, in some people no specific cause of death is found other than dementia, thus it can be listed as sole or main cause of death, or a contributory factor.[5] In England and Wales the mortality rates reported for Alzheimer's disease have increased greatly from 1979 to 1996 (from about 1 to 20 per 100,000 aged over 65 years) (Figure 4).[23] However, senile dementia still remains three-times more common than Alzheimer's disease as an underlying cause of death on death certificates. Given its greater prevalence, many cases of Alzheimer's disease are thus being misclassified at death as senile dementia.

Pathology and aetiology

The aetiology of Alzheimer's disease is unknown.[11] Amyloid plaques and neurofibrillary tangles are commonly associated with Alzheimer's disease and are probably related to the cause, development and course of the

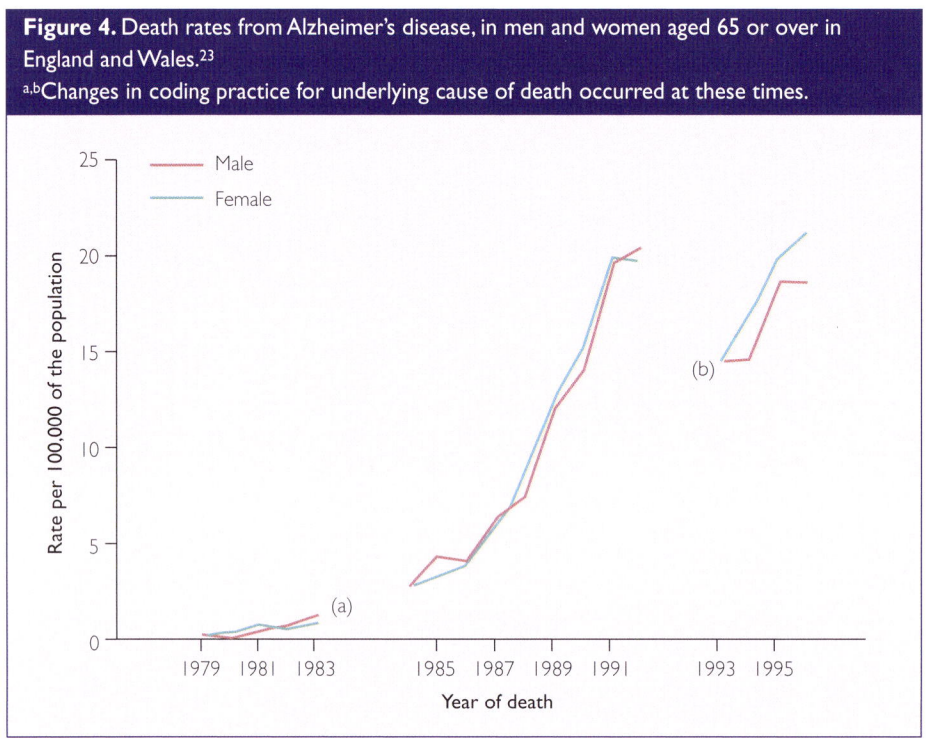

Figure 4. Death rates from Alzheimer's disease, in men and women aged 65 or over in England and Wales.[23]
[a,b]Changes in coding practice for underlying cause of death occurred at these times.

disease. However, these pathological markers are not exclusive to Alzheimer's disease and may occur in other dementias and as a result of the normal ageing process.

Amyloid plaques are composed of β-amyloid polypeptides, and seem to form as a result of disorders in processing β-amyloid and its precursor protein, APP, for which a combination of genetic predisposition and environmental factors are probably responsible.[24] Subclinical ischaemia represents one such environmental factor, particularly as patients with hypertension and elevated cholesterol tend to be at increased risk of developing Alzheimer's disease.[25] In reaction to amyloid, the microglia are stimulated to intense metabolic activity, and the resulting increase in cellular respiration consumes oxygen and generates highly reactive oxygen-containing free radicals.[12] These can cause oxidative damage to the cell, the by-products of which can cause further microglial activation that is associated with neurodegeneration.

Neurofibrillary tangles are essentially biochemical modifications of the natural neuronal cytoskeleton; when neurons die in Alzheimer's disease neurofibrillary tangles are found between surviving neurons, and have thus been likened to neuronal 'gravestones'.[12] A key component of the tangles is derived from a naturally occurring microtubule protein, tau. In Alzheimer's

> When neurons die in Alzheimer's disease neurofibrillary tangles are found between surviving neurons, and have thus been likened to neuronal 'gravestones'.

disease tau is hyperphosphorylated or glycated, and thus much more likely to form tangles.[12] It is unclear whether these tangles are linked to senile plaque formation, but their ultimate effect is to compromise microtubular function, leading to the eventual destruction of neurons.[24]

In addition to the actions of β-amyloid, oxidative neuronal damage and pathobiology of tau proteins' conversion to neurofibrillary tangles, neurotransmitter depletion also plays a central role in Alzheimer's disease.[26] Alzheimer's disease is associated with deficits in acetylcholine, noradrenaline, serotonin and glutamate. The cognitive decline associated with Alzheimer's disease is primarily attributed to the loss of cholinergic neurons in the cortex and hippocampus, and cholinergic deficiencies are also implicated in the formation of amyloid plaques and neurofibrillary tangles.[22,27] Abnormalities of the cholinergic system, including the upregulation of the cholineacetyltransferase enzyme, ChAT, and abnormal neuronal sprouting, characterise early disease progression. Cholinergic deficits are also correlated with the cognitive decline and behavioural symptoms associated with Alzheimer's disease.[28,29]

In light of the accumulated evidence for the role of a cholinergic deficit in Alzheimer's disease, early symptomatic treatment focuses on the restoration of this function. Acetylcholinesterase inhibitors are approved in the UK for the treatment of mild-to-moderate Alzheimer's dementia. Individual members of this pharmacological class exert non-cholinergic actions which may be relevant to their efficacy, such as:
- binding to the allosteric activator site on nicotinic receptors
- increasing non-cholinergic neurotransmitter release
- inhibiting β-amyloid toxicity
- increasing soluble β-amyloid precursor protein release
- modulating the effects of oestrogens.[30]

Risk factors

There are multiple risk factors for Alzheimer's disease. However, there is some controversy over which elements are true risk factors, though the strongest evidence is for increased age (the disease is rare in those younger than 60 years but increases to about 24% of those aged ≥85 years).[31] Other risk factors are:
- a family history of dementia (children, brothers or sisters of a person with Alzheimer's disease are three- or four-times more likely to develop this disease than someone with no affected relatives)
- Mutations of genes for familial Alzheimer's disease (e.g. presenilin 1 and 2, amyloid precursor protein)

- Mutations of susceptibility genes for sporadic Alzheimer's disease (e.g. apolipoprotein E4)
- low educational attainment (Alzheimer's disease is less common in those with higher levels of education)
- longstanding alcohol abuse
- cardiovascular disease and risk factors
- the presence of Down syndrome, as those who survive to late adulthood develop Alzheimer's disease, probably due to genetic disturbances (90% of people with Down syndrome have amyloid plaques, neurofibrillary tangles and cholinergic deficits at 30 years of age; 75% exhibit dementia by the age of 60 years).[17,31–35]

Older people with depression may also be at an increased risk of developing Alzheimer's disease, but whether depression is simply an early symptom or increases susceptibility through another mechanism remains to be determined.[36]

Treatment

Treatments for Alzheimer's disease address cognitive and behavioural symptoms as the disease itself is, at present, irreversible. Traditional approaches involving the manipulation of the patient's environment and the introduction of structured behaviours and activities may be useful.[2] Support group activities, hobbies and outings may reduce anger, depression and anxiety in patients with mild Alzheimer's disease.[2] As the disease progresses changes to patients' immediate surroundings, including the alteration and simplification of living spaces, may also be helpful.[2,3] There are limited data to suggest that some preventative measures may be effective in Alzheimer's disease, such as eating oily fish at least once a week or increasing the intake of antioxidants from food (e.g. vitamins C and E).[37–40]

To date, pharmacological treatments have addressed the cholinergic deficit associated with Alzheimer's disease, usually by preventing its breakdown. The cholinesterase inhibitors donepezil, galantamine and rivastigmine are the current recommended standard of care for the treatment of mild-to-moderately severe Alzheimer's dementia.[41] Treatment with cholinesterase inhibitors can stabilise and in some cases improve cognition and disruptive behaviour. Furthermore, nursing home placement has been shown to be delayed by almost 2 years following donepezil treatment in comparison with placebo.[35] The N-methyl-D-aspartate (NMDA) antagonist, memantine, is also indicated for moderately severe-to-severe Alzheimer's dementia. Memantine allows the physiological activation of NMDA receptors during memory formation but blocks the effects of the toxic accumulation of glutamate that may be responsible for neuronal dysfunction.[42,43] However, there is a relative paucity of published data for the use of memantine in comparison with that for the cholinesterase inhibitors. Some guidelines (excluding the National Institute for Clinical Excellence [NICE] UK guidelines) still recommend the use of vitamin E for treating Alzheimer's disease. Vitamin E has been shown to delay patients' disability, placement in a nursing home, but does not improve cognitive deficits.[24,44]

The treatment of common concurrent disorders such as depression should also be undertaken, as these can add to patients' burden of disability.[17] In these cases a selective serotonin reuptake inhibitor is normally given as first-line treatment. Typical antipsychotic compounds are generally avoided, as they are not only more likely to induce extrapyramidal side-effects, but also because their anticholinergic effects may add to the confusion, restlessness, agitation and akathisia experienced by some patients with Alzheimer's disease.[17]

Key points

- Alzheimer's dementia is defined clinically by a gradual decline in memory, plus a reduction in at least one other area of higher intellectual function (i.e. cognition, daily functioning and behaviour).
- In the UK, the prevalence of dementia is about 1%, and there are currently over 775,000 cases of dementia. Its prevalence increases sharply with advancing age amongst those in their 70s and 80s.
- Dementia costs the UK £6.1 billion a year, although the costs of effective treatment need to be offset against savings accrued in delaying the requirement for nursing care.
- Risk factors for Alzheimer's disease include a family history of dementia, mutations in specific genes, mutations in susceptibility genes, low educational attainment, cardiovascular disease and risk factors, longstanding alcohol abuse and Down syndrome.
- The development of amyloid plaques and neurofibrillary tangles in the brains of patients with Alzheimer's disease are probably related to the cause, development and course of the disease.
- The symptoms of Alzheimer's disease start gradually, so patients are often unaware of their own health problems.
- Despite the difficulty in assessing treatment benefit in patients who are chronically declining, symptoms of Alzheimer's disease can be ameliorated by pharmacological intervention.
- Early treatment is vital in order to achieve maximum clinical benefit to the patient.
- The manipulation of the patient's environment and the introduction of structured behaviours and activities can help to address their behavioural and psychological symptoms.
- Cholinesterase inhibitors (donepezil, galantamine and rivastigmine) are the current recommended standard of care for the treatment of mild-to-moderately severe Alzheimer's dementia.

References

1. *International Statistical Classification of Diseases and Related Health Problems, tenth revision (ICD-10)*. Geneva: World Health Organization, 1992.
2. Grossberg GT. The ABC of Alzheimer's disease: behavioral symptoms and their treatment. *Int Psychogeriatr* 2002; **14(Suppl 1)**: 27–49.
3. Potkin SG. The ABC of Alzheimer's disease: ADL and improving day-to-day functioning of patients. *Int Psychogeriatr* 2002; **14(Suppl 1)**: 7–26.
4. Dementia: diagnosis and management in primary care. http://www.alzheimers.org.uk/
5. Alzheimer's Society website. *http://www.alzheimers.org.uk/*
6. Alzheimer's Disease International website. *http://www.alz.co.uk*
7. *World Health Organization guide to mental and neurological health in primary care, 2nd edition.* London: Royal Society of Medicine Press, 2004.
8. Prince M, Jorm A. Alzheimer's Disease International website. Factsheet 3. The prevalence of dementia. http://www.alz.co.uk
9. Jorm AF, Korten AE, Henderson AS. The prevalence of dementia: a quantitative integration of the literature. *Acta Psychiatr Scand* 1987; **76**: 465–79.
10. Audit Commission. *Forget me not*. Portsmouth: Holbrooks, 2000.
11. O'Brien JT, Ballard CG. Drugs for Alzheimer's disease. *BMJ* 2001; **323**: 123–4.
12. Whalley L, Breitner J. *Dementia*. Oxford: Oxford Health Press, 2002.
13. Lopez O, Becker J, Wisniewski S *et al*. Cholinesterase inhibitor treatment alters the natural history of Alzheimer's disease. *J Neurol Neurosurg Psychiatry* 2002; **72**: 310–14.
14. National Institute for Clinical Excellence. Guidance on the use of donepezil, rivastigmine and galantamine for the treatment of Alzheimer's disease. Technology Appraisal Guideline No.19 (2001). www.nice.org.uk
15. Murman D, Chen Q, Powell M *et al*. The incremental direct costs associated with behavioral symptoms in AD. *Neurology* 2002; **59**: 1721–9.
16. Small G, McDonnell D, Brooks R, Papadopoulos G. The impact of symptom severity on the cost of Alzheimer's disease. *J Am Geriatr Soc* 2002; **50**: 321–7.
17. Ahmed MB. Alzheimer's disease: recent advances in etiology, diagnosis, and management. *Tex Med* 2001; **97**: 50–8.
18. Larrieu S, Letenneur L, Orgogozo J *et al*. Incidence and outcome of mild cognitive impairment in a population-based prospective cohort. *Neurology* 2002; **59**: 1594–9.
19. Celsis P. Age-related cognitive decline, mild cognitive impairment or preclinical Alzheimer's disease? *Ann Med* 2000; **32**: 6–14.
20. Data on file. Pfizer.
21. Interventions in the Management of Behavioural and Psychological Aspects of Dementia. Edinburgh: Scottish Intercollegiate Guidelines Network, 1998. www.sign.ac.uk
22. Dooley M, Lamb HM. Donepezil: a review of its use in Alzheimer's disease. *Drugs Aging* 2000; **16**: 199–226.
23. Kirby L, Lehmann P, Majeed A. Dementia in people aged 65 years and older: a growing problem? *Population Trends* 1998; **92**: 23–8.
24. DeLaGarza VW. Pharmacologic treatment of Alzheimer's disease: an update. *Am Fam Physician* 2003; **68**: 1365–72.
25. Kivipelto M, Helkala EL, Hanninen T *et al*. Midlife vascular risk factors and late-life mild cognitive impairment: a population-based study. *Neurology* 2001; **56**: 1683–9.
26. DeKosky ST. Pathology and pathways of Alzheimer's disease with an update on new developments in treatment. *J Am Geriatr Soc* 2003; **51**: S314–20.
27. Doody RS. Clinical profile of donepezil in the treatment of Alzheimer's disease. *Gerontology* 1999; **45(Suppl 1)**: 23–32.
28. Shinotoh H, Namba H, Fukushi K *et al*. Progressive loss of cortical acetylcholinesterase activity in association with cognitive decline in Alzheimer's disease: a positron emission tomography study. *Ann Neurol* 2000; **48**: 194–200.
29. Cummings JL, Back C. The cholinergic hypothesis of neuropsychiatric symptoms in Alzheimer's disease. *Am J Geriatr Psychiatry* 1998; **6**: S64–78.
30. Imbimbo BP. Pharmacodynamic-tolerability relationships of cholinesterase inhibitors for Alzheimer's disease. *CNS Drugs* 2001; **15**: 375–90.
31. Stewart R. Risk factors for dementia. Alzheimer's Disease International website; Factsheet 9: *http://www.alz.co.uk*
32. Lindsay J, Laurin D, Verreault R *et al*. Risk factors for Alzheimer's disease: a prospective analysis from the Canadian Study of Health and Aging. *Am J Epidemiol* 2002; **156**: 445–53.
33. Wisniewski KE, Wisniewski HM, Wen GY. Occurrence of neuropathological changes and dementia of Alzheimer's disease in Down's syndrome. *Ann Neurol* 1985; **17**: 278–82.
34. Lemere CA, Blusztajn JK, Yamaguchi H *et al*. Sequence of deposition of heterogeneous amyloid beta-peptides and APO E in Down syndrome: implications for initial events in amyloid plaque formation. *Neurobiol Dis* 1996; **3**: 16–32.
35. Roman GC, Rogers SJ. Donepezil: a clinical review of current and emerging indications. *Expert Opin Pharmacother* 2004; **5**: 161–80.
36. Devanand D, Sano M, Tang M *et al*. Depressed mood and the incidence of Alzheimer's disease in the elderly living in the community. *Arch Gen Psychiatry* 1996; **53**: 175–82.
37. Barberger-Gateau P, Letenneur L, Deschamps V *et al*. Fish, meat, and risk of dementia: cohort study. *BMJ* 2002; **325**: 932–3.
38. Morris M, Evans D, Bienias J *et al*. Dietary intake of antioxidant nutrients and the risk of incident Alzheimer disease in a biracial community study. *JAMA* 2002; **287**: 3230–7.
39. Morris M, Evans D, Bienias J *et al*. Consumption of fish and n-3 fatty acids and risk of incident Alzheimer disease. *Arch Neurol* 2003; **60**: 940–6.
40. Engelhart M, Geerlings M, Ruitenberg A *et al*. Dietary intake of antioxidants and risk of Alzheimer disease. *JAMA* 2002; **287**: 3223–9.

41 Doody RS. Current treatments for Alzheimer's disease: cholinesterase inhibitors. *J Clin Psychiatry* 2003; **64(Suppl 9)**: 11–17.

42 Reisberg B, Doody R, Stoffler A *et al*. Memantine in moderate-to-severe Alzheimer's disease. *N Engl J Med* 2003; **348**: 1333–41.

43 Ferris SH. Evaluation of memantine for the treatment of Alzheimer's disease. *Expert Opin Pharmacother* 2003; **4**: 2305–13.

44 Sano M, Ernesto C, Thomas RG *et al*. A controlled trial of selegiline, alpha-tocopherol, or both as treatment for Alzheimer's disease. The Alzheimer's Disease Cooperative Study. *N Engl J Med* 1997; **336**: 1216–22.

3. Angina

Dr Richard Clark
CSF Medical Communications Ltd

Summary

Approximately 2 million people in the UK have experienced angina.[1] Angina pectoris, usually termed angina, is a pain or discomfort in the chest that occurs when part of the heart does not receive enough blood. It is a common symptom of coronary heart disease (CHD) and is usually caused by the narrowing of blood vessels to the heart due to atherosclerosis. Angina feels like a tightness, heaviness or dull ache in the chest that can spread to the arms, neck and body, and is often precipitated by exertion or emotional stress, but is usually relieved within a few minutes by resting or by taking appropriate medicine.[2] About 25% of all patients presenting with a first myocardial infarction (MI) have a history of stable angina, thus it is important as a marker for CHD as well as being a cause of disability *per se*. The accurate diagnosis and selection of appropriate treatment is crucial for the effective management of stable angina.

Prevalence and impact

Approximately 2 million people in the UK have experienced angina, and every year there are approximately 335,000 new cases.[1] Angina is the most common form of cardiovascular disease, itself the leading cause of death in the UK.[1] About 5% of men and 4% of women in the UK have had angina, whilst its prevalence increases with increasing age.[1] Of those aged 55–64 years, 9 and 5% of men and women, respectively, have had angina, compared with 14 and 8% of men and women, respectively, aged 65–74 years.[1]

There are huge numbers of people living with heart disease in the UK. Whilst mortality from heart disease is falling rapidly, the burden of morbidity associated with heart and circulatory disease is not falling. For example, in the UK mortality rates for CHD have reduced dramatically since the early 1980s – by 41% over the last 10 years for adults under 65 years – but morbidity rates for angina have not decreased to the same extent.[1] The British Regional Heart Survey has shown only a 1.8% decrease

> Approximately 2 million people in the UK have experienced angina, and every year there are approximately 335,000 new cases.

in the prevalence of angina in British men under 65 years between 1978 and 1996.[1] Furthermore, statistics gathered from general practice in 1981–2 and 1991–2 showed increases in the prevalence of angina of 60 and 69% for men and women, respectively, in England and Wales (Figure 1).[1] Although this increase may be partly due to improved awareness and reporting of angina, this is still a worrying trend. Moreover, angina has a profound effect on patients' quality of life and their employment status, and there is a strong link between employment status and the severity of angina.[3]

Angina can exist in a number of forms (see the following section), but this review will focus primarily on stable angina. Despite its name, stable angina should be taken very seriously since people with this condition have a three-fold increased risk of developing unstable angina, MI or sudden cardiac death within 2 years of presentation.[4] About 25% of all patients presenting with a first MI have a history of stable angina.[5] Therefore, stable angina can be important as a marker for CHD, in addition to being a cause of disability.[5] However, the prognosis for patients with stable angina is reasonably good, with a mortality rate of about 2–3% per annum and a further 2–3% per year sustaining a non-fatal MI.[6] As people with stable angina are both easily identifiable and are at much higher risk of experiencing an adverse cardiac event than those without angina, they constitute an important group to target with effective treatment.[7]

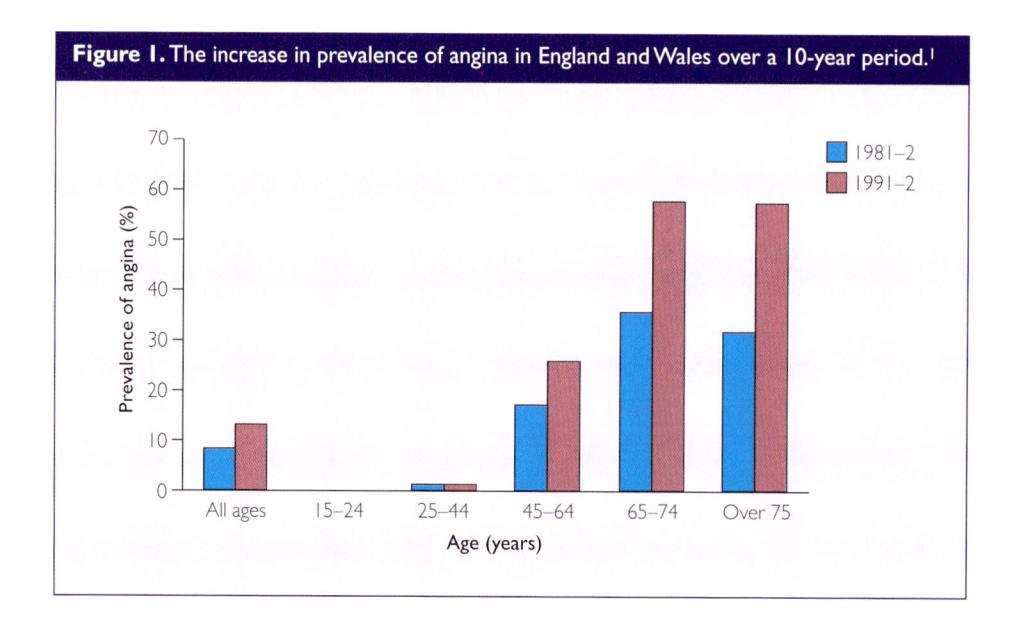

> People with this condition have a three-fold increased risk of developing unstable angina, MI or sudden cardiac death within 2 years of presentation.

Figure 1. The increase in prevalence of angina in England and Wales over a 10-year period.[1]

Classification

Angina should be clearly differentiated from MI. Angina is an indication that part of the myocardium is at times not receiving enough oxygen (e.g. during exercise, when the heart has to work harder). In contrast, MI occurs when the blood flow to part of the heart is suddenly cut off, causing permanent damage to the myocardium. Typically, chest pain associated with MI lasts longer and is more severe than angina, and does not dissipate after rest or with angina medication. The most commonly used classification of angina symptom severity is that devised by the Canadian Cardiovascular Society.[8]

Angina can be classified as:
- stable angina
- unstable angina
- variant (or Prinzmetal's or vasospastic) angina
- cardiac syndrome X/microvascular angina.

Stable angina is the most common form of angina, and is also called exertional or typical angina. The underlying pathology is usually an atherosclerotic obstruction of the coronary blood vessels. Unstable angina, in contrast, is generally associated with more intense chest pain, which lasts longer, is brought on by less effort and may occur spontaneously at rest.[9] Whilst stable angina has an established and fairly stable pattern of symptoms, unstable angina may appear as a first very severe episode or as a sharp change in the established pattern of angina.[2] There is no universally accepted definition of unstable angina, but it has been described as a clinical syndrome lying between stable angina and acute MI.[10] Unstable angina is caused by an acute but reversible increase in coronary obstruction, usually secondary to the rupture or fissuring of the fibrous cap of an atheromatous plaque with subsequent thrombus formation.[9] As such, unstable angina is often grouped with other acute MI states (e.g. ST-segment elevation MI and non-ST-segment elevation MI) as acute coronary syndrome.[10]

Variant angina and cardiac syndrome X are far less common than stable or unstable angina. Variant angina is characterised by chest discomfort at rest, which is relieved by sublingual nitroglycerin, and by ST-segment elevation on electrocardiography (ECG) during an attack. However, between anginal attacks – which usually occur with regularity and at certain times of day – the ECG may be normal.[9] This type of angina is caused by a spasm occurring within 1 cm of an obstruction of the proximal portion of a major coronary artery.[9] Cardiac syndrome X is angina – or an angina-like

Stable angina is the most common form of angina, and is also called exertional or typical angina.

chest pain – relieved by rest or by sublingual nitroglycerin, in patients who have an abnormal ECG during an exercise test but a normal angiogram (i.e. no obvious coronary atherosclerotic legion).[2,9] The cause of this syndrome is not clear, but it is likely to represent a heterogeneous set of changes characterised by a reduced capacity of the coronary circulation to increase blood flow when an increase in oxygen demand occurs.[9] One cause of cardiac syndrome X can be the narrowing of the smaller coronary arteries through atherosclerosis (microvascular angina) which has not been detected by a coronary angiogram.

Pathophysiology of atherosclerosis and atherothrombosis

The presence of stable angina indicates that there is underlying CHD, and these patients are at greater risk of acute MI than those without symptoms of CHD.[2] Underlying CHD is usually caused by the progression of a stable atherosclerotic plaque, though a minority of patients with unstable angina or non-ST elevation MI have no obvious angiographic lesion.[11] Stable atherosclerotic plaques are the precursors for chronic stable angina. Atherosclerosis is a long-term process that causes structural changes in the intima and media walls of major arteries, initially resulting in endothelial abnormalities and, ultimately, atherosclerotic plaques.[12] Despite large increases in atherosclerotic plaque size, blood flow is not always compromised because compensatory vascular enlargement (remodelling) can occur during plaque growth.[13] The progression from atherosclerosis to atherothrombosis (atherosclerosis with superimposed thrombosis) usually occurs due to the rupture of the fibrous cap or superficial erosion of the endothelial layer.[14] The plaque composition rather than the severity of stenosis may be the most important determinant of plaque disruption and subsequent thrombosis.[13] In general, vulnerable or high-risk plaques are characterised by the following features:

- a thin, fibrous cap with disorganised collagen
- a large atheromatous, lipid core containing high concentrations of cholesteryl esters
- infiltration by large numbers of macrophages and other inflammatory cells, such as T-lymphocytes
- a scarcity of smooth muscle cells
- a high concentration of tissue factor.[13–15]

In contrast, stable plaques are characterised by a small lipid core covered by a thick fibrous cap.

Passive plaque rupture tends to occur more frequently at the shoulders of a plaque, possibly as a consequence of physical forces, blood flow or even due to the high concentrations of macrophages located in these areas. The abundant activated macrophage population within a vulnerable atheroma may be involved in plaque destabilisation through the secretion of proteolytic enzymes, particularly matrix metalloproteinases, which degrade the extracellular matrix components of the fibrous cap.[13] A variety of local, mechanical and haemodynamic forces subject plaques to constant stresses that may trigger disruption of vulnerable plaques (Figure 2).[16] Changes in blood flow due to arterial stenosis, hypertension, dyslipidaemia and irritants in tobacco smoke can also accelerate the process of plaque vulnerability and rupture.[12]

The rupture or erosion of the plaque results in the abrupt exposure of thrombogenic plaque components (e.g. lipid core, collagen, macrophages and tissue factor). These components stimulate platelet attachment and aggregation, thrombin generation and fibrin accretion – events that lead to the formation of a thrombus.[14,16] Furthermore, the lipid-rich core of the plaque contains a procoagulant tissue factor, thought to be produced by macrophages, that activates the extrinsic clotting cascade leading to the generation of thrombin.[16] Thus, inflammatory cells such as macrophages play a critical role in determining the thrombogenicity of an atherosclerotic plaque.

Although disrupted coronary plaques are frequently found in the arteries of patients who have died of acute coronary disease, plaque rupture or erosion does not always result in a lumen-occluding thrombus and a subsequent clinical coronary event.[14,16] In fact, most plaque disruptions probably do not cause any coronary symptoms.[17] When the prevailing fibrinolytic mechanisms outweigh the procoagulant pathways this leads to the formation of a limited mural thrombus rather than an occlusive and sustained blood clot.[17] However, though resorption of the mural thrombus can occur, the healing process can lead to fibrous tissue formation, thickening the fibrous cap and causing further expansion of the intima in an inwards direction, thus causing a constriction in the lumen.[17] Stenotic lesions produced by the luminal encroachment of a fibrosed plaque may restrict blood flow, particularly during strenuous exercise, with the resulting ischaemia leading to symptoms such as angina.[17] It is also possible to stabilise vulnerable plaques to yield a more stable plaque with a thick fibrous cap and preserved lumen diameter (Figure 3). Plaque stabilisation may be achieved through some of the following measures:

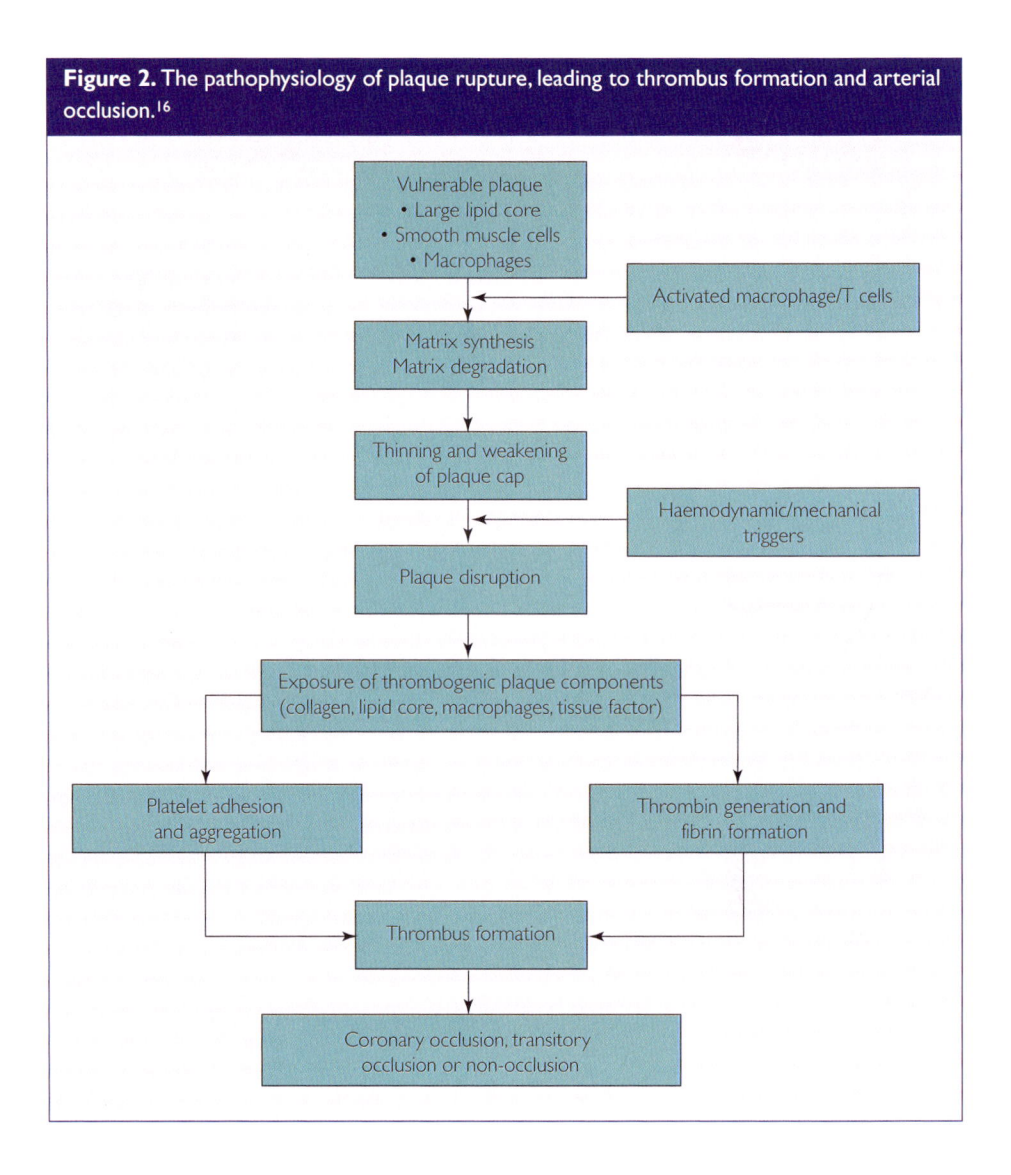

Figure 2. The pathophysiology of plaque rupture, leading to thrombus formation and arterial occlusion.[16]

- lipid-lowering therapies (e.g. statins)
- dietary and lifestyle changes
- cessation of smoking
- angiotensin converting enzyme (ACE) inhibition.[16]

Risk factors

The following risk factors for stable angina should be considered when making a diagnosis:
- increased age
- male gender
- family history of angina

Figure 3. Atherosclerosis can result in atherothrombosis, leading to either a coronary event or healing of the ruptured plaque, followed by fibrous tissue formation causing a constriction in the lumen, reduced blood flow and angina during times of increased oxygen demand.[17]

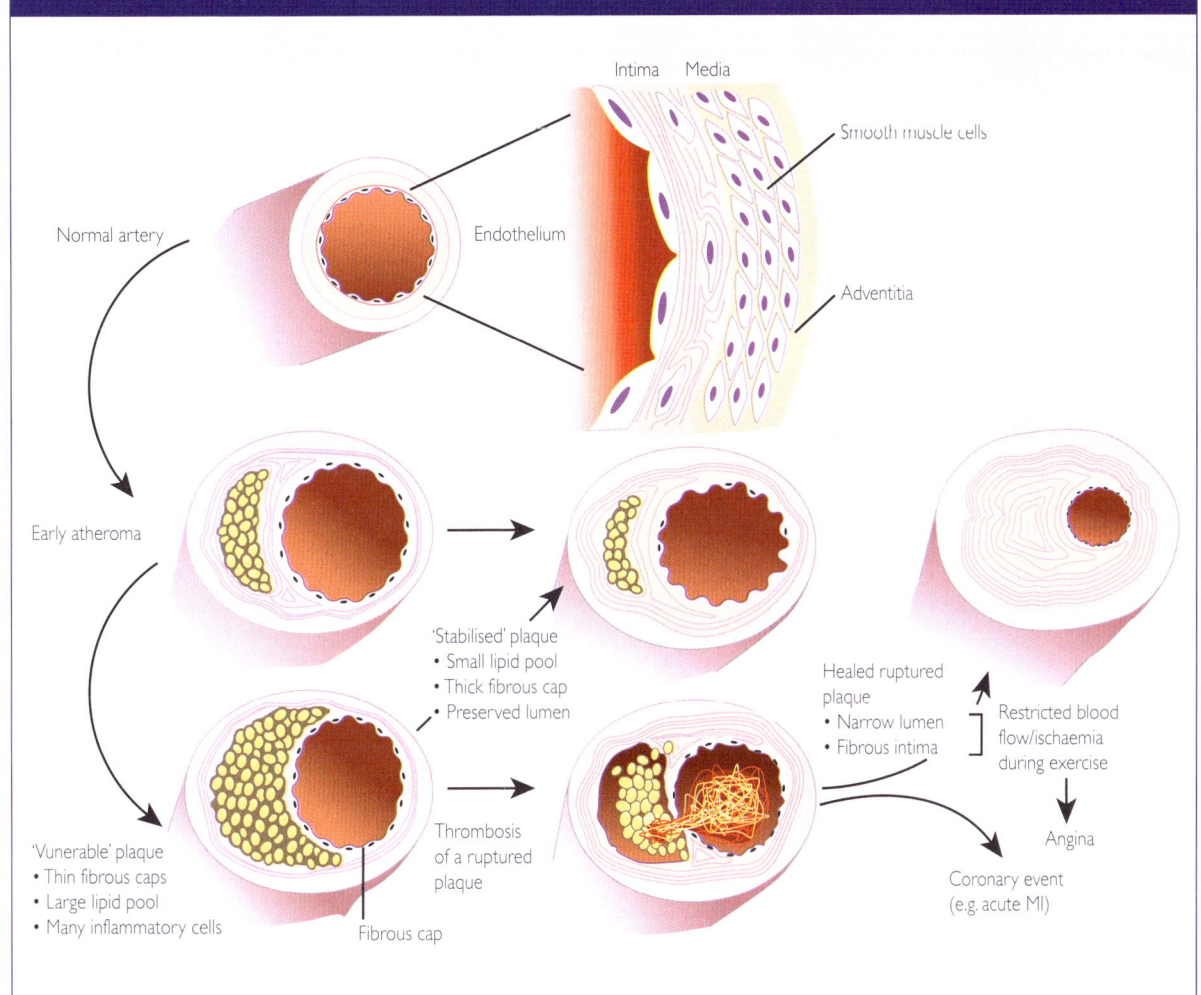

- smoking
- Indo-Asian ethnicity
- dietary factors, including excess alcohol consumption
- high body-mass index (BMI)
- raised serum cholesterol, low density lipoprotein cholesterol (LDL-C) and triglycerides, and lowered high density lipoprotein cholesterol (HDL-C) levels
- low levels of physical activity
- concomitant hypertension, diabetes, anaemia or other disorders
- psychological factors.[6,18,19]

> Control of risk factors in patients with angina leads to an improved outcome.

There is evidence that effective control of risk factors in patients with angina leads to an improved outcome in terms of a reduced incidence of ischaemic events and improved survival.[18] Recommendations include advice on the cessation of smoking, control of hypertension by following British Hypertension Society guidelines, lowering of plasma cholesterol by dietary or pharmacological means, regular exercise, weight reduction towards ideal BMI and the control of diabetes.[18,20]

Diagnosis

The following key evaluations should usually be offered to patients presenting with angina:
- clinical history
- clinical examination
- full blood count
- thyroid function test
- fasting lipoprotein profile
- fasting blood glucose level
- blood pressure
- 12-lead resting ECG
- exercise ECG test.[4,21]

The initial evaluation of stable angina can be performed within the primary-care setting and should always include patients' clinical history, a physical examination and a resting ECG.[6] The resting ECG provides evidence on cardiac rhythm, presence of heart block, previous MI and myocardial hypertrophy and ischaemia. It should be stressed that though patients with angina and an abnormal ECG should be considered for urgent referral and investigation, a normal ECG does not necessarily exclude CHD.[19,22] A patient's history should include investigations into:
- precipitants of anginal attacks
- stability of symptoms
- smoking history
- occupation
- the intensity, length and regularity of exercise undertaken
- diet
- alcohol intake
- family history of CHD.[18,19]

The physical examination should record:
- weight and height (to calculate BMI) or waist circumference (to calculate waist/hip ratio)
- blood pressure
- presence of murmurs, particularly from aortic stenosis
- evidence of hyperlipidaemia
- evidence of peripheral vascular disease.[19]

This is frequently supplemented by some form of functional test(s), such as exercise testing with ECG or myocardial perfusion imaging (MPI), to determine if myocardial ischaemia is present, and if so, to what extent (Figure 4). In patients with significant functional abnormalities this may be followed by coronary angiography to assess whether coronary intervention is indicated, and which intervention would be most appropriate.[6] Furthermore, if a patient is considered to be 'high risk' (i.e. severe symptoms of angina, unstable angina, early symptoms of angina after a previous coronary intervention or early post-infarction angina) it may be advisable to perform angiography as soon as possible.[6,18]

It is important to differentiate angina from other causes of chest pain. Other likely cardiac causes of chest pain are MI, pericardial pain or an arrhythmia.[23] Non-cardiac causes of chest pain include:
- oesophageal disorders (e.g. gastro-oesophageal reflux)
- musculoskeletal pain (e.g. Tietze's syndrome)
- acute cholecystitis
- pleural pain
- psychological causes (anxiety, hyperventilation, panic attacks or depression).[23]

Specialist referral

Patients who have suspected or confirmed angina secondary to CHD may be referred to a cardiologist if they are likely to benefit from early specialist investigation or revascularisation. These are patients who:
- are known to have had a previous MI, coronary artery bypass graft (CABG) or percutaneous transluminal coronary angioplasty (PTCA)
- appear to have had a previous MI on their initial ECG, or other anomaly that the GP considers may be clinically significant
- fail to respond to medical treatment, and who have had an exercise test
- have an ejection systolic murmur, suggesting aortic stenosis.[19]

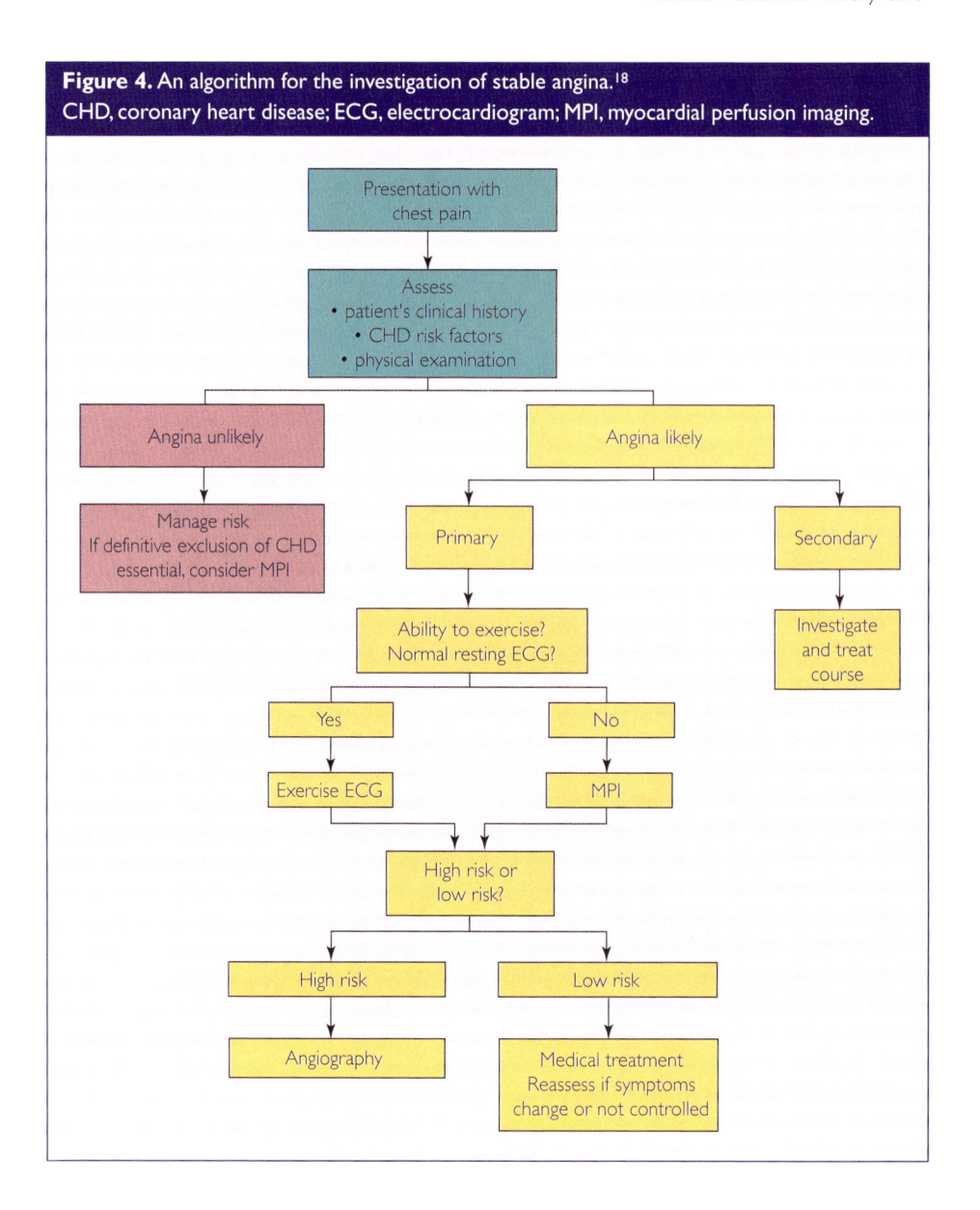

Figure 4. An algorithm for the investigation of stable angina.[18]
CHD, coronary heart disease; ECG, electrocardiogram; MPI, myocardial perfusion imaging.

Further clinical scenarios in which to consider immediate referral of a patient to a cardiologist include:
- suspected unstable angina
- to confirm or refute a diagnosis in patients with atypical symptoms
- a strong family history of CHD
- high risk or the presence of comorbid disorders such as diabetes
- refractory to therapy and/or the modification of risk factors.[19]

It is important not to delay treatment whilst awaiting referral and to consider the wishes of individual patients. Some patients may not want to be referred, and others may wish to be referred at an early stage.[19,23] In addition, the new Gencral Medical Services (GMS) contract specifically requires specialist confirmation of angina diagnosis.

Managing risk factors

Many risk factors can be modified or controlled. Cigarette smoking should be strongly discouraged as cessation greatly improves the symptoms of CHD and patients' prognosis.[6] Patients should be encouraged to adopt a diet in line with healthy eating advice – increasing fruit and vegetable consumption to five portions per day and eating at least one portion of oily fish per week. Those who are overweight should be encouraged to adopt a low-fat diet, increasing the proportion of monosaturated and non-hydrogenated polyunsaturated fats.[6,23] Serum cholesterol levels should be reduced using appropriate medications. Daily alcohol intake should be moderated to three units for men and two units for women.[19] Advice and treatment should be given to manage concomitant disorders that increase the risk of CHD progression.[6,21] Patients should be encouraged to undertake aerobic exercise within the limits set by their disease state, as it can increase their exercise tolerance, reduce symptoms of angina and have a favourable effect on weight, serum cholesterol levels and blood pressure.[6,19]

Treatment options

The aims of treatment are to relieve symptoms, to prolong life and minimise cardiac risk.[21] Chronic stable angina can be treated medically or by revascularisation. Drug therapy in patients with stable angina can be divided into three main categories:
- secondary prophylactic treatment (i.e. the prevention of cardiovascular diseases secondary to angina by the use of antiplatelet agents)
- immediate relief of angina symptoms
- long-term prevention of angina symptoms.[19]

Secondary prophylactic treatment

Patients with stable angina should be treated with a daily dose of aspirin, 75 mg, in the absence of contra-indications.[6,19,21,23] When used at low doses, aspirin can greatly reduce the risk of first MI in patients with stable angina, however, there is no evidence that doses in excess of 75 mg are likely to provide greater benefits.[19,24,25] Aspirin can reduce vascular events by 23%.[23,26] One of the most common side-effects related to aspirin use is dyspepsia; if persistent, this can be treated with antacids, H_2 antagonists or proton pump inhibitors or another antiplatelet agent (e.g. clopidogrel) can be used.[19] Enteric-coated aspirin is not recommended when used at this dose as the risks of gastric or duodenal bleeding are similar to standard aspirin.[19] Patients who are hypersensitive to aspirin (i.e. those for whom aspirin induces angioedema or bronchospasm) or who are generally unable to tolerate aspirin should be given clopidogrel as an alternative antiplatelet agent.[19,23]

Patients with stable angina should be treated with a daily dose of aspirin, 75 mg, in the absence of contra-indications.

Immediate relief of angina symptoms

Sublingual nitroglycerin is indicated for the immediate relief of pain associated with acute attacks of angina.[19,23,27,28] Patients should be urged to seek urgent medical help if the pain persists after three doses over 15 minutes.[23]

Sublingual nitroglycerin is indicated for acute attacks of angina.

Long-term prevention of angina symptoms

The main classes of agents available as maintenance therapy for the prevention of anginal symptoms are β-blockers, calcium-channel blockers, long-acting nitrates and potassium channel activators. β-blockers (e.g. atenolol, bisoprolol, metoprolol, pindolol and propanolol) decrease sinus rate, slow atrioventricular (AV) conduction and decrease myocardium contractility, which in combination reduces myocardial oxygen demand (MVO_2).[27,29] Furthermore, the reduction in heart rate results in prolonged diastolic perfusion and so can improve myocardial oxygen delivery.[27,29] The calcium-channel blockers include the dihydropyridines (e.g. nifedipine, amlodipine and felodipine) and the non-dihydropyridines, diltiazem and verapamil. These primarily cause coronary arterial vasodilation, and so improve myocardial oxygen supply, but also decrease MVO_2 through reductions in systemic vascular resistance and negative inotropism. Furthermore, diltiazem and verapamil can also reduce heart rate through reductions in AV conduction. Nitrates are vasodilators that possess venous selectivity, and so reduce cardiac work by reducing MVO_2 through veno- and arterial dilation, and increase myocardial oxygen supply through coronary vasodilation.[29] The potassium-channel activator nicorandil also produces 'nitrate-like' venodilation effects. It relaxes vascular smooth muscle in coronary arteries, systemic veins and peripheral arteries, thereby increasing coronary blood flow and reducing vascular resistance, preload and afterload.[27]

All of these drugs have been shown to be effective as monotherapy in relieving the symptoms of angina, increasing treadmill-based measurements of exercise capacity and reducing silent myocardial ischaemia on ambulatory ECG during normal daily activities.[27] Although a mortality benefit for anti-anginals has not yet been established rigorously in patients with stable angina, a recent large outcomes trial has shown that nicorandil reduces cardiovascular events in this population.[18,27,30] However, β-blockers do have outcomes data in post-MI patients, and this evidence has generally been extrapolated to include all patients in CHD.

As the majority of angina attacks are preceded by an increase in heart rate it has become an 'article of faith' that patients should be treated with a negative chronotropic agent. There is some evidence to suggest that, for this reason, a β-blocker is frequently the agent of first choice for stable angina.[27] Indeed, β-blocker monotherapy is recommended as first-line medication (unless contra-indicated) for stable angina by numerous guidelines.[18,19,23,28] However, β-blockers can be associated with severe bradycardia, hypotension, bronchospasm and, more rarely, heart failure.[6] Alternatives to β-blockers are rate-limiting calcium-channel blockers (diltiazem or verapamil), long-acting dihydropyridines (e.g. amlodipine or felodipine), long-acting nitrates (e.g. isosorbide mononitrate [ISMN]) or the potassium-channel activator nicorandil.[19,23] Calcium-channel blockers should be used with caution in patients with heart failure, poor left ventricular function and elderly patients, though some long-acting dihydropyridines may be safer in this context.[6] Long-acting nitrates are associated with tolerance in some patients, though this can be reduced or avoided by the use of asymmetric dosing regimens (e.g. 8 am and 2 pm), though they are generally given once daily in the morning, and are of particular use in patients with heart failure who are contra-indicated β-blockers.[6,23] The potassium-channel activator nicorandil does not appear to cause tolerance with chronic dosing, though it is associated with a similar spectrum of side-effects as nitrates.[6,23] In addition, a recently published large outcomes trial in patients with stable angina has demonstrated that nicorandil reduces cardiovascular events in this population.[30]

If symptom control is poor during monotherapy, dual therapy should be considered.[18,19,23] In patients receiving a β-blocker, a long-acting dihydropyridine calcium-channel blocker is recommended (e.g. modified-release nifedipine).[23] Alternatively, ISMN or the potassium-channel activator nicorandil may be added.[19,23] Dual therapy of a calcium-channel blocker/ISMN, calcium-channel blocker/nicorandil or nitrate/nicorandil may also be effective.[23] There is no firm evidence that the addition of a third agent improves symptom control.[19,23,27]

Surgery and alternative treatments

Patients with refractory angina despite adequate medical therapy (two anti-ischaemic agents) should be referred for angiography.[27] Revascularisation is indicated for the relief of symptoms refractory to medical therapy. As yet, however, there is no conclusive evidence that revascularisation – with or without stenting – offers prognostic benefit in patients with chronic stable angina.[27] CABG is still the treatment of choice in patients with disease of the left coronary artery, multi-vessel disease involving the proximal left anterior descending artery or three-vessel disease, as long-term survival is increased in these cases.[6,23] However, PTCA allows patients to be treated as day cases, avoids the risks of general anaesthesia, uncomfortable sternotomy and the complications of major surgery associated with CABG.[31] Although PTCA may result in greater relief from angina compared with medical treatment, there is no firm evidence that PTCA reduces the incidence of non-fatal MI, death or repeated angioplasty.[32] Comparisons of patients undergoing PTCA or medical treatment have shown that patients undergoing PTCA derived greater symptom relief, but required more subsequent revascularisation procedures and had more complications, including non-fatal MI.[31]

Increasing numbers of patients have chronic stable angina that is unresponsive to maximal drug treatment or even revascularisation techniques.[31] In these cases emerging treatments to palliate angina include neurostimulation using transcutaneous electrical nerve stimulation (TENS) or spinal cord stimulation (SCS). SCS, in particular, has been shown to be equivalent to CABG in terms of pain relief.[32] There is also limited evidence that acupuncture may be useful in some patients with angina that is refractory to medical treatment.[32,33]

An algorithm for the management of patients with stable angina is shown in Figure 5.

Immunisation

The 'Green Book' recommends that patients with chronic heart disease are protected by annual influenza vaccinations and single pneumococcus vaccination.[34]

Figure 5. An algorithm for the management of patients with stable angina.[21]
[a]Medical therapy may be the only option if there is very poor ventricular function or extensive distal coronary artery disease.

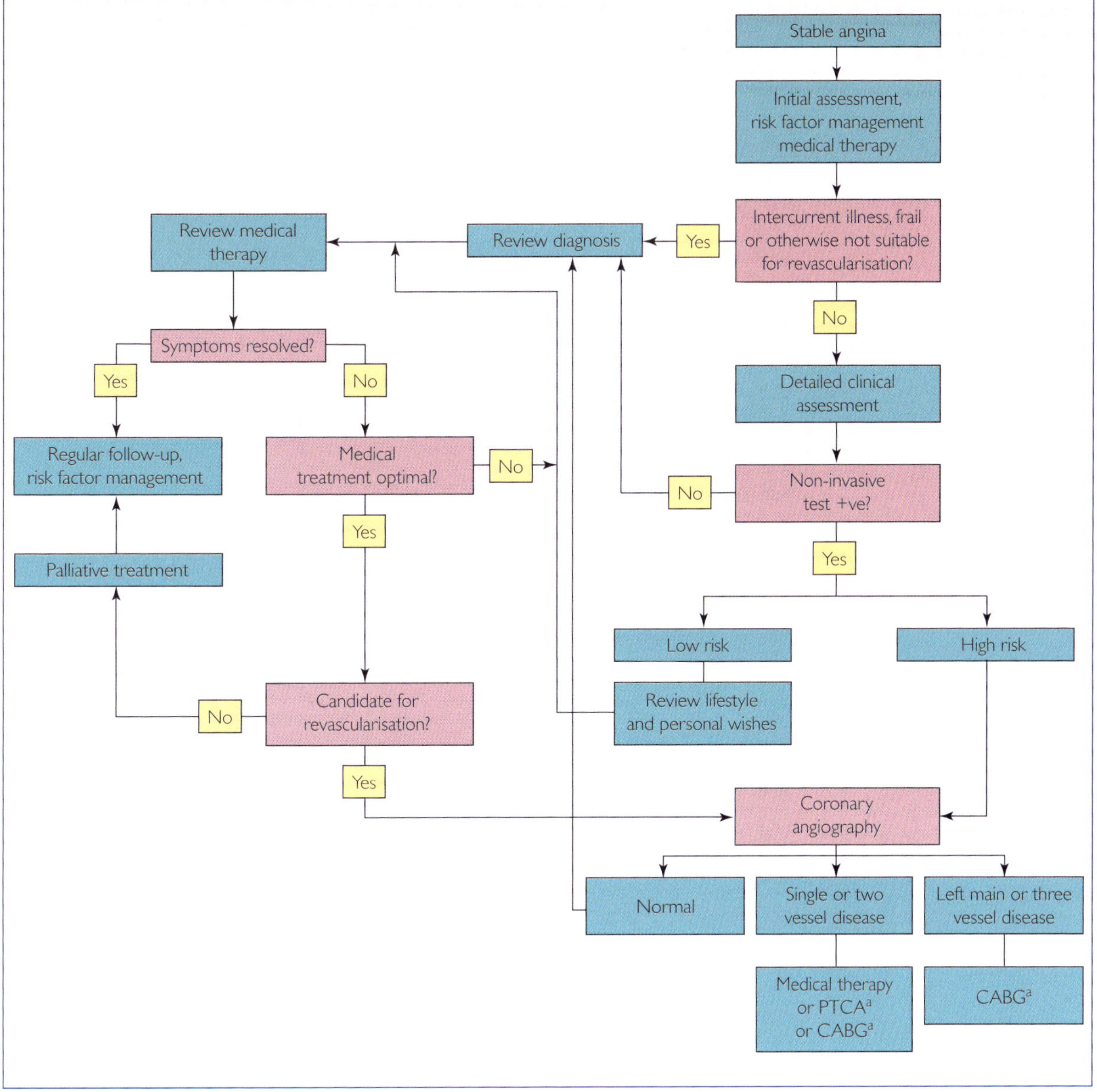

Key points

- Approximately 2 million people in the UK have angina, with approximately 335,000 new cases reported every year.
- Whilst mortality due to CHD is falling year on year, morbidity associated with CHD, particularly angina, is static or increasing.
- Stable angina is the most common form of angina, is precipitated by exertional or emotional stress, and is usually relieved within a few minutes by rest; it has an established, fairly stable pattern, such that a predictable level of stress or activity provokes angina.
- Patients with stable angina have a three-fold increased risk of developing unstable angina, MI or sudden cardiac death within 2 years of presentation.
- Stable angina is a symptom of underlying CHD, thus atherosclerotic plaque stabilisation measures such as lipid-lowering therapies, dietary and lifestyle changes may help to prevent the onset of angina.
- The diagnosis of stable angina in the primary-care setting should always include the patient's clinical history, a physical examination and a resting ECG, and often may be supplemented by exercise testing with ECG or MPI to determine if myocardial ischaemia is present.
- Treatment of stable angina includes the management of risk factors (e.g. cessation of smoking, adopting a healthy diet, a sensible level of alcohol intake and regular aerobic exercise), pharmacological and surgical options.
- Secondary prophylaxis treatment should be undertaken; an antiplatelet agent such as low-dose aspirin is suitable in most cases.
- Acute relief of angina is provided by sublingual nitroglycerin, whilst long-term prevention of symptoms is provided by β-blockers, calcium-channel blockers, long-acting nitrates and potassium-channel activators.

References

1. British Heart Foundation website. *http://www.bhf.org.uk* Accessed in September 2003.
2. National Heart, Lung and Blood Institute, National Institutes of Health. Facts about angina. Accessed in September 2003. *http://www.nhlbi.nih.gov/health/public/heart/other/angina.htm*
3. Pocock SJ, Henderson RA, Seed P, Treasure T, Hampton JR. Quality of life, employment status, and anginal symptoms after coronary angioplasty or bypass surgery. 3-year follow-up in the Randomized Intervention Treatment of Angina (RITA) trial. *Circulation* 1996; **94**: 135–42.
4. MacDermott A. Reducing symptoms and improving outcomes in patients with angina. *Prof Nurse* 2001; **17**: 103–6.
5. Gandhi MM. Clinical epidemiology of coronary heart disease in the UK. *Br J Hosp Med* 1997; **58**: 23–7.
6. Management of stable angina pectoris. Recommendations of the Task Force of the European Society of Cardiology. *Eur Heart J* 1997; **18**: 394–413.
7. Baker S, Petticrew M, Press P *et al*. Management of unstable angina. *Effective Health Care* 1997; **3**: 1–8.
8. Campeau L. The Canadian Cardiovascular Society grading of angina pectoris revisited 30 years later. *Can J Cardiol* 2002; **18**: 371–9.
9. Reiner Z. Pathophysiology and classification of cardiovascular diseases caused by atherosclerosis. *J Int Fed Clin Chem Lab Med* 2003; **13**: 1–4.
10. Grech E, Ramsdale D. ABC of interventional cardiology. Acute coronary syndrome; unstable angina and non-ST segment elevated myocardial infarction. *BMJ* 2003; **326**: 1259–61.
11. Sheridan PJ, Crossman DC. Critical review of unstable angina and non-ST elevation myocardial infarction. *Postgrad Med J* 2002; **78**: 717–26.
12. Leys D. Atherothrombosis: a major health burden. *Cerebrovasc Dis* 2001; **11 (Suppl 2)**: 1–4.
13. Fuster V, Badimon JJ, Chesebro JH. Atherothrombosis: mechanisms and clinical therapeutic approaches. *Vasc Med* 1998; **3**: 231–9.
14. Libby P. Multiple mechanisms of thrombosis complicating atherosclerotic plaques. *Clin Cardiol* 2000; **23 (Suppl 6)**: VI-3–7.
15. Willeit J, Kiechl S. Biology of arterial atheroma. *Cerebrovasc Dis* 2000; **10 (Suppl 5)**: 1–8.
16. Shah PK. New insights into the pathogenesis and prevention of acute coronary syndromes. *Am J Cardiol* 1997; **79**: 17–23.
17. Libby P. Inflammation in atherosclerosis. *Nature* 2002; **420**: 868–74.
18. de Bono D. Investigation and management of stable angina: revised guidelines 1998. Joint Working Party of the British Cardiac Society and Royal College of Physicians of London. *Heart* 1999; **81**: 546–55.
19. Scottish Intercollegiate Guidelines Network (SIGN) guideline on the management of stable angina. April 2001. *www.sign.ac.uk*
20. Ramsay L, Williams B, Johnston G *et al*. Guidelines for management of hypertension: report of the third working party of the British Hypertension Society. *J Hum Hypertens* 1999; **13**: 569–92.
21. National Service Framework for Coronary Heart Disease. March 2000.
22. Norell M, Lythall D, Coghlan G *et al*. Limited value of the resting electrocardiogram in assessing patients with recent onset chest pain: lessons from a chest pain clinic. *Br Heart J* 1992; **67**: 53–6.
23. Prodigy Guidance – Angina. April 2003. *http://www.prodigy.nhs.uk/guidance.asp?gt=Angina*
24. Ridker PM, Manson JE, Gaziano JM, Buring JE, Hennekens CH. Low-dose aspirin therapy for chronic stable angina. A randomized, placebo-controlled clinical trial. *Ann Intern Med* 1991; **114**: 835–9.
25. Eccles M, Freemantle N, Mason J. North of England evidence based guideline development project: guideline on the use of aspirin as secondary prophylaxis for vascular disease in primary care. North of England Aspirin Guideline Development Group. *BMJ* 1998; **316**: 1303–9.
26. Collaborative meta-analysis of randomised trials of antiplatelet therapy for prevention of death, myocardial infarction, and stroke in high risk patients. *BMJ* 2002; **324**: 71–86.
27. Staniforth AD. Contemporary management of chronic stable angina. *Drugs Aging* 2001; **18**: 109–21.
28. Gibbons RJ, Chatterjee K, Daley J *et al*. ACC/AHA/ACP-ASIM guidelines for the management of patients with chronic stable angina: executive summary and recommendations. A Report of the American College of Cardiology/American Heart Association Task Force on Practice Guidelines (Committee on Management of Patients with Chronic Stable Angina). *Circulation* 1999; **99**: 2829–48.
29. Anderson JR, Khou S, Nawarskas JJ. Ranolazine: a potential new treatment for chronic stable angina. *Heart Dis* 2001; **3**: 263–9.
30. Effect of nicorandil on coronary events in patients with stable angina: the Impact Of Nicorandil in Angina (IONA) randomised trial. *Lancet* 2002; **359**: 1269–75.
31. O'Toole L, Grech ED. Chronic stable angina: treatment options. *BMJ* 2003; **326**: 1185–8.
32. Bucher HC, Hengstler P, Schindler C, Guyatt GH. Percutaneous transluminal coronary angioplasty versus medical treatment for non-acute coronary heart disease: meta-analysis of randomised controlled trials. *BMJ* 2000; **321**: 73–7.
33. Kim MC, Kini A, Sharma SK. Refractory angina pectoris: mechanism and therapeutic options. *J Am Coll Cardiol* 2002; **39**: 923–34.
34. *Immunisation Against Infectious Disease 1996.* 'The Green Book'. *http://www.doh.gov.uk/greenbook*

4. Asthma

Dr Eleanor Bull
CSF Medical Communications Ltd

Summary

Asthma is a chronic inflammatory disorder of the airways associated with airway hyper-responsiveness, reversible airflow limitation and other respiratory problems. Characteristically, the symptoms of asthma are variable in nature and worsen at night or following exposure to recognised triggers. In this manner, asthma is distinguished from other respiratory disorders. Asthma is one of the most common chronic diseases worldwide, affecting between 100 and 150 million people – thus it imposes a substantial economic burden on healthcare resources. For the individual, asthma can impact greatly on quality of life through the periodic limitation of everyday activities. The causes of asthma are multifactorial and many relate to an inherited predisposition. Environmental factors, including animal allergens, tobacco smoke and air pollution, may aggravate the condition. There is no current cure for asthma, and once established, no intervention can prevent the natural course of disease development, although steroidal agents may slow the rate of progression. In general, available treatments provide symptomatic relief of varying degrees and may reduce the frequency of exacerbations, but do not address the underlying cause of disease.

Introduction

Asthma is characterised by widespread but variable airflow obstruction that is mostly reversible, either spontaneously or with treatment. A dynamic condition, the severity of asthma varies with time such that episodic worsening of airflow is a major feature of the disease. Exacerbations of asthma (attacks or worsening of symptoms and lung function) can be rapid in onset or occur gradually. Severe exacerbations can be fatal if not treated appropriately, although the mortality rate for asthma has decreased to some extent, thanks largely to improved treatment options and patient education.

Symptoms

The main symptoms of asthma are shared with other respiratory disorders, including chronic obstructive pulmonary disease, bronchiectasis, cystic fibrosis and obliterative bronchiolitis. What differentiates asthma from these other diseases is the frequency of occurrence and aetiology of the symptoms. In addition, there will commonly be a personal or family history of asthma or other atopic conditions (allergic rhinitis and eczema), in which abnormal amounts of IgE antibodies are produced in response to common environmental allergens. The principal, non-specific symptoms of asthma include:

- wheeze
- cough
- shortness of breath
- chest tightness.

When these symptoms are related specifically to asthma, they tend to be:
- variable in severity
- intermittent
- worse at night
- provoked by triggers including exercise and allergen exposure in susceptible individuals.

Epidemiology

It has been estimated that asthma affects between 100 and 150 million people worldwide, and its prevalence is on the increase.[1] There are insufficient data to determine the likely causes of this growth, although factors associated with a western lifestyle are thought to contribute. The socioeconomic status of an individual is a recognised factor that contributes to disease severity. Inner-city living is associated with a greater prevalence of asthma, which may be related to higher levels of environmental pollution, dampness and poor ventilation.[2,3] Alternatively, in westernised countries the surrounding environment is more sterile and infants' immune systems may fail to develop appropriately as a result of reduced microbial exposure in early life, thereby increasing susceptibility to atopic disease development, a concept known as the 'hygiene hypothesis'.[4,5]

An International Study of Asthma and Allergies in Childhood (ISAAC) survey reported that in children aged 13–14 years, the UK has the fifth highest prevalence of asthma (20.7%; Table 1) out of 56 countries worldwide.[6] In the UK, out of a population of 59 million, over 5 million people are currently receiving treatment and 8 million people have been diagnosed as having asthma at some point in their lives. Furthermore, in

Table 1. International comparison of asthma prevalence in children aged 13–14 years – a selection of countries with the highest and lowest prevalence.[6]

Country	Percentage diagnosed with asthma
Australia	28.2
Peru	28.0
New Zealand	24.4
Singapore	20.9
UK	20.7
South Korea	2.4
Russia	2.4
Uzbekistan	1.7
Indonesia	1.6
Albania	1.6

2000, over 18,000 first or new episodes of asthma presented every week to GPs in the UK.[7] Although mortality rates are decreasing, around 1500 people still die from asthma each year in the UK. The majority of these deaths are in the elderly, but in 1999, 25 children and over 500 adults under the age of 65 died as a result of asthma.[7]

Pathophysiology

Asthma is a chronic inflammatory disorder of the airways in which many cells and mediators play a role (Table 2). The pathophysiological features of the asthmatic response are illustrated in Figure 1.

Airway hyper-responsiveness

In patients with asthma, the smooth muscle of the airway is hyper-reactive to various spasmogens, resulting in the exaggerated narrowing of the airways in response to normally non-inflammatory stimuli. Ultimately, this leads to an increased variation in airway calibre and increased basal airway tone. Airway hyper-responsiveness can be elicited by the infiltration and accumulation of activated inflammatory cells, including eosinophils, T-lymphocytes, mast cells and macrophages. These cells produce chemical mediators (leukotrienes, cytokines, histamine) which perpetuate airway hyper-responsiveness and exacerbate tissue damage.[8]

T-lymphocytes are differentiated into Th1 and Th2 phenotypes. An imbalance of these cells in favour of the Th2 phenotype commonly occurs in patients with allergic asthma.[9] Following exposure to an allergen, Th2 cells stimulate the secretion of IgE antibodies from B-lymphocytes and

Table 2. Summary of the inflammatory cells and mediators involved in asthma.

	Role in asthma
Inflammatory cell type	
Eosinophils	Induce airway epithelial damage through release of basic proteins and oxygen-derived free radicals
Mast cells	Acute response to allergen
	Multiple roles: histamine release, airway remodelling
Neutrophils	Induce airway obstruction and epithelial damage through release of lipid mediators and oxygen-derived free radicals
T-lymphocytes	Release IgE antibodies and cytokines, resulting in recruitment and maintenance of eosinophils
Macrophages	Release cytokines
Inflammatory mediator	
Histamine, prostaglandins, leukotrienes	Contract airway smooth muscle, increase microvasculature leakage, mucus secretion and chemotaxis of inflammatory cells
Platelet-activating factor	Increases vascular permeability, chemotaxis of inflammatory cells
Substance P, neurokinin A, calcitonin gene-related peptide	Inflammatory neurotransmitters: increase and extend inflammatory response
Cytokines	Chronic inflammation, multiple roles
Endothelins	Vasoconstriction, bronchoconstriction, airway smooth muscle proliferation fibrosis

produce a distinct profile of cytokines (specifically interleukins 4, 5 and 13) that are strongly associated with the pathophysiology of asthma and other atopic diseases.[10] Interleukin 5 in particular is responsible for the recruitment and activation of eosinophils. Eosinophil infiltration into the airways is considered to be a defining feature of asthma, and the mediators released following eosinophil activation – major basic protein and eosinophilic cationic protein – are thought to be integral to the epithelial damage that is characteristic of asthma pathophysiology.

Airway epithelial shedding

Damage to, or loss of, the cells forming the bronchial epithelium further contributes to airway hyper-responsiveness. Many factors can initiate epithelial shedding, including chemical sensitisers, viral infection, allergen exposure and inflammatory mediators released from inflammatory cells, in particular, eosinophils.[11] As a consequence, clumps of epithelial cells aggregate in the lumen of the airways of asthmatics, where they may obstruct airflow. Furthermore, epithelial damage also results in the loss of

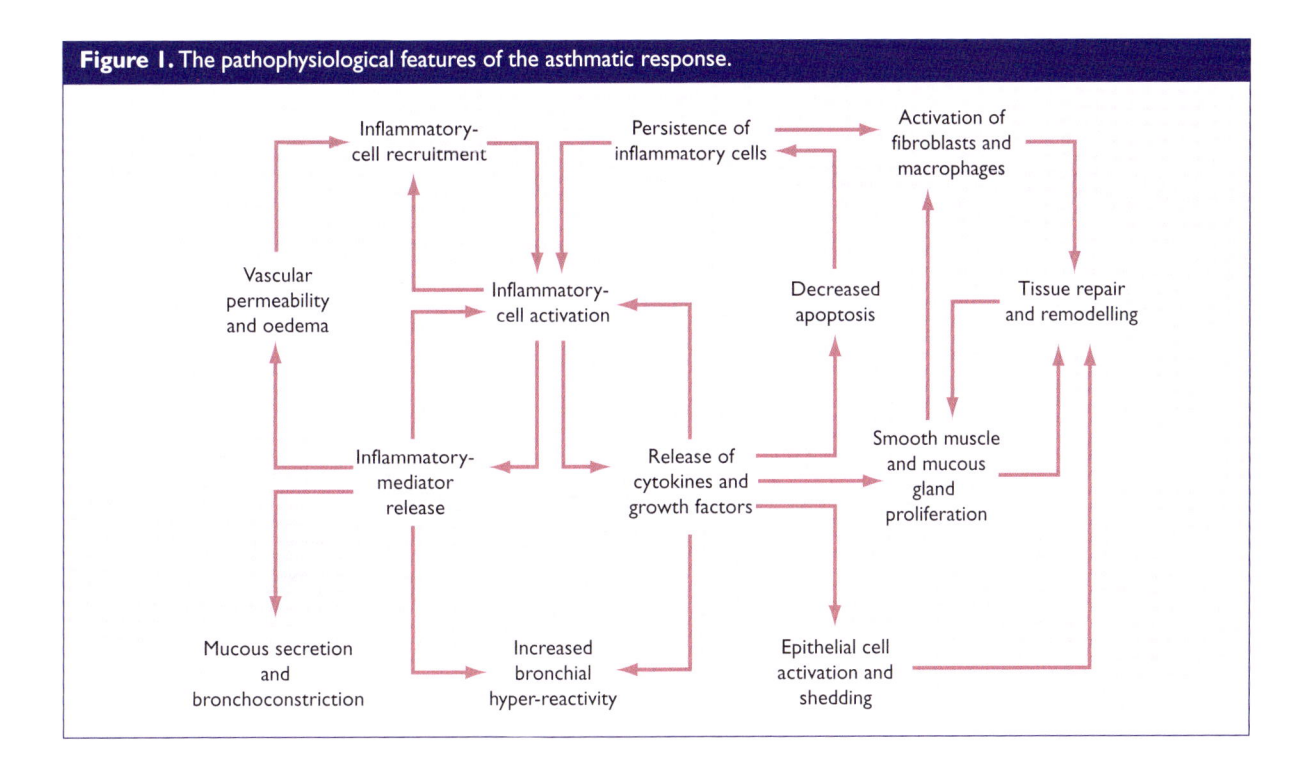

Figure 1. The pathophysiological features of the asthmatic response.

enzymes, relaxant properties and protective barrier functions attributed to the bronchial epithelium.

Occlusion of airways by mucus plugs

In patients with asthma, the epithelial goblet cells responsible for mucus production in the airways proliferate rapidly, causing mucus hypersecretion. Excess mucus may form obstructive plugs in the airways and accumulates cellular debris from necrotic epithelial cells. Increased microvascular leakage can be evoked by many of the inflammatory mediators implicated in asthma and may also lead to mucosal oedema of the airway wall and increased airway secretions.[12]

Activation of airway sensory nerve endings

The exposure of sensory nerves as a result of epithelial damage may elicit reflex neural effects in asthmatics, including cough and chest tightness. In addition, the release of the inflammatory neuropeptides, substance P, neurokinin A and calcitonin gene-related peptide from sensitised inflammatory nerves in the airways further impacts on the overall inflammatory response.[13]

Airway wall remodelling

Patients with chronic asthma may undergo long-term structural changes in their airways caused by the accumulation of collagen in subepithelial tissue (subepithelial fibrosis).[14] Airway integrity is further modified by smooth muscle hypertrophy and hyperplasia, leading to an overall increase in airway smooth muscle.[15] Both of these factors result in an exaggerated degree of airway wall narrowing which has a profoundly reduces air supply to the patient, particularly in instances of airway smooth muscle contraction.

Airway smooth muscle contraction

Patients with asthma exhibit increased shortening in measurements of isotonic contraction of airway smooth muscle.[16,17] The enhanced contractility observed in asthma seems to be associated with an increased velocity of shortening.[18] It is thought that the reorganisation of contractile filaments and the plasticity of smooth muscle cells may underlie chronic airway hyper-responsiveness.[19]

Aetiology

The causes of asthma are multifactorial and differ according to individual patients. Asthma is a heritable condition and in the majority of cases the individual is predisposed to disease development as a result of pre-existing, innate characteristics.[20,21] Environmental factors contribute to the manifestation of disease symptoms in a predisposed individual.

A number of host factors influence the likelihood of predisposing a patient to asthma. These factors include:
- atopy
- airway hyper-responsiveness
- gender
- race/ethnicity.

Environmental factors influence the susceptibility of a predisposed individual to develop asthma. Such factors include:
- indoor allergens (house dust mites, animal allergens, fungi, moulds, yeast)
- outdoor allergens (pollens, fungi, moulds, yeast)
- occupational sensitisers (requiring special assessment)
- tobacco smoke
- air pollution
- respiratory infection
- parasitic infection

- socioeconomic status
- diet
- drugs
- obesity
- increasingly sterile environment with reduced microbial exposure: the 'hygiene hypothesis'.

Furthermore, a number of environmental factors precipitate asthma exacerbations, and include:
- indoor and outdoor allergens
- indoor and outdoor air pollutants
- respiratory and viral infections
- exercise
- weather changes
- sulphur dioxide
- foods, additives, drugs (e.g. aspirin, non-steroidal anti-inflammatory drugs, paracetamol)
- extreme emotional suppression
- tobacco smoke (inhaled passively or actively).

The onset of asthma may occur at any stage of life, although the factors that influence onset may differ between individuals. In infants, asthma is primarily related to atopy, which predisposes the airways to sensitisation by allergens, and is characterised by a predominance of Th2 lymphocytes. There is evidence to suggest that children living in affluent societies may be exposed to lower levels of pathogens and that, as a result, their immune systems may polarise towards a Th2 rather than Th1 phenotype and hence increase the chances of developing allergic disease.[5] Exposure to pathogens in early life may confer protection against allergic diseases through the suppression of Th2-mediated immunity. In older children, allergy is the predominant feature associated with asthma. In adults, asthma can result from the occupational sensitisation of the airways and from the development of atopy in later life.

Diagnosis

Asthma is under-diagnosed throughout the world and as a consequence it is under-treated. The principal underlying reason behind this is that many patients tolerate intermittent respiratory symptoms before seeking medical advice. Diagnosis can be made on the basis of presenting symptoms; however, measurements of lung function greatly enhance diagnostic accuracy.

Lung function tests measure the peak expiratory flow rate (PEFR), forced vital capacity (FVC) and forced expiratory volume in 1 second (FEV$_1$). These measurements depend on airflow limitation relating directly to the luminal size of airways and the elastic properties of the surrounding lung tissue, and will be markedly decreased in asthmatic patients, with a pronounced variability of function. Lung function tests should be conducted in both the presence and absence of symptoms. If function is normal in the presence of symptoms, a diagnosis of asthma is unlikely. Considering the diurnal variation of symptoms in asthma, patient self-monitoring is particularly important. Patients are encouraged to maintain a diary card of their expiratory peak flow and to record any reduction in peak flow following exposure to a recognised trigger (including exercise).

In short, a diagnosis of asthma should be considered if there is a:
- history of classic symptoms (e.g. cough, wheeze, shortness of breath, tightness, exercise-induced symptoms)
- 15–20% or greater variability in lung function as measured by changes in PEFR, FVC and FEV$_1$ between morning and evening
- response to asthma treatment (i.e. an increase in lung function after inhalation of a short-acting β_2-agonist or after a trial of corticosteroid tablets)
- a decrease in lung function after 6 minutes of exercise (e.g. running).

The severity of asthma can be judged on the basis of the severity and frequency of symptoms and the level of medication required for their adequate control, as well as the degree to which the patient's lifestyle is limited. The aetiology and the pattern of airflow limitation are also useful indicators of the severity of the disease.

Treatment of asthma

The main aims of asthma treatment are the control of symptoms, the prevention of exacerbations and achievement of best possible pulmonary function with minimal side-effects. Although pharmacological interventions are effective in controlling symptoms and improving quality of life in the majority of patients, the prevention of asthma exacerbations by non-pharmacological means is of great importance in the management of the disease. By limiting exposure to risk factors such as allergens and environmental pollutants, the likelihood of asthma exacerbations can be greatly reduced. Additional lifestyle changes should also be implemented.

Prophylactic lifestyle changes that reduce the impact of asthma include:
- dietary manipulations
- weight reduction

- smoking cessation
- self-management plans
- breathing retraining in patients with symptoms suggestive of dysfunctional breathing.

Pharmacological treatment

Pharmacological intervention should be selected on the basis of disease severity in the individual patient and in accordance with clearly defined treatment guidelines. These guidelines advocate a stepwise approach, in which treatment is started at the step most appropriate for the individual patient (Table 3). Many patients can be treated adequately with inhaled corticosteroids but an important number require additional therapy. Representative large-scale surveys in the UK have revealed that 1 in 10 people living with asthma have severe or moderately severe asthma that

> Treatment guidelines advocate a stepwise approach, in which treatment is started at the step most appropriate for the individual patient.

Table 3. Recommended guidelines for the treatment of asthma in adults according to the severity of symptoms, adapted from the Global Initiative for Asthma, Workshop Report, 2002 and the British Guideline for the Treatment of Asthma.[23,24] It should be noted that guidelines differ for children and pregnant women.

Level of severity	Daily preventer medications	Other treatment options
Step 1 Mild intermittent asthma	None necessary	Inhaled short-acting β_2-agonist as required
Step 2 Mild persistent asthma	Inhaled corticosteroid (200–800 mg/day)	Sustained-release theophylline, or cromone, or leukotriene receptor antagonist
Step 3 Moderate persistent asthma	Inhaled corticosteroid (200–800 mg/day)	*Add* sustained-release theophylline, or *add* long-acting oral β_2-agonist, or *add* leukotriene receptor antagonist, or increase dose of corticosteroid
Step 4 Severe persistent asthma	Inhaled corticosteroid plus long-acting inhaled β_2-agonist, plus one or more of: • sustained-release theophylline • leukotriene receptor antagonist • long-acting oral β_2-agonist • oral corticosteroid	

NB. At all steps, a rapidly acting inhaled β_2-agonist should be taken as needed for the relief of symptoms. Once control of asthma, in terms of clinical symptoms and lung function measurements, has been maintained for at least 3 months, therapy should be gradually stepped down.

is not effectively controlled.[22] Newly developed therapies should aim to improve symptom control in severe cases, minimise side-effects and improve patient compliance. The current treatments of choice and the recommended treatment guidelines are described below.

Medications for asthma are usually administered by inhalation, the advantage of this being that drugs are delivered directly to the airways where they are needed at high concentrations and the onset of action is accelerated. However, inhaler devices can be associated with reduced compliance and localised side-effects.

When treating paediatric patients, the basic treatment principles remain the same as those for adults. However, in children under 3 years of age, the only recommended controller medications are the inhaled corticosteroids. Oral formulations are preferable in this age group, since difficulties may be encountered with inhaler devices. The use of nebulisers and face masks is also advocated.

Short-acting β_2-agonists

β_2-agonists (e.g. salbutamol and terbutaline) are effective bronchodilators and as such are commonly prescribed for the relief of the acute asthmatic response, with maximum effects achieved within 30 minutes and maintained for 4–6 hours. They relax airway smooth muscle, increase mucociliary clearance, inhibit mediator release from mast cells and decrease vascular permeability. Side-effects are limited but can include tremor, palpitations and tachycardia at high doses. Tolerance, associated with a loss of bronchodilator activity, may also occur.[25]

Low-dose inhaled corticosteroids

Corticosteroids (e.g. beclometasone, fluticasone, mometasone and budenoside) are currently the most effective anti-inflammatory medication for asthma at all levels of severity. They act by directly inhibiting a range of inflammatory cells, particularly eosinophils, and by activating glucocorticoid receptors leading to the altered regulation of transcription of target genes.[26] This leads to dramatic improvements in airway hyper-responsiveness, lung function and a reduction in the frequency of exacerbations. In the short term, side-effects commonly include dysphonia and oral candidiasis, although this may be prevented by the use of spacer devices and the 'gargling' of water following drug administration. However, it is the long-term systemic consequences of exposure that are of most concern, with bruising, reduced bone mineral density and suppression of the adrenocortical axis reported, albeit rarely, in both paediatric and adult patients and usually in those receiving high doses.[27,28] As a result, guidelines recommend that the maximum dose of beclometasone, or equivalent, does not exceed 400 µg per day in children and 800 µg per day in adults.

Cromones

Cromones (e.g. sodium cromoglycate and nedocromil sodium) are occasionally used in conjunction with corticosteroids. Although their mechanism of action is not fully understood, it is thought to involve the suppression of the IgE-mediated inflammatory response.[29] Side-effects are minimal although an inconvenient dosing regimen and a lack of effectiveness in adults limit the widespread use of these agents.

Long-acting β_2-agonists

Compounds in this class (e.g. salmeterol, formoterol) act in the same manner as the short-acting β_2-agonists but efficacy is sustained for up to 12 hours. This extended duration of action warrants their use in the treatment of moderate persistent asthma as a means of improving asthma control and reducing exacerbations, rather than the immediate symptomatic relief of the acute asthma response. Inhaled steroids are the recommended intervention for both adults and children for the effective control of asthma.

Leukotriene receptor antagonists

A recently developed oral asthma therapy, the leukotriene receptor antagonists (e.g. montelukast and zafirlukast) act by blocking the inflammatory effects of leukotrienes. In this way they remain active over a wide spectrum of asthma severity and exhibit both anti-inflammatory and bronchodilator activity.[30] Initial findings indicate that these drugs are not as effective as the corticosteroids, although, in contrast, they are well tolerated, with few side-effects reported. As such they are commonly employed as add-on therapy to an existing inhaled corticosteroid treatment regimen.

Methylxanthines

Theophylline is a bronchodilator with possible anti-inflammatory activity, employed as preventer therapy and as an adjunct to corticosteroids. However, it has a very low therapeutic index and its use is limited by side-effects including gastrointestinal upset, nausea and vomiting, tachycardia, arrhythmia and tremor.[31]

Socioeconomic impact

The treatment of asthma places a particularly high burden on the primary healthcare system, with almost 4 million consultations for asthma each year in the UK and estimated annual healthcare costs of over £850 million.[7,32,33]

The morbidity associated with asthma is such that a high proportion of patients are hospitalised for treatment. In the UK in 1999 there were 80,000 admissions to hospital due to asthma, with over 30,000 of these accounted for by children.[7] Over 18 million working days are lost due to asthma each year.[32] In the UK, asthma is a major cause of work and school absence, with consequent repercussions in professional and educational attainment. Recent findings suggest that the perception of the severity of asthma-related lifestyle restrictions differs between paediatric patients and healthcare professionals such that lifestyle limitation is underestimated by the latter group (Figure 2).[34] Measures should be taken to address this discrepancy in order to improve patient outcomes.

Clearly, reducing the number and severity of attacks will improve both patients' quality of life and the efficiency of the healthcare system.

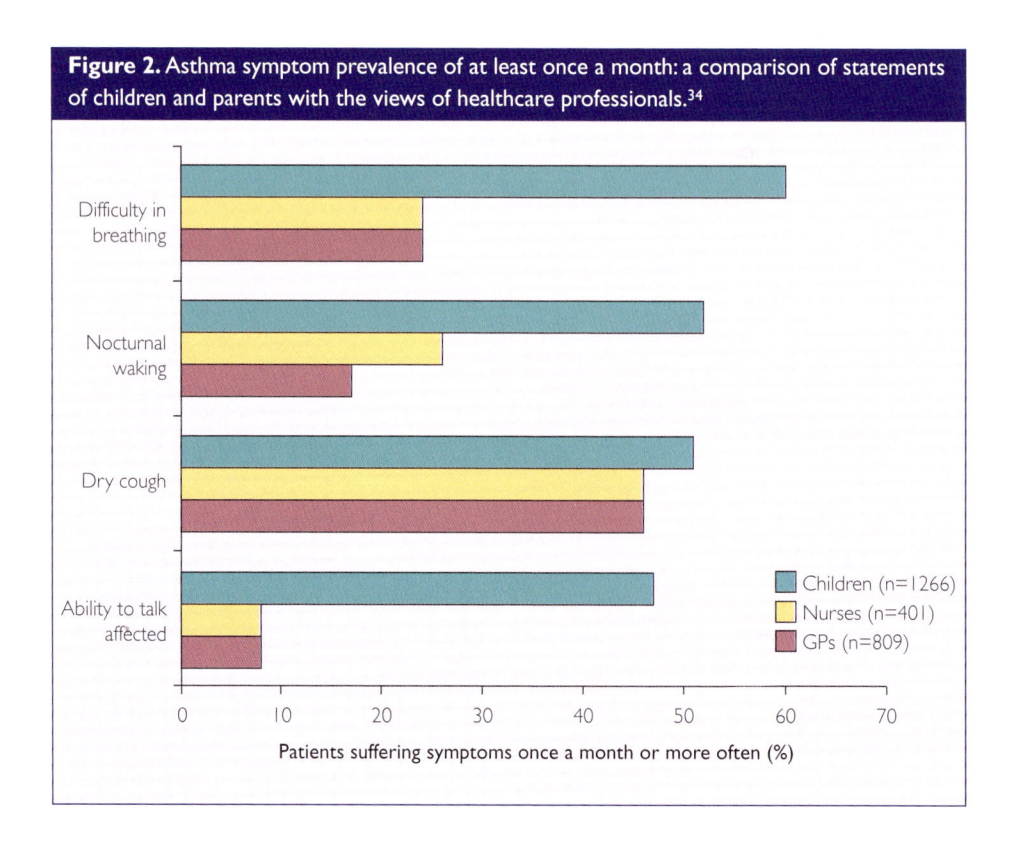

Figure 2. Asthma symptom prevalence of at least once a month: a comparison of statements of children and parents with the views of healthcare professionals.[34]

Key points

- Asthma is a chronic inflammatory disorder of the airways with recurrent exacerbations.
- The increasing worldwide incidence of asthma exerts significant pressure on healthcare resources.
- The main symptoms are wheeze, cough, shortness of breath and chest tightness; these are intermittent, worsen at night and are provoked by recognised triggers.
- Asthma is characterised by airway hyper-responsiveness, airway obstruction, epithelial damage and long-term structural remodelling of the airways.
- The causes of asthma are multifactorial with genetic and environmental contributions, including tobacco smoke, air pollution and animal allergens.
- Current asthma therapy is directed at treating chronic inflammation and improving lung function through bronchodilation, although non-pharmacological preventative measures should be taken where possible to avoid exacerbations.
- Inhaled corticosteroids remain the cornerstone of treatment, with the addition of add-on therapy if symptoms continue.

References

1. World Health Organization. WHO Factsheet No. 206: Bronchial Asthma. 2000.
2. Shapiro G, Stout J. Childhood asthma in the United States: urban issues. *Pediatr Pulmonol* 2002; **33**: 47–55.
3. Cesaroni G, Farchi S, Davoli M, Forastiere F, Perucci C. Individual and area-based indicators of socioeconomic status and childhood asthma. *Eur Respir J* 2003; **22**: 619–24.
4. Strachan D. Hay fever, hygiene, and household size. *BMJ* 1989; **299**: 1259–60.
5. Strachan D. Family size, infection and atopy: the first decade of the "hygiene hypothesis". *Thorax* 2000; **55**: S2–10.
6. Worldwide variations in the prevalence of asthma symptoms: the International Study of Asthma and Allergies in Childhood (ISAAC). *Eur Respir J* 1998; **12**: 315–35.
7. National Asthma Campaign. Out in the open: a true picture of asthma in the United Kingdom today. *The Asthma Journal* 2001; **6**: 1–14.
8. Fireman P. Understanding asthma pathophysiology. *Allergy Asthma Proc* 2003; **24**: 79–83.
9. Umetsu D, DeKruyff R. TH1 and TH2 CD4+ cells in human allergic diseases. *J Allergy Clin Immunol* 1997; **10**: 1–6.
10. Tattersfield A, Knox A, Britton J, Hall I. Asthma. *Lancet* 2002; **360**: 1313–22.
11. Barnes P. Pathophysiology of asthma. *Br J Clin Pharmacol* 1996; **42**: 3–10.
12. Barnes P, Chung K, Page C. Inflammatory mediators and asthma. *Pharmacol Rev* 1988; **40**: 49–84.
13. Barnes P. Sensory nerves, neuropeptides, and asthma. *Ann N Y Acad Sci* 1991; **629**: 359–70.
14. Djukanovic R, Roche W, Wilson J *et al*. Mucosal inflammation in asthma. *Am Rev Respir Dis* 1990; **142**: 434–57.
15. Ebina M, Yaegashi H, Chiba R, Takahashi T, Motomiya M, Tanemura M. Hyperreactive site in the airway tree of asthmatic patients revealed by thickening of bronchial muscles. A morphometric study. *Am Rev Respir Dis* 1990; **141**: 1327–32.
16. Bai T. Abnormalities in airway smooth muscle in fatal asthma. *Am Rev Respir Dis* 1990; **141**: 552–7.
17. Thomson R, Bramley A, Schellenberg R. Airway muscle stereology: implications for increased shortening in asthma. *Am J Respir Crit Care Med* 1996; **154**: 749–57.
18. Mitchell R, Ruhlmann E, Magnussen H, Leff A, Rabe K. Passive sensitization of human bronchi augments smooth muscle shortening velocity and capacity. *Am J Physiol* 1994; **267**: L218–22.
19. Gunst S, Tang D. The contractile apparatus and mechanical properties of airway smooth muscle. *Eur Respir J* 2000; **15**: 600–16.
20. Holgate S. Genetic and environmental interaction in allergy and asthma. *J Allergy Clin Immunol* 1999; **104**: 1139–46.
21. Palmer L, Burton P, James A, Musk A, Cookson W. Familial aggregation and heritability of asthma-associated quantitative traits in a population-based sample of nuclear families. *Eur J Hum Genet* 2000; **8**: 853–60.
22. National Asthma Campaign. Greater expectations? Findings from the National Asthma Campaign's representative study of the Needs of People with Asthma (NOPWA) in the UK. *The Asthma Journal* 2000; **5**(3).
23. Global Initiative for Asthma. GINA Workshop Report, Global Strategy for Asthma Management and Prevention, 2002.
24. British Guideline on the Management of Asthma. *Thorax* 2003; **58(Suppl 1)**: 1–94.
25. O'Connor B, Aikman S, Barnes P. Tolerance to the nonbronchodilator effects of inhaled beta 2-agonists in asthma. *N Engl J Med* 1992; **327**: 1204–8.
26. Green R, Brightling C, Pavord I, Wardlaw A. Management of asthma in adults: current therapy and future directions. *Postgrad Med J* 2003; **79**: 259–67.
27. Clark D, Lipworth B. Adrenal suppression with chronic dosing of fluticasone propionate compared with budesonide in adult asthmatic patients. *Thorax* 1997; **52**: 55–8.
28. Israel E, Banerjee T, Fitzmaurice G, Kotlov T, LaHive K, LeBoff M. Effects of inhaled glucocorticoids on bone density in premenopausal women. *N Engl J Med* 2001; **345**: 941–7.
29. Diaz P, Gallegguillos F, Gonzalez M, Pantin C, Kay A. Bronchoalveolar lavage in asthma: the effect of disodium cromoglycate (cromolyn) on leukocyte counts, immunoglobulins, and complement. *J Allergy Clin Immunol* 1984; **74**: 41–8.
30. Lipworth B. Leukotriene-receptor antagonists. *Lancet* 1999; **353**: 57–62.
31. Pollard S, Spector S, Yancey S, Cox F, Emmett A. Salmeterol versus theophylline in the treatment of asthma. *Ann Allergy Asthma Immunol* 1997; **78**: 457–64.
32. National Asthma Campaign. National Asthma Audit: Direct Publishing Solutions Ltd, 1999/2000.
33. Hoskins G, McCowan C, Neville R, Thomas G, Smith B, Silverman S. Risk factors and costs associated with an asthma attack. *Thorax* 2000; **55**: 19–24.
34. Price D, Ryan D, Pearce L *et al*. The burden of paediatric asthma is higher than health professionals think: results from the Asthma in Real Life (AIR) study. *Prim Care Respir J* 2002; **11**: 30–3.

5. Atherothrombosis

Dr Scott Chambers
CSF Medical Communications Ltd

Dr Jonathan Morrell
GP, Hastings, East Sussex

Summary

Cardiovascular disease (CVD) is responsible for 40% of all deaths in the UK each year, and consequently, it represents a huge and growing burden on NHS resources. Atherothrombosis (thrombus formation superimposed on disrupted or eroded atherosclerotic plaques) is the underlying pathology responsible for the majority of cases of CVD, and it is the common, final pathway resulting in the clinical manifestations of myocardial infarction (MI), stroke, transient ischaemic attacks (TIA) and critical limb ischaemia. Platelets are intimately involved in the process of atherothrombosis, and play a critical role in the development and progression of atherosclerotic plaques, resulting in the clinical manifestations of CVD.

CVD can be prevented and delayed in many instances. However, such intervention requires effective risk stratification, lifestyle modification and the use of appropriate pharamacological treatments. The mainstay of pharmacological therapy in the management of acute atherothrombotic events and prevention of subsequent events is the use of antiplatelet agents such as aspirin. Indeed, the majority of clinical guidelines place antiplatelet therapy at the forefront of patient management. The availability of new generation antiplatelet agents such as clopidogrel and dipyridamole may provide further improvements in patient management, either given as monotherapy, or in combination with aspirin.

Introduction

Atherothrombosis is the underlying pathology responsible for the majority of cases of CVD. It transforms previously stable atherosclerotic disease into acute, life-threatening clinical manifestations: MI and unstable angina (collectively referred to as acute coronary syndrome [ACS]), ischaemic stroke, TIA and peripheral arterial disease (PAD). As atherothrombosis affects multiple vascular beds, individuals with any one of its clinical manifestations are at a significantly increased risk of additional events at different sites within the vascular tree.

Platelets play a central role in the pathophysiology of atherothrombosis, in which three critical platelet-dependent steps – platelet adhesion, platelet activation and platelet aggregation – occur at the sites of disrupted or eroded atherosclerotic plaques within a principal arterial wall. These events result in the exposure of highly thrombogenic substances (e.g. tissue factor) within the plaque to the circulating blood, ultimately leading to thrombus formation, complete or partial occlusion of the artery, or embolisation and subsequent microvascular obstruction at distal sites.

Antiplatelet therapies remain the cornerstone of treatment strategies in the secondary prevention of a variety of acute ischaemic events in patients at risk of recurrent, major cardiovascular and cerebrovascular events. Whilst our greatest experience has been with aspirin, newer and more effective agents have come to the fore over the past decade, and have the potential to offer advances in the clinical management of the disease.

Epidemiology

CVD, predominantly comprising coronary heart disease (CHD) and stroke, is a principal cause of premature death worldwide, accounting for over 15 million deaths every year.[1] Globally, ischaemic heart disease (IHD) and cerebrovascular disease were responsible for 51% of all deaths in 2001.[2] CVD is also associated with a growing burden of morbidity, with stroke in particular being the principal cause of disability in western industrialised countries.[3] Consequently, CVD has a major and spiralling impact upon global healthcare resources.

In the UK in 2001, CVD was the main cause of death, accounting for more than 240,000 deaths, and representing nearly 40% of total mortality.[4] The principal manifestations of CVD – CHD and stroke – were responsible for approximately half and one-quarter of all deaths from CVD, respectively.[4] CHD alone was the most common cause of death, usually from MI, and accounted for more than 120,000 deaths (one death in five), whilst strokes accounted for one in ten deaths.[4] In addition, more than 2 million individuals in the UK are currently diagnosed with angina, the most common form of CHD.[4]

In addition to these extremely high fatality rates, CVD also accounts for an enormous burden of morbidity (Table 1).[4–9] This is likely to increase in the future, due to an ageing population and the rapidly increasing prevalence of diabetes.

These epidemiological data illustrate the huge burden of CVD, and the

Table 1. The incidence of new patients per year presenting with vascular disease or type 2 diabetes in the UK population and in a theoretical GP list of 2000 patients.[4–9]

Condition	UK	Per 2000 patients
Vascular disease	632,920	21.2
Stroke[5,6]	155,000	5.2
Myocardial infarction (MI)[4]	274,000	9.2
Unstable angina/non-ST-segment elevation MI (ACS)[7]	180,000	6.0
Peripheral artery disease (PAD)[8]	23,920	0.8
Type 2 diabetes[9]	100,000[a]	3.3[a]

[a]Incidence of diabetes represents an estimate assuming a UK population of 59.8 million.

challenge that faces clinicians in managing this disease. Nevertheless, it should be remembered that CVD can be postponed in many instances, as many of its common risk factors are modifiable either by lifestyle interventions or by pharmacotherapy.

The burden of vascular disease: key facts

MI

- 25% of patients die in the period immediately following MI.[10]
- 10% of survivors die within the first year and 5% per year thereafter.[10]
- 18% of male and 35% of female survivors have a recurrent MI within 6 years.[11]
- 20% of patients are disabled by heart failure within 6 years of an index event.[12]
- The 5-year rate of stroke in MI survivors is 8.1%.[13]

Non-ST-segment elevation ACS

- Patients have a one-in-three chance of death, MI, refractory angina or readmission for unstable angina over 3 months.[14]

Stroke

- 20% of patients die within 1 month, 31% within 1 year.[15]
- 70% of the survivors become disabled.[16]
- 16% of patients die from recurrent stroke.[15]
- 35% die from another (non-stroke) cardiovascular event.[15]
- 12% of TIAs lead to stroke within one year.[17]

PAD

- PAD increases with increasing age, affecting 7% of patients aged 50–75 years.[18]
- 15% of male patients die within 5 years of diagnosis.[18]
- 25% of deaths result from stroke or abdominal vascular disease.[18]
- 50% of deaths are due to CHD.

Diabetes mellitus

- Mortality rates from CHD and stroke are three- to five-times higher for patients with diabetes.[19]

A glance at these key facts underlines the considerable overlap between the different clinical manifestations of ischaemic vascular disease within individual patients. This overlap reflects the disseminated and generalised nature of atherosclerotic disease, which often affects more than one vascular bed.[20] Thus, it is not uncommon for a patient who has presented with one manifestation of vascular disease to present subsequently with either a recurrent or a different manifestation (Figure 1).[21] The culprit lesions are

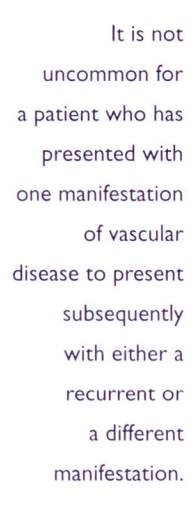

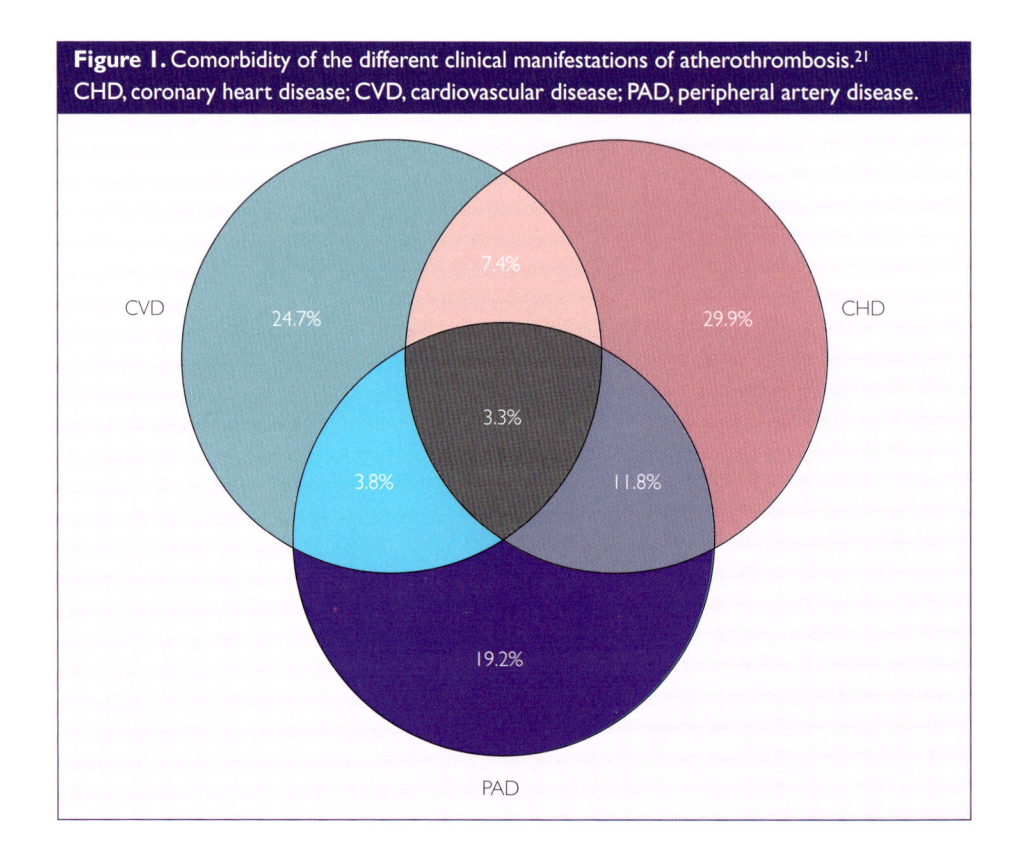

> It is not uncommon for a patient who has presented with one manifestation of vascular disease to present subsequently with either a recurrent or a different manifestation.

Figure 1. Comorbidity of the different clinical manifestations of atherothrombosis.[21] CHD, coronary heart disease; CVD, cardiovascular disease; PAD, peripheral artery disease.

atherosclerotic plaques which, in western society, are present from the teens and increase steadily with advancing age and exposure to risk factors.

Pathophysiology of atherothrombosis

Atherothrombosis is a generalised disease process, characterised by thrombus formation that is superimposed on disrupted or eroded atherosclerotic plaques in major arterial walls.[22] Thrombus formation is associated with the occlusion of major or minor arteries, together with embolisation and downstream occlusive events in the microvasculature. It is these mechanisms that are responsible for the majority of ischaemic events and their subsequent clinical manifestations, and ultimately for the major burden of mortality observed with CVD.

Plaque progression

Atherosclerosis begins with structural changes in the intima and media of the walls of large and medium sized arteries, predominantly the aorta and the coronary, cervical and iliac arteries. These structural changes arise from injuries in the endothelium generated by the combined impact of multiple risk factors.[3] Injury may also arise from disturbances in blood flow in particularly susceptible regions. Subsequently, endothelial dysfunction results in the accumulation of lipoproteins (mostly derived from plasma low density lipoprotein cholesterol [LDL-C], including highly atherogenic oxidised LDL-C particles), leading to the recruitment of monocytes into the vessel wall. These cells differentiate into macrophages, which imbibe the modified lipoproteins and are then converted into foam cells. These macrophages can also liberate a large number of vasoactive products that may lead to further damage in the endothelium, resulting in vasoconstriction. Smooth muscle cells become activated and invade these early atherosclerotic lesions and generate connective tissue fibrils which encapsulate the lipid core.[22]

Plaque stability

The arterial wall will frequently remodel itself by increasing its diameter, thereby accommodating the development of plaques without reducing the size of the lumen. Thus, the size of a plaque is not necessarily a predictor of acute ischaemic events; rather it is the intrinsic vulnerability of a plaque to rupture or erode that is responsible for the clinical manifestations of atherosclerosis.

A number of factors determine the stability of a plaque and its likelihood to rupture or erode.[22] In particular, intrinsic structural features ('passive

> It is the intrinsic vulnerability of a plaque to rupture or erode that is responsible for the clinical manifestations of atherosclerosis.

disruption') of a plaque can act in concert with active processes ('active disruption') to destabilise the lesion. In general, vulnerable or high-risk plaques are characterised by the following features:

- a thin, fibrous cap with disorganised collagen
- a large atheromatous lipid core containing high concentrations of cholesteryl esters
- significant infiltration by macrophages and other inflammatory cells, such as T-lymphocytes
- a scarcity of smooth muscle cells
- a high concentration of tissue factor.[22–24]

In contrast, stable plaques are characterised by a small lipid core covered with a thick fibrous cap.

Passive plaque rupture tends to occur more frequently at the shoulders of a plaque, possibly as a consequence of physical forces and blood flow. It may also arise due to the high concentration of macrophages located within these regions, since these are intrinsically involved in the active processes of plaque destabilisation, mediated by phagocytosis or by the secretion of proteolytic enzymes (in particular the matrix metalloproteinases) that act to degrade the extracellular matrix components of the fibrous cap.[22]

Finally, changes in blood flow due to arterial stenosis, hypertension, dyslipidaemia and irritants in tobacco smoke can also accelerate the process of plaque vulnerability and rupture.

Platelet adhesion, activation and aggregation

Platelets play a critical role in the initiation and propagation of the events involved in thrombosis (Figure 2). The development of a thrombus at the site of a ruptured or eroded atherosclerotic plaque proceeds via three critical platelet-dependent steps.

- *Platelet adhesion.* Adhesion of platelets occurs shortly after an atherosclerotic plaque has ruptured, eroded or become disrupted.[23,25] This step is mediated by the binding of von Willebrand factor and thrombospondin to the glycoprotein (GP) Ib receptor on the platelet membrane, and leads to the formation of a monolayer of platelets at the rupture site.
- *Platelet activation.* Platelet shape changes dramatically during platelet activation, from a smooth discoid to a spiculated form, increasing the surface area of the membrane for thrombin generation. This is followed by degranulation of the alpha granules and dense granules within the platelet, and the release of various prothrombotic, inflammatory and

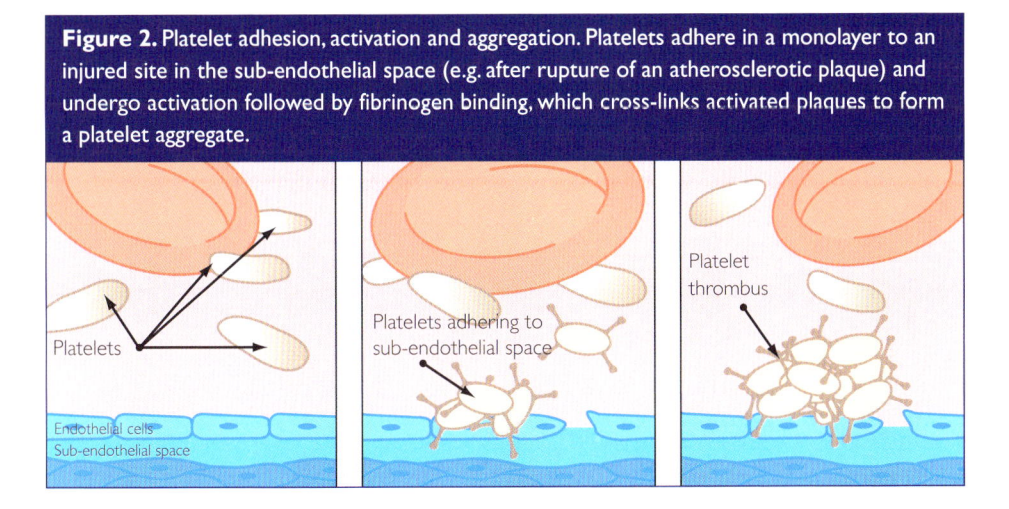

Figure 2. Platelet adhesion, activation and aggregation. Platelets adhere in a monolayer to an injured site in the sub-endothelial space (e.g. after rupture of an atherosclerotic plaque) and undergo activation followed by fibrinogen binding, which cross-links activated plaques to form a platelet aggregate.

chemoattractant molecules, such as adenosine diphosphate (ADP), fibrinogen and thromboxane A_2 (via the activation of cyclo-oxygenase).[23]

- *Platelet aggregation.* Platelet aggregation is mediated by conformational changes in the GP IIb/IIIa receptor on the platelet surface, which allow it to bind fibrinogen with a high affinity. Fibrinogen's multivalent nature facilitates platelet cross-linking, thereby creating a platelet aggregate or 'plug' and, with enmeshed blood cells and coagulation factors, the formation of a mature, potentially occlusive thrombus proceeds. Degranulated platelets release ADP, which binds to the ADP receptor on neighbouring platelets and serves to amplify the activation response.[23]

Inflammation and atherosclerosis

From a histological perspective, atherosclerosis shares many of the features of an inflammatory process. Indeed, over the past decade, there has been a growing awareness of the prominent role of chronic inflammation and the immune response in the various stages of the atherosclerosis, not only in its initiation and progression, but also in its thrombotic complications.[26,27] The source of the chronic inflammation leading to atherosclerosis is unclear, but it may have an infectious origin (e.g. *Chlamydia pneumoniae*) or alternatively may arise from non-infectious sources (e.g. cigarette smoke, obesity, or hyperglycaemia).

As alluded to previously, leukocytes are associated with the earliest atherosclerotic lesions. Chemokines attract monocytes and T-lymphocytes from the blood stream where they adhere to the vessel wall via interactions with selective adhesion molecules expressed by the endothelium in response to various factors, including ingestion of an atherogenic diet. Fluctuations in blood flow and in wall stresses also augment the expression of adhesion molecules, increasing the interaction of leukocytes with the vessel wall. Monocytes are stimulated via various chemoattractants to migrate into the intima, where they differentiate into macrophages which imbibe modified lipoproteins and develop into foam cells. These foam cells produce a number of cytokines which stimulate smooth muscle cell migration and the subsequent generation of a fibrous cap over the nascent atheroma. This cap can be disrupted by the secretion of macrophage-derived matrix metalloproteinases, which digest the extracellular matrix, weakening it and thereby making the plaque increasingly prone to rupture. Inflammatory cells may also inhibit smooth muscle cell protein synthesis and induce smooth muscle cell apoptosis, thereby destabilising the plaque further, leading to its rupture and ultimately thrombus formation. However, episodes of plaque rupture can also induce recruitment of new vascular smooth muscle cells via mitogens present in a thrombus. These reparative processes can drive the formation of a new fibrous cap covering the thrombus, thereby stabilising the plaque but resulting in an increase in size of the lesion.[26,27]

Serum markers of the acute phase of inflammation, such as C-reactive protein (CRP) and serum amyloid A, have generated significant interest in their utility as markers of cardiovascular risk. CRP is now viewed as a particularly robust marker of risk and is also a predictor of outcome in patients with ACS. Therefore, CRP is likely to be a useful marker in future risk stratification to identify those most likely to benefit from appropriate clinical intervention.[26,27]

Risk factors for atherothrombosis

The initiation and progression of atherosclerosis is influenced by the presence of multiple risk factors within a single individual.[20] These factors initiate events that begin with endothelial injury, and progress to endothelial dysfunction and ultimately atherothrombosis.

Different individuals have differing levels of cardiovascular risk, with different individual risk factors impacting on cardiovascular outcome to varying extents. However, the influence of one risk factor on clinical outcome is profoundly influenced by the coexistence of other risk factors.[20] Therefore, in order to modify the risk and tailor treatment appropriately, an assessment of the impact of each risk factor, set in the context of an overall risk profile, is necessary to give an indication of the urgency of treatment.[20] Risk factors for atherothrombosis include:
- left ventricular dysfunction
- dyslipidaemia

- congestive heart failure
- diabetes mellitus
- hypertension
- thrombogenic factors
- family history
- increased age
- male gender
- inactivity
- smoking
- poor diet and obesity
- excessive alcohol consumption.

Diagnosis

ACS

A physical examination generally elicits normal results in patients with ACS.[28] However, examination is still useful to exclude any possible non-cardiac causes of chest pain and non-ischaemic causes, and to search for any other signs of haemodynamic instability or ventricular dysfunction.

An electrocardiogram (ECG) taken at rest is a critical diagnostic assessment in patients with ACS.[28] The most reliable changes in the ECG which relate to ischaemic events in ACS are ST-segment depression, T-wave inversion and flat T-waves.[28,29] Despite its value, a completely normal ECG does not necessarily exclude the presence of an ACS.

Biochemical markers such as cardiac troponin T and troponin I are useful in detecting myocardial damage, and are specific markers of irreversible cellular necrosis and thus MI.[29] Due to this specificity, these biochemical markers are now considered to be the gold standard for diagnosis of ACS.[28] Raised levels of troponins are also useful in detecting damage in patients with ACS in the absence of elevated creatinine kinase, a less specific marker of cardiac damage.

PAD

Clinically, the most common symptom of PAD is intermittent claudication, though the majority of patients presenting in clinical practice remain asymptomatic.[30,31] Consequently, PAD is grossly under-diagnosed, leading to an unnecessarily increased burden of cardiovascular risk.

In addition to a patient history and physical examination, the ankle/brachial pressure index (ABPI) is a simple, effective screening method useful in identifying PAD in patients. The ABPI is measured by taking the ankle and brachial blood pressure measurements using a hand-held Doppler

> The ABPI is an independent predictor of morbidity and mortality.

device. An ABPI ratio of less than 0.9 is strongly associated with an increase in cardiovascular events in middle-aged and older patients.[30–32] In addition to being an important diagnostic marker, the ABPI is also an independent predictor of morbidity (non-fatal MI, unstable angina) and mortality (cardiovascular death).[30–32]

Stroke

Brain imaging via computed tomography (CT) or magnetic resonance imaging (MRI) is the principal diagnostic tool used to identify stroke.[33] A specific type of MRI imaging – diffusion weighted imaging – is particularly useful for detecting early ischaemic changes in the brain, and these appear as bright white lesions ('lightbulbs') on the MRI scan. More ischaemic strokes show up with diffusion weighted imaging than on a CT scan or conventional MRI within the first few hours of an event and up to 8 weeks after a stroke.[34] Such techniques also allow the detection of intracerebral or subarachnoid haemorrhage and can exclude other potential causes of stroke. This is particularly important in determining which treatment strategy to employ, and should be performed before any anticoagulant is administered.[33]

Pharmacological treatment

> Patients with atherosclerosis should be managed within a comprehensive programme of care that includes lifestyle modifications and pharmacological intervention.

Patients with atherosclerosis should be managed within a comprehensive programme of care that includes lifestyle modifications (e.g. smoking cessation, cholesterol reduction, blood pressure control, exercise and blood sugar control) and pharmacological intervention.[35] Antiplatelet therapy represents the mainstay of pharmacological treatment in the management of patients with established atherosclerosis, regardless of the disease origin.[35] The evidence base for a variety of antiplatelet agents, such as aspirin, thienopyridines, GP IIb/IIIa antagonists and dipyridamole, is discussed below. These diverse agents target multiple pathways in the platelet adhesion–activation–aggregation axis (Figure 3).

The evidence base for antiplatelet agents

In 1994, the publication of the Antiplatelet Trialists' Collaboration (ATC) provided the most compelling evidence for the benefits of antiplatelet therapy.[36] This meta-analysis included 145 randomised trials conducted before 1990, and involved more than 100,000 patients, over two-thirds of whom were treated with aspirin, and demonstrated a relative reduction in vascular events of 25% compared with placebo.[36]

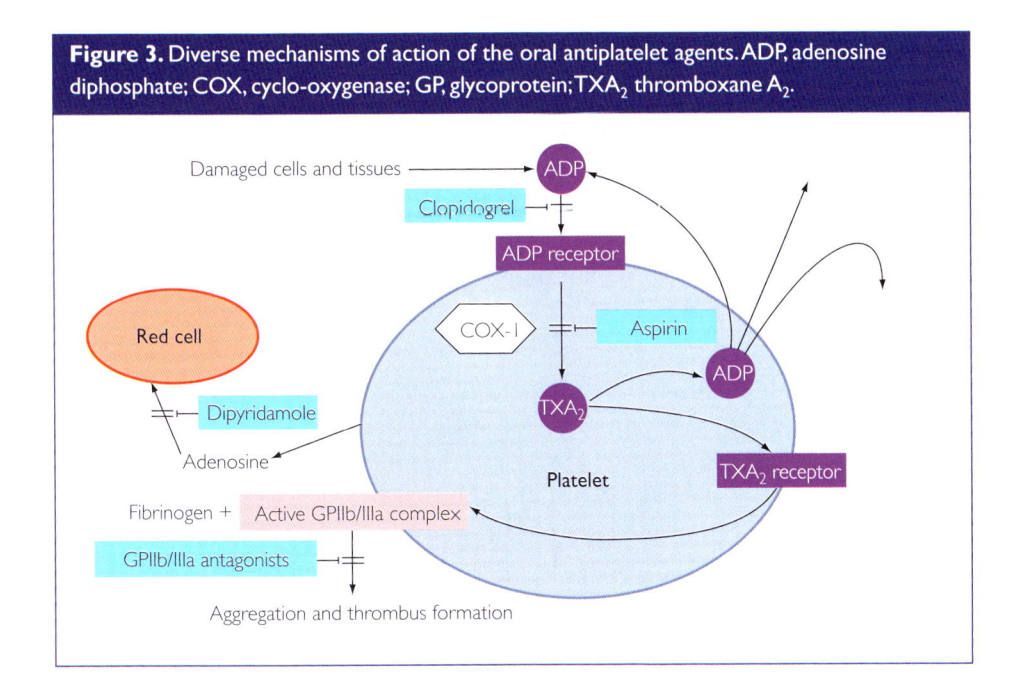

Figure 3. Diverse mechanisms of action of the oral antiplatelet agents. ADP, adenosine diphosphate; COX, cyclo-oxygenase; GP, glycoprotein; TXA$_2$ thromboxane A$_2$.

In 2002, the ATC updated the evidence base to 1997, expanding the database to 195 randomised trials of vascular events involving aspirin, and 89 trials in which another antiplatelet agent was used.[37] Again there was a significant overall benefit of antiplatelet therapy compared with placebo, with a reduction in the odds ratio (OR) of 22% in terms of vascular events (Table 2).

Table 2. Odds reductions of a variety of vascular events with antiplatelet therapy in the Antiplatelet Trialists Collaboration (ATC) meta-analysis.[37]

Vascular event	Odds reduction (%)
Acute MI	30
MI (secondary prevention)	25
Acute stroke	11
Stroke (secondary prevention)	22
Unstable angina	46
PTCA	53
Stable angina	33
Peripheral arterial disease	23

MI, myocardial infarction; PTCA, percutaneous transluminal coronary angioplasty.

For aspirin specifically, the reduction in vascular events was 23%. Overall, no significant difference in benefit was seen between different doses of aspirin used (daily doses in this analysis ranged from <75 to 1500 mg). Within a few days of beginning aspirin, 75 mg/day, platelet cyclo-oxygenase is almost completely inhibited. Doses higher than 150 mg/day are more gastrotoxic. Indeed, doses of 75–150 mg/day appear at least as effective as higher doses, although the effects of doses lower than 75 mg/day are less certain. This means that the common practice of increasing the dose of aspirin after a second vascular event has no supportive evidence base.

For the long-term prevention of vascular events, the evidence supports the use of aspirin across the 75–150 mg dose range. For acute events, such as acute stroke, MI or unstable angina, where more rapid inhibition of cyclo-oxygenase is desirable, a loading dose of 150–300 mg may be given.

Although aspirin can prevent up to a quarter of vascular events there are many events which still occur. Hence, antiplatelet regimes are needed that are more effective than aspirin alone. In the ATC, agents such as clopidogrel and ticlopidine reduced serious vascular events by 10–12% compared with aspirin, whilst other antiplatelet regimens, such as the addition of dipyridamole to aspirin, failed to provide any further reduction in vascular events compared with aspirin alone. However, with smaller differences between different antiplatelet agents than between an individual agent and placebo, very large trials are necessary to demonstrate clinically significant superiority.

Adding aspirin to another antiplatelet agent that targets an alternative platelet aggregation pathway could in theory produce a further reduction in vascular events. However, except in the case of a combination of aspirin and intravenous GP IIb/IIIa antagonists, used in percutaneous coronary intervention (PCI), no clear benefit of adding a second agent was found up to 1997. In particular, the combination of dipyridamole and aspirin was not found to confer any additional benefit, except in one trial involving patients with stroke and TIA.[38]

Aspirin

Clinical practice has utilised the analgesic and anti-inflammatory properties of this remarkable drug for over 100 years. The discovery that additional benefits were conferred via aspirin's inhibition of platelet cyclo-oxygenase led to its ubiquitous use in vascular disease. However, whilst there is considerable evidence that many patients with CHD are routinely given treatment with aspirin, many patients with ischaemic stroke, PAD and other high-risk conditions such as diabetes are not.

Aspirin costs very little and, with a particularly favourable risk–benefit ratio in high-risk cases, the net benefits of aspirin treatment are effectively cost–neutral. Inevitably, clinical recommendations and guidelines for the prevention of vascular disease all include aspirin as the first-line antiplatelet agent.

Despite this, aspirin causes adverse events in about one-in-seven patients, and up to 15% are unable to tolerate it.[39,40] Three-quarters of such patients have gastric intolerance due to the inhibition of cyclo-oxygenase within the gastric mucosa and the resultant impairment of gastric cyto-protective mechanisms. Dyspepsia, peptic ulceration and gastrointestinal haemorrhage are all common and familiar adverse events associated with aspirin therapy. As a result, aspirin is often co-prescribed with proton pump inhibitors or H_2-receptor antagonists, thereby increasing the overall cost of treatment. In other patients, particularly atopic individuals, bronchospasm and nasal or skin reactions are a problem and a few patients may experience major bleeds, such as cerebral haemorrhage.

More recent concerns have emerged regarding potential interactions between aspirin and other non-steroidal anti-inflammatory drugs (NSAIDs). Apart from increasing the potential for gastrointestinal intolerance when both are used together, there is some evidence that other NSAIDs may reduce the cardiovascular protective effects of aspirin. In addition, there is a potential interaction between aspirin and angiotensin-converting enzyme (ACE) inhibitors that may diminish the effects of ACE inhibition.[41] Part of the action of ACE inhibitors stems from a decrease in the breakdown of bradykinin, which, in turn, stimulates prostaglandin-mediated vasodilatation, a process that may be impaired by aspirin.[40] In the case of both potential interactions, the cases are not fully proven and further research is needed to conclusively demonstrate them.

Aspirin in primary prevention

Whilst the use of aspirin in the secondary prevention of vascular events in patients with CHD, ischaemic stroke, TIA and PAD is well established,[36,37] recommendations for its use in high-risk primary prevention have been slow to crystallise. Three trials form the evidence base for current recommendations: the Hypertension Optimal Treatment (HOT) trial, the Medical Research Council (MRC) Thrombosis Prevention trial and the Primary Prevention Project (PPP).[42–44] The results of these studies are summarised in Table 3. In all three trials, the number of clinically significant bleeding episodes caused by aspirin was similar to the number of cardiovascular events prevented, underlining that the margin between benefit and risk is significantly narrower in lower risk populations. Taking

Table 3. Summary of the results from the primary prevention trials of aspirin.[42–44]

Clinical trial	Reduction in cardiovascular events (%)	Reduction in MI (%)
Hypertension Optimal Treatment (HOT)	15	36
MRC Thrombosis Prevention trial	16	20
Primary Prevention Project (PPP)	23	31

MI, myocardial infarction.

benefit and risk into account, a 10-year CHD risk threshold of 15% or greater would indicate the need for the introduction of aspirin. However, due to the increased risk of cerebral haemorrhage associated with high blood pressure, it is recommended that aspirin should be initiated only when blood pressure is adequately controlled. Many primary prevention patients with hypertension, dyslipidaemia or diabetes can now be identified who exceed this risk threshold and who would therefore receive additional therapeutic benefit.

ADP-receptor antagonists – the thienopyridines

Thienopyridines, such as ticlopidine and clopidogrel, inhibit the early stages in the process of platelet activation by irreversibly blocking the receptor for ADP, which promotes platelet aggregation via the GP IIb/IIIa receptor (Figure 3). These agents also inhibit platelet degranulation, and thereby reduce the release of other prothrombotic and inflammatory markers. Consequently, they reduce the probability of thrombus formation at the site of a disrupted atherosclerotic plaque.

Clopidogrel has proven to be about six-times more effective than ticlopidine in preventing platelet aggregation, and, with fewer serious haematological side-effects and a mounting evidence base, it is now the thienopyridine of choice in antiplatelet therapy.

The Clopidogrel *vs* Aspirin in Patients at Risk of Ischaemic Events (CAPRIE) study identified a significant, incremental benefit of clopidogrel over aspirin in a large population of patients with atherosclerotic disease (relative risk reduction [RRR] 8.7%; $p=0.043$).[45] As in many clinical trials, the vascular event rate was lower than predicted, and therefore its results may mask greater benefits in populations at higher risk. *Post hoc* subgroup analyses of the CAPRIE data have supported this hypothesis, with greater benefits observed in patients with hyperlipidaemia, diabetes and previous cardiac surgery.[45–48]

The Clopidogrel in Unstable Angina to Prevent Recurrent Events (CURE) trial utilised the complementary actions of aspirin and clopidogrel in combination in patients with non-ST-segment elevation ACS.[49] Despite this condition being primarily the province of secondary care, the survival curves from the trial were still separating 1 year after the index event, and GPs therefore need to continue prescribing both agents for at least this time in such patients. The same applies to patients who have undergone a PCI.[50] The evidence from the Clopidogrel for the Reduction of Events During Observation (CREDO) trial also suggests continuing benefits from long-term therapy in such patients.[51]

In these major trials, clopidogrel was shown to be well tolerated. In CAPRIE (albeit an aspirin-tolerant population), discontinuations for gastrointestinal side-effects, including haemorrhage, were significantly less than with aspirin. The incidence of major gastrointestinal bleeds was also reduced with clopidogrel. In the CURE study there was an increase in the number of major bleeds, though there was no significant increase in life-threatening bleeding events.

Therapeutic uses of clopidogrel

- *Vascular disease*. Whilst aspirin is accepted as the 'gold standard' antiplatelet agent, it fails to prevent over 75% of vascular events. Therefore, the small advantage with clopidogrel may be useful for the patient who suffers a recurrent ischaemic event whilst taking aspirin.
- *Very high-risk patients*. Secondary prevention patients whose cardiovascular risk is still very high by virtue of the multiplicative effect of other risk factors, such as dyslipidaemia, hypertension or diabetes.
- *Non-ST-segment elevation ACS and PCI*. Clopidogrel has established benefit in these settings, particularly when given as a loading dose of 300 mg, and in combination with aspirin for at least 1 year.
- *Aspirin intolerance*. The use of clopidogrel as an alternative to aspirin in patients intolerant or allergic to aspirin is gaining widespread acceptability.

Other ongoing clinical trials are focusing on the combination of clopidogrel and aspirin in a variety of other clinical settings (e.g. acute MI and stroke; MI, stroke and TIA secondary prevention; high-risk primary prevention; heart failure; atrial fibrillation; PAD).

Dipyridamole

Dipyridamole works through a phosphodiesterase-mediated pathway leading ultimately to the activation of the GP IIb/IIIa receptor (Figure 3). Whilst its mechanism is not fully clear, it is thought to block the re-uptake of adenosine into red blood cells. This increases the plasma concentration of adenosine, which inhibits platelet aggregation through an interaction with cyclic adenosine monophosphate (cAMP). Until the publication of the European Stroke Prevention Study 2 (ESPS2), dipyridamole, either alone or in combination with aspirin, was not conclusively shown to produce a significant reduction in vascular events.[36] ESPS2 showed a reduction in non-fatal stroke and TIA, but no significant effect on fatal stroke, total mortality or MI.[38] The positive outcome may have arisen due to a reformulation of dipyridamole, rendering it more bioavailable with demonstrable antiplatelet activity *in vivo*. It is also possible that the results may have arisen due to chance, due to an inadequate dose of aspirin being used (25 mg twice daily), or due to an antihypertensive effect of dipyridamole. The new formulation of dipyridamole is being tested again with aspirin in stroke, and one trial (Prevention Regimen for Effectively Avoiding Second Strokes [PROFESS]) will compare dipyridamole and low-dose aspirin (the ESPS2 combination) with clopidogrel.

GP IIb/IIIa inhibitors

The activated GP IIb/IIIa receptor on the platelet surface promotes platelet aggregation via the binding of fibrinogen. This is considered to be the final pathway of platelet aggregation. Thus, inhibitors of the GP IIb/IIIa receptor directly block platelet aggregation, thereby reducing the likelihood of thrombus formation. Three GP IIb/IIIa inhibitors are currently approved for clinical use: abciximab, eptifibatide and tirofiban. These parenteral agents are used as adjuncts to aspirin and heparin to prevent early MI in patients with unstable angina or non-ST-segment elevation MI, or in high-risk patients undergoing angioplasty to prevent arterial occlusion or restenosis. However, they are not indicated for longer term use. Indeed, a number of clinical trials and meta-analyses have indicated a trend towards increased mortality when oral GP IIb/IIIa receptor antagonists are used for longer durations (>24 hours) in patients with a wide range of atherosclerotic disease.[25]

Clinical guidelines – antiplatelet therapy
ACS
The American College of Cardiology/American Heart Association (ACC/AHA) guidelines for the management of ACS (unstable angina and non-ST-segment elevation MI) now recommend the use of parenteral GP IIb/IIIa receptor antagonists in patients with ACS who undergo PCI, but

question their use in patients not undergoing the procedure.[52] These revised guidelines state that antiplatelet therapy should be initiated promptly after presentation and continued indefinitely, and also emphasise a more prominent role for clopidogrel in the management of ACS, particularly in those unable to take aspirin due to insensitivity or intolerance.[52] Based on the results of CURE and PCI-CURE studies, the use of clopidogrel as an adjunct to standard therapy, including aspirin, is now recommended for patients with ACS, including those with varying levels of cardiovascular risk and those undergoing PCI.

The European Society of Cardiology (ESC) guidelines for the management of ACS recommend that patients should receive baseline treatment, including aspirin, low molecular weight heparin, clopidogrel, β-blockers and nitrates, in addition to aggressive management of cardiovascular risk factors.[53] In addition, high-risk patients should also receive infusion of a GP IIb/IIIa inhibitor followed by coronary angiography. Where PCI is indicated, patients should also receive clopidogrel unless there is a likelihood of urgent surgery within 5 days of dose administration.[53]

Ischaemic stroke

The Royal College of Physicians has produced national clinical guidelines for the secondary prevention of stroke in the UK.[33] In addition to standard blood pressure control with long-acting ACE inhibitors and thiazide diuretics, the guidelines indicate that all patients with ischaemic stroke should be treated with aspirin (75–325 mg/day) or clopidogrel (75 mg/day), or a combination of a low-dose aspirin and dipyridamole. In those patients intolerant of aspirin, clopidogrel or dipyridamole (200 mg, twice daily) should be given. Addition of a statin should also be considered for all patients with a history of IHD and with elevated baseline total cholesterol levels (>5 mmol/L) following stroke.[33]

PAD

A recent consensus statement has provided evidence-based recommendations on the use of antiplatelets in the management of patients with PAD.[54] These recommendations focus on a number of common clinical scenarios that face clinicians dealing with PAD, and emphasise the central importance of antiplatelet agents in patient management. It is recommended that long-term antiplatelet therapy with either aspirin, 75–325 mg/day, or clopidogrel, 75 mg/day, be given to patients with symptomatic intermittent claudication or critical limb ischaemia who have had previous vascular interventions.[54] Long-term therapy is also recommended in patients undergoing angioplasty or stenting in peripheral arteries and in those undergoing peripheral artery bypass surgery, unless contra-indicated. In these cases, aspirin should be continued peri-operatively in the absence of any concerns over increased bleeding. However, consideration should be given to stopping clopidogrel 5 days prior to elective surgery.[54] Finally, in patients with PAD who have had recurrent vascular events whilst receiving antiplatelet therapy, consideration should be given to the addition of another antiplatelet agent, or to substituting the existing agent (e.g. clopidogrel for aspirin) or switching to an anticoagulant.[54]

Further guidelines

Further evidence-based guidelines may assist in the appropriate selection of antiplatelet therapy.[35] These indicate that antiplatelet agents should be widely used to prevent thrombosis and ischaemic vascular events in patients with established atherosclerosis. They also argue that clopidogrel is the treatment of choice in patients with established PAD. Aspirin or clopidogrel should be used in all patients with a history of previous MI, with clopidogrel favoured in patients who experience recurrent cardiovascular events whilst taking aspirin, in those who are intolerant of it, and/or in those who are at particular risk of further cardiovascular events. Finally, antiplatelet agents are also of benefit in the management of ischaemic stroke, again with clopidogrel favoured in those with recurrent events on aspirin.[35] In addition, the results from the ESPS2 study show that dipyridamole (in combination with aspirin or as monotherapy in those intolerant of aspirin) is also a useful antiplatelet agent for the management of ischaemic stroke.[33]

Economic impact of CHD

CHD alone cost the NHS about £1750 million in terms of direct healthcare in 1999 (Figure 4).[55] Only a minute fraction of these direct costs is spent on primary prevention of the disease (<1%), which, if effectively implemented, would reduce direct and indirect costs in the longer term.

In addition to the direct costs of CHD, a large economic burden is placed on society by the impact of the disease on the productivity of affected individuals. CHD is essentially a disease affecting people in their most productive years. It has been estimated that its cost to the UK economy in terms of days lost due to death, illness and dependent care is about £5300 million.[55] In total, therefore, the annual costs of the CHD-related burden can be estimated at about £7 billion, which represents the

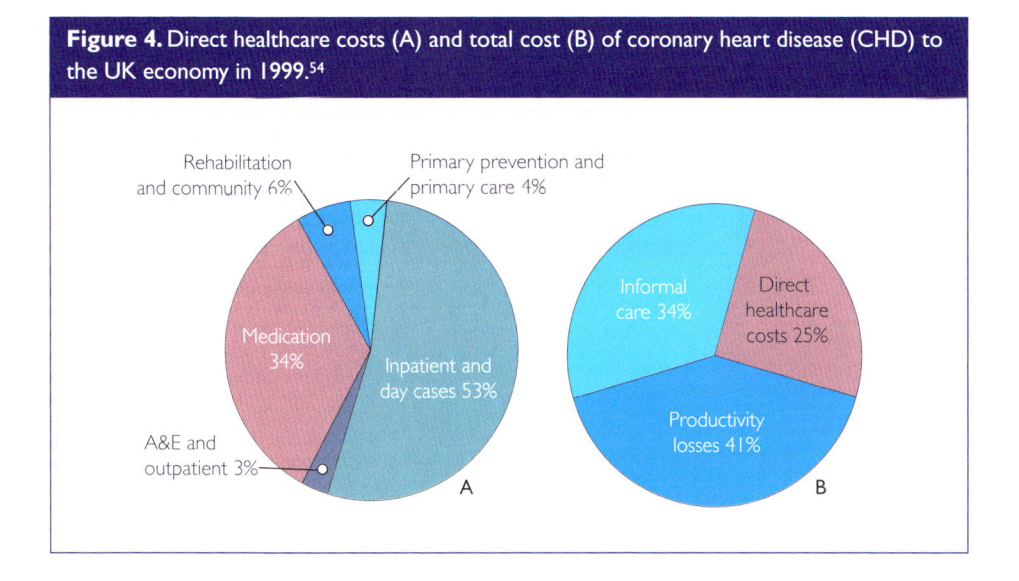

Figure 4. Direct healthcare costs (A) and total cost (B) of coronary heart disease (CHD) to the UK economy in 1999.[54]

- Rehabilitation and community 6%
- Primary prevention and primary care 4%
- Medication 34%
- Inpatient and day cases 53%
- A&E and outpatient 3%

A

- Informal care 34%
- Direct healthcare costs 25%
- Productivity losses 41%

B

highest cost of all diseases in the UK for which comparable analyses have been done.

In conclusion, CHD, and CVD in general, is a leading public health problem in the UK, not only in terms of morbidity and mortality but also in terms of its associated economic burden.

CHD is a leading public health problem in the UK, not only in terms of morbidity and mortality but also in terms of its associated economic burden.

Key points

- CVD is a leading cause of global mortality and in the UK is responsible for more than 40% of deaths.
- Atherothrombosis is the principal pathophysiology underlying CVD, and is characterised by thrombus formation superimposed on disrupted or eroded atherosclerotic plaques located in major arterial walls.
- Platelets play a central role in the development of atherothrombosis via three critical steps – platelet adhesion, activation and aggregation.
- Subsequent thrombus formation at the sites of disrupted plaques leads to arterial lumen compromise and occlusion, or embolisation and subsequent microvascular obstruction at distal sites, ultimately manifesting clinically as MI, unstable angina, stroke, TIA, PAD or death.
- Patient management involves lifestyle modification and pharmacological intervention, with antiplatelet therapy the principal pharmacological approach in patients with established atherosclerosis.
- The widest experience with antiplatelet therapy has been with aspirin which has been well documented to show considerable benefit in terms of secondary prevention of vascular events.
- Despite this evidence, many cardiovascular events still occur in patients receiving aspirin. Consequently, newer agents, such as clopidogrel and dipyridamole, which target alternative pathways in platelet aggregation may provide additional benefit, either as monotherapy or in combination with aspirin.

References

1. The World Health Organization. *The World Health Report 1997. Conquering suffering, enriching humanity*. Geneva: World Health Organization, 1997.
2. The World Health Organization. *The World Health Report 2002. Reducing risk promoting healthy life*. Geneva: World Health Organization, 2002.
3. Leys D. Atherothrombosis: a major health burden. *Cerebrovasc Dis* 2001; **11(Suppl 2)**: 1–4.
4. British Heart Foundation. Coronary heart disease statistics. British Heart Foundation Statistics Database 2003. *www.heartstats.org*.
5. Department of Health. National Service Framework for older people, March 2001. London Stationery Office.
6. Scottish Intercollegiate Guidelines Network. Guideline 13: Management of Patients with Stroke Part 1. Edinburgh: SIGN, 1997.
7. McDonagh MS, Bachmann LM, Golder S *et al*. A rapid and systematic review of the clinical effectiveness and cost-effectiveness of glycoprotein IIb/IIIa antagonists in the medical management of unstable angina. *Health Technol Assess* 2000; **4**: 1–95.
8. Vascular Surgical Society of Great Britain and Ireland. Critical limb ischaemia: management and outcome – report of a national survey. *Eur J Vas Endovasc Surg* 1995; **10**: 108–13.
9. Annual Incidence of Diabetes and Diabetic Complications. *www.diabetes-healthnet.ac.uk/dnew/feb2001/incidence.htm*
10. Mehta RH, Eagle KA. Secondary prevention in acute myocardial infarction. *BMJ* 1998; **316**: 838–42.
11. Heart and stroke statistical update. Dallas: American Heart Association and American Stroke Association, 2002.
12. Petrie M, McMurray J. *Prescriber* 1998; **9**: 75–88.
13. Loh E, Sutton MS, Wun CC *et al*. Ventricular dysfunction and the risk of stroke after myocardial infarction. *N Engl J Med* 1997; **336**: 251–7.
14. Collinson J, Flather MD, Fox KA *et al*. Clinical outcomes, risk stratification and practice patterns of unstable angina and myocardial infarction without ST elevation: Prospective Registry of Acute Ischaemic Syndromes in the UK (PRAIS-UK). *Eur Heart J* 2000; **21**: 1450–7.
15. Dennis MS, Burn JP, Sandercock PA *et al*. Long-term survival after first-ever stroke: the Oxfordshire Community Stroke Project. *Stroke* 1993; **24**: 796–800.
16. Wolfe C, Rudd A, Beech R. *Stroke services and research*. An overview with recommendations for future research. London: Stroke Association, 1996.
17. Dennis MS, Burn JP, Sandercock PA. Prognosis of transient ischaemic attacks in Oxfordshire Community Stroke Project. *Stroke* 1990; **21**: 848–53.
18. Golledge J. Lower-limb arterial disease. *Lancet* 1997; **350**: 1459–65.
19. Department of Health. National Service Framework for diabetes: standards. 2001. London Stationery Office.
20. Kannel WB. Risk factors for atherosclerotic cardiovascular outcomes in different arterial territories. *J Cardiovasc Risk* 1994; **1**: 333–9.
21. Coccheri S. Distribution of symptomatic atherothrombosis and influence of atherosclerotic disease burden on risk of secondary ischaemic events: results from CAPRIE. *Eur Heart J* 1998; **19(Supp)**: 1288.
22. Fuster V, Badimon JJ, Chesebro JH. Atherothrombosis: mechanisms and clinical therapeutic approaches. *Vasc Med* 1998; **3**: 231–9.
23. Libby P. Multiple mechanisms of thrombosis complicating atherosclerotic plaques. *Clin Cardiol* 2000; **23(Suppl 6)**: VI-3–7.
24. Willeit J, Kiechl S. Biology of arterial atheroma. *Cerebrovasc Dis* 2000; **10(Suppl 5)**: 1–8.
25. Mehta SR, Yusuf S. Short- and long-term oral antiplatelet therapy in acute coronary syndromes and percutaneous coronary intervention. *J Am Coll Cardiol* 2003; **41**: S79–88.
26. Libby P. Inflammation in atherosclerosis. *Nature* 2002; **420**: 868–74.
27. Libby P, Ridker PM, Maseri A. Inflammation and atherosclerosis. *Circulation* 2002; **105**: 1135–43.
28. Mehta SR. Appropriate antiplatelet and antithrombotic therapy in patients with acute coronary syndromes: recent updates to the ACC/AHA Guidelines. *J Invasive Cardiol* **14(Suppl E)**: 27–35.
29. Grech ED, Ramsdale DR. Acute coronary syndrome: unstable angina and non-ST segment elevation myocardial infarction. *BMJ* 2003; **326**: 1259–61.
30. Newman AB, Shemanski L, Manolio TA *et al*. Ankle-arm index as a predictor of cardiovascular disease and mortality in the Cardiovascular Health Study. The Cardiovascular Health Study Group. *Arterioscler Thromb Vasc Biol* 1999; **19**: 538–45.
31. Papamichael CM, Lekakis JP, Stamatelopoulos KS *et al*. Ankle-brachial index as a predictor of the extent of coronary atherosclerosis and cardiovascular events in patients with coronary artery disease. *Am J Cardiol* 2000; **86**: 615–18.
32. Sikkink CJ, van Asten WN, van 't Hof MA, van Langen H, van der Vliet JA. Decreased ankle/brachial indices in relation to morbidity and mortality in patients with peripheral arterial disease. *Vasc Med* 1997; **2**: 169–73.
33. Royal College of Physicians. National clinical guidelines for stroke – an update. Concise guide. 2002.
34. Wardlaw JM, Farrall AJ. Diagnosis of stroke on neuroimaging. *BMJ* 2004; **328**: 655-6.
35. Zusman RM, Chesebro JH, Comerota A *et al*. Antiplatelet therapy in the prevention of ischemic vascular events: literature review and evidence-based guidelines for drug selection. *Clin Cardiol* 1999; **22**: 559–73.
36. Antiplatelet Trialists' Collaboration. Collaborative overview of randomised trials of antiplatelet therapy–I: prevention of death, myocardial infarction, and stroke by prolonged antiplatelet therapy in various categories of patients. *BMJ* 1994; **308**: 81–106.
37. Antiplatelet Trialists' Collaboration. Collaborative meta-analysis of randomised trials of antiplatelet therapy for prevention of death, myocardial infarction, and stroke in high risk patients. *BMJ* 2002; **324**: 71–86.

38. Diener HC, Cunha L, Forbes C *et al*. European Stroke Prevention Study 2. Dipyridamole and acetylsalicylic acid in the secondary prevention of stroke. *J Neurol Sci* 1996; **143**: 1–13.
39. Wilcox D, Webster J, Forrest D. Secondary prevention of occlusive vascular disease using low dose (75–325mg) daily aspirin. *Audit Trends* 1996, **4**: 102–6.
40. Garcia-Dorado D, Theroux P, Tornos P *et al*. Previous aspirin use may alleviate the severity of the manifestations of acute ischaemic syndromes. *Circulation* 1995; **92**: 1743–8.
41. Peterson JG, Topol EJ, Sapp SK *et al*. Evaluation of the effects of aspirin combined with angiotensin-converting enzyme inhibitors in patients with coronary artery disease. *Am J Med* 2000; **109**: 371–7.
42. Hansson L, Zanchetti A, Carruthers SG *et al*. Effects of intensive blood-pressure lowering and low-dose aspirin in patients with hypertension: principal results of the Hypertension Optimal Treatment (HOT) randomised trial. HOT Study Group. *Lancet* 1998; **351**: 1755–62.
43. Elwood PC. British studies of aspirin and myocardial infarction. *Am J Med* 1983; **74**: 50–4.
44. de Gaetano G. Low-dose aspirin and vitamin E in people at cardiovascular risk: a randomised trial in general practice. Collaborative Group of the Primary Prevention Project. *Lancet* 2001; **357**: 89–95.
45. CAPRIE Steering Committee. A randomised, blinded, trial of clopidogrel versus aspirin in patients at risk of ischaemic events (CAPRIE). *Lancet* 1996; **348**: 1329–39.
46. Bhatt DL, Foody JM, Hirsch AT *et al*. Complementary, additive benefit of clopidogrel and lipid-lowering therapy in patients with atherosclerosis. *J Am Coll Cardiol* 2000: **35(Suppl A)**: 326.
47. Bhatt DL, Chew DP, Hirsch AT *et al*. Superiority of clopidogrel versus aspirin in patients with prior cardiac surgery. *Circulation* 2001; **103**: 363–8.
48. Bhatt DL, Marso SP, Hirsch AT *et al*. Amplified benefit of clopidogrel versus aspirin in patients with diabetes mellitus. *Am J Cardiol* 2002; **90**: 625–8.
49. Yusuf S, Zhao F, Mehta SR *et al*. Effects of clopidogrel in addition to aspirin in patients with acute coronary syndromes without ST-segment elevation. *N Engl J Med* 2001; **345**: 494–502.
50. Mehta SR, Yusuf S, Peters RJ *et al*. Effects of pretreatment with clopidogrel and aspirin followed by long-term therapy in patients undergoing percutaneous coronary intervention: the PCI-CURE study. *Lancet* 2001; **358**: 527–33.
51. Steinhubl SR, Berger PB, Mann JT *et al*. Early and sustained dual oral antiplatelet therapy following percutaneous coronary intervention: a randomized controlled trial. *JAMA* 2002; **288**: 2411–20.
52. Braunwald E, Antman EM, Beasley JW *et al*. ACC/AHA guideline update for the management of patients with unstable angina and non-ST-segment elevation myocardial infarction – 2002: summary article: a report of the American College of Cardiology/American Heart Association Task Force on Practice Guidelines (Committee on the Management of Patients With Unstable Angina). *Circulation* 2002; **106**: 1893–900.
53. Bertrand ME, Simoons ML, Fox KA *et al*. Management of acute coronary syndromes in patients presenting without persistent ST-segment elevation. *Eur Heart J* 2002; **23**: 1809–40.
54. Peripheral Arterial Diseases Antiplatelet Consensus Group. Antiplatelet therapy in peripheral arterial disease. Consensus statement. *Eur J Vasc Endovasc Surg* 2003; **26**: 1–16.
55. Liu JL, Maniadakis N, Gray A, Rayner M. The economic burden of coronary heart disease in the UK. *Heart* 2002; **88**: 597–603.

Acknowledgements

Figure 1 is adapted from Coccheri, 1998.[21]
Figure 4 is adapted from Liu *et al.*, 2002.[55]

6. Atopic eczema

Dr Eleanor Bull and Dr Scott Chambers
CSF Medical Communications Ltd

Summary

Atopic eczema is a chronic skin condition that presents predominantly in childhood, affecting 10–20% of school children in developed countries. The majority of cases are associated with atopy which is associated with an elevation of serum IgE concentrations as a result of the abnormal production of IgE antibodies in response to common environmental allergens. Symptoms of atopic eczema consist principally of dry skin and an itchy rash, often with flexural involvement, and a characteristic distribution pattern that varies with the age of the patient. Commonly, the disease first presents during early infancy and childhood but can persist into adulthood in a small proportion of patients. Atopic eczema is strongly associated with the other atopic diseases (e.g. allergic rhinitis and asthma – the so-called atopic triad), and there is some suggestion that eczema may be a precursor to the development of these other atopic conditions in later life. The clinical emergence of atopic eczema results from a combination of genetic and environmental factors. The disease is associated with higher social class and is encountered more frequently in urban settings. The prevalence of atopic eczema has rapidly increased in recent years, particularly in the UK, Scandinavia and Japan. The 'hygiene hypothesis' relates the increased prevalence in atopic disease to reduced exposure to microbial allergens and the widespread increase in the use of antibiotics. The condition places a substantial economic burden on healthcare resources, whilst an individual patient's quality of life is severely compromised by the condition. Current pharmacological treatments, such as the use of emollient creams and topical corticosteroids are largely effective in relieving symptoms. However, prolonged use of more potent topical corticosteroids is not recommended in view of the potential for local and systemic side-effects.

Introduction

Eczema denotes an inflammation of the skin or dermatitis. It can derive from multiple causes, and its main types are allergic, irritant, atopic and contact. The most common form of the condition is atopic eczema.

The term atopic describes the abnormal production of IgE antibodies in response to common environmental allergens including house-dust mites, grass, pollen, animal allergens and certain foodstuffs. Atopic eczema is a chronic inflammatory skin condition, the occurrence of which is strongly associated with other atopic diseases such as asthma and allergic rhinitis. Substantial evidence suggests that eczema may predispose the individual to the development of these other conditions in later life. Indeed, up to 80% of children with atopic eczema will develop allergic rhinitis or asthma later in childhood.[1] There are two recognised types of atopic eczema, extrinsic, which involves IgE antibody-mediated sensitisation and affects 70–80% of the patient population, and intrinsic, which is non-IgE-mediated, affecting 20–30% of patients.[2] A highly heritable disease, atopic eczema commonly presents during early infancy and childhood, and represents the most common disease in individuals within this age group, but it may also persist into adulthood, albeit only in a proportion of patients.

Symptoms

The clinical features of atopic eczema are highly variable, occurring with different skin rash morphology, in different places and over a variable time period. However, in general terms, atopic eczema is characterised by patches of red, dry, itchy skin, often starting on the face and spreading to the outside of the limbs and body, usually in the bends of the elbows or behind the knees (antecubital and popliteal fossae). Scaling and crusting on the scalp, cheeks and skin folds of the neck may also occur. Lichenification, or thickening of the skin, is normally observed in children after the ages of 3–4 years, primarily as a result of excessive and repeated scratching. In adults, exacerbations of atopic eczema are more often located on the hands. The itching, or pruritus, may worsen at night, leading to sleep deprivation which can impact profoundly and negatively on patients' quality of life.

Atopic eczema may be complicated by recurrent viral skin infections including warts and eczema molluscatum.[3] Proliferation of *Staphylococcus aureus* may also occur on the eczematous skin of 90% of patients,[4] a feature which may exacerbate or maintain skin inflammation and further predisposes the patient to skin infection.[4] Frequently, it leads to impetigo – lesions that develop suddenly and grow with brown crusts.[5] Occasionally, *Streptococcus pyogenes* can exacerbate eczema. Oozing from an eczematous site is an indication of infection.

Aside from the clearly visible clinical symptoms of atopic eczema, there are a number of significant psychological issues associated with the condition. As the visible manifestations of the condition commonly occur at a critical stage in the social development of a child, they may give rise to

> Atopic eczema is characterised by patches of red, dry, itchy skin, often starting on the face and spreading to the outside of the limbs and body, commonly on the creases of the limbs.

teasing and heightened self-consciousness which may ultimately result in educational problems due to school absence and sleep deprivation.

Pathophysiology

The characteristic appearance of atopic eczema, on a microscopic level, is of excess fluid between the cells in the epidermis (spongiosis). As the build-up of fluid ensues, adjacent cells can become disrupted, leading to the formation of vesicles. Blood stem cells carrying the abnormal genetic expression of atopy, infiltrate and remain in the mucosal surfaces and the skin, leading to chronic sensitisation.[6] During the chronic phase, pruritus and associated scratching cause thickening of the epidermis (acanthosis), increased risk of infection and irritation.

Factors that contribute to atopic eczema include:
- family history of atopy, allergic rhinitis, or asthma
- immunoglobulin E (IgE) antibody imbalance
- microbial colonisation
- lipid and barrier impairment
- aeroallergens
- food allergy or hypersensitivity
- psychosomatic factors.[7]

There is strong evidence to show that susceptibility to atopic eczema exists in families.[8] This inheritance pattern causes cytokine gene activation and among the 20 or so genes involved in atopic eczema, the locus 5q31-33, which contains the cytokine genes for interleukin (IL)-3, -4, -5, -13 and GM-CSF, appears to be particularly influential.[9] Thus, a genetic predisposition to a variety of allergenic triggers may exist in those with atopic eczema.

Immunological investigations have found that a large percentage (80–85%) of patients have an elevated serum level of IgE.[7] Heightened levels of IgE indicate an imbalance in T-cell immunity, namely, a predominance of Th2 in acute lesions. This also affects Th1 secretions of IL-2, tumour necrosis factor (TNF)-β and interferon (IFN)-γ in chronic phase with an increased activation of macrophages, T-cell growth and monocytes. Th2 cells secrete IL-4, which stimulates IgE synthesis. The predominance of IgE, affecting cell defences during both acute and chronic phases of disease, can lead to a higher risk of relapse from secondary fungal or viral infection.[10]

Immune stimulation resulting in skin reaction can also be caused by certain microbial organisms, for example, *S. aureus*.[11] This organism appears to be a persistent irritant with inflammatory potency on atopic skin. Studies suggest the release of superantigens, caused by the production of enterotoxins from *S. aureus*, induce marked immune stimulation.[11]

The dry, scaling skin indicative of atopic eczema suggests an impaired skin barrier function, with enhanced transepidermal water loss and reduced skin surface water content directly reflecting this theory.[12] The lipid composition within the *stratum corneum*, which maintains the barrier function, appears different in eczematous skin compared with normal skin.[12]

The role of food allergies in the aggravation of atopic eczema is variable in adults. Specific IgE antibodies to food, microbes and various allergens have been found (Figure 1).[13,14] Instigating dietary changes in children and infants, for instance, eliminating cow's milk, seems to relieve symptoms.[7] Serum IgE levels in infants and children with atopic eczema are higher in response to food substances such as milk, nuts and wheat,[7] compared with healthy participants.

Some aeroallergens may have induced eczematous skin lesions, as identified with atopy patch testing (APT). These allergens include the house-dust mite and pollen or animal dander.[15,16] However, further exacerbation of symptoms in sufferers can occur from stressful emotional events; similarly, the effects of coping with chronic disease also need to be considered.

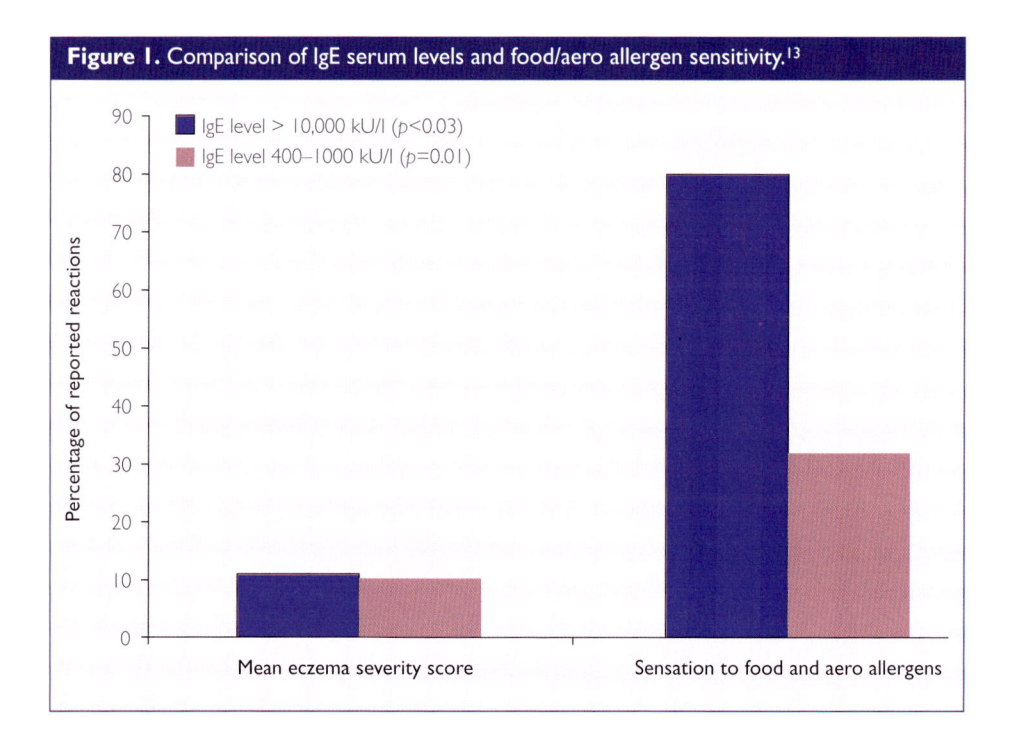

Figure 1. Comparison of IgE serum levels and food/aero allergen sensitivity.[13]

- IgE level > 10,000 kU/l ($p<0.03$)
- IgE level 400–1000 kU/l ($p=0.01$)

Diagnosis

Owing to the broad and variable spectrum of its symptoms, there is no unique diagnostic test that is specific for all patients with atopic eczema. Therefore, diagnosis is largely made by the subjective assessment of the principal presenting clinical symptoms. The skin condition itself will generally exhibit exacerbations and remissions. Pruritus is the predominant feature of atopic eczema, and, as such, a non-itching rash generally excludes a diagnosis of atopic eczema. In addition, the patient will characteristically have a family history of atopic disease.

A UK-specific revision of the Hanifin and Rajka diagnostic criteria[17] for atopic eczema specifies a check-list of clinical symptoms.[18] Thus, patients with atopic eczema will have experienced an itchy skin condition in the previous 12 months, plus three or more of the following criteria:

- onset below the age of 2 years
- history of flexural involvement
- past involvement of the skin creases, such as the bends of the elbows or behind the knees
- history of a generally dry skin
- personal or family history of other atopic disease
- visible flexural dermatitis.

Epidemiology

Atopic eczema is the most common disease of childhood, occurring most frequently in the first 5 years of life and affecting 10–20% of schoolchildren in western Europe and the United States.[19,20] The prevalence in adults is much reduced, with only about 1–3% of the general population affected.[20] However, the disease tends to be more persistent and severe among the adult population.

The prevalence of atopic eczema has dramatically increased over the past 30 years[21] and currently verges on epidemic proportions, for reasons that are largely unexplained. In industrialised countries, in particular the UK, Scandinavia and Japan, the incidence of atopic disease has increased by 2–3 fold over the last three decades, but it remains less common in agricultural regions including China, Eastern Europe and rural Africa.[4,22] The worldwide prevalence of atopic eczema symptoms, as determined by the International Study of Asthma and Allergies in Childhood (ISAAC) survey, is illustrated in Figure 2.

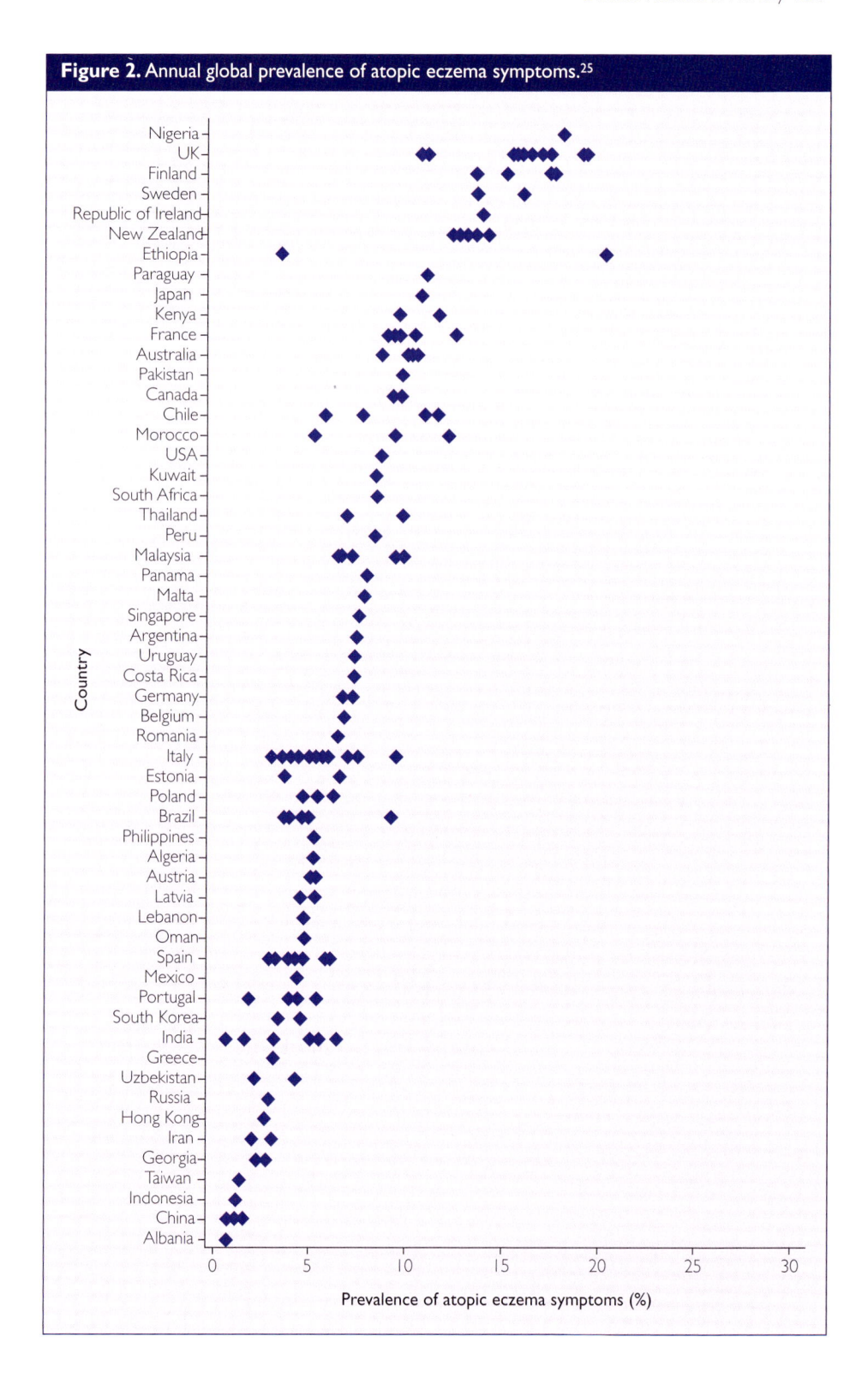

Figure 2. Annual global prevalence of atopic eczema symptoms.[25]

Aetiology

In common with the other atopic diseases, the clinical expression of atopic eczema in the individual is thought to result from a combination of genetic and environmental factors. Whilst an individual may be genetically predisposed to atopy, it is the interaction of these factors with widespread environmental elements that may lead to the development and clinical manifestation of the disease.

Genetic components

Atopic eczema has a strong familial basis, such that the perinatal risk of developing the disease is almost double for those children with a parental history of eczema compared with those without such history.[23] Studies conducted in twins have shown that monozygotic twins have an 86% risk of having atopic eczema if the twin partner has the disease, whereas the 21% disease risk in dizygotic twins does not differ from the frequency seen in ordinary siblings.[24] As a consequence of our growing understanding of the genetic basis for the condition, the identification of specific genes underlying atopic eczema is likely within the next few years.

Environmental components

A number of environmental factors have also been implicated in the onset and/or exacerbation of atopic eczema. Table 1 lists some of the environmental elements which are known to contribute to disease activity. Limited evidence suggests that factors such as lower maternal age and exclusive breast-feeding during the first 3 months of life may be associated with a lower incidence of atopic eczema in children with a family history of atopy.[26]

In line with the increased incidence of atopic eczema observed in developed countries, it is thought likely that environmental factors associated with family lifestyle such as socioeconomic status, allergen exposure, family size, early childhood infections and dietary habits, may prove to be of greatest relevance. Indeed, atopic eczema is more common in wealthier families,[27] a finding that has been linked to aspects of the home environment, including double glazing, fitted carpets, pets, increased exposure to soaps and decreased air circulation as a result of good insulation. Migrant populations, moving from rural, undeveloped environments to towns and cities, exhibit increased rates of atopic disease as a result of changes in allergen exposure. Overcrowding, exposure to industrial pollution, automobile exhausts, housing and bedding, central heating, and eradication of parasites, may all contribute to the observed

Table 1. Factors known to elicit disease activity in patients with atopic eczema.[5]

Physical factors
• Warm surroundings
• Physical irritation of the skin
• Climate
Psychological factors
• Stress (e.g. work-related, school examinations)
Foods
• Tomato and orange juice
• Handling of certain fresh vegetables
• Juice from fish and meat
Allergens
• House-dust mites
• Animal hair and fur, pollen, plants
Other
• *Staphylococcus aureus*

differences in disease frequency between industrialised and developing nations.[28]

The 'hygiene hypothesis' has been proposed in an attempt to rationalise the increase in the prevalence of atopic disease observed in recent years, which was not thought to be solely attributable to increases in mite and other allergen exposures.[29,30] It is based on the premise that in developed countries, an infant's immune system fails to develop appropriately as a result of reduced microbial exposure early in life in conjunction with an overuse of antibiotics, thereby increasing susceptibility to atopic disease development. The inverse association between atopic eczema and family size adds weight to this principle, by suggesting a protective effect conferred by increased cross-infection from siblings.[30]

Treatment

There are many available treatment options currently available for atopic eczema. These treatments focus on hydration of the skin, the reduction of inflammation and the relief of eczema-related symptoms, particularly pruritus. However, poor patient compliance as a result of a poor understanding of the chronic nature of the disease, together with an irrational fear of the hazards associated with long-term use of topical corticosteroids, are significant obstacles to the effective treatment of this disease. Patient education is therefore critical for the effective management of atopic eczema.

Currently, emollients and topical corticosteroids represent the first-line treatment options for mild to-moderate atopic eczema, providing effective symptomatic relief of itching and inflammation. Certain anti-histamines, by virtue of their central sedative effects, may also be useful in preventing sleep deprivation, but their use in the long term should be avoided. Allergen avoidance and phototherapy are also valuable adjunctive treatment tools, whilst systemic and topical immunomodulatory agents are also effective in short-term treatment and long-term exacerbations.

Skin care

Simple yet effective measures can be taken to avoid skin dryness and excessive trans-epidermal water loss via the use of appropriate emollients and soap substitutes with neutral pH and minimum de-fatting activity.[4] Emollients constitute the preventive background therapy in all stages of eczema. Dressings can be applied as a protective barrier against scratching and infection, and cooling of the skin may relieve itching.

Topical corticosteroids

Drugs of this class (e.g. hydrocortisone, betametasone, fluticasone propionate, mometasone furoate) represent the first-line treatment option for atopic eczema and have been used for almost 40 years. However, the more potent members of this drug class, such as betametasone, are generally reserved for more severe disease or in disease that is refractory to treatment with less potent topical corticosteroids.

Administered topically, corticosteroids control acute exacerbations through their anti-inflammatory activity, and whilst they do not offer a cure for atopic eczema, they can suppress symptoms for short periods whilst they are applied. However, corticosteroid use should be limited to only a few days a week for acute eczema and up to 4–6 weeks to gain initial remission from chronic eczema, and care should be taken to match drug potency to the disease severity.[31] In addition, repeated application of these agents is not generally recommended when applying to certain sensitive areas of the body, particularly around the eyes.

The long-term use of corticosteroids is associated with symptom rebound upon treatment discontinuation, resistance to therapy (tachyphylaxis) and suppressive effects on the connective tissue, which manifests clinically as skin atrophy. Patients should be monitored closely for signs of both local and systemic side-effects, which may include contact dermatitis, irreversible striae atrophicae, telangiectasia, spread or worsening of untreated infections, suppression of the pituitary–adrenal axis, growth retardation and Cushing's syndrome. In general terms, the potency of the topical corticosteroid applied, together with the extent of body surface area affected and the duration of application, dictate the probability of experiencing a systemic adverse event. Thus, with increased and prolonged application of high-potency corticosteroids, there is a greater risk of systemic side-effects.

Anti-histamines

The oral H_1 receptor antagonists (e.g. levocetirizine, fexofenadine and loratadine) block the activation of H_1 receptors located on dermal mast cells and in this way may relieve histamine-mediated aspects of the itch response. Consequently, these compounds are of limited use if the cause of the itch is not histamine related. However, the central sedative effects of certain agents such as chlorpheniramine may help to avoid the sleep deprivation associated with eczema-related itch.

Allergen avoidance

Selective allergy tests, including the skin prick test, serum tests for allergen-specific IgE antibodies and controlled food challenges, can aid in the identification of eczema-triggering factors. Once known, these allergens may be avoidable, insofar as is possible, and an improvement in symptoms may thereby result.

Phototherapy

Patients with mild atopic eczema have reported symptomatic improvement following exposure to natural sunlight, whilst clinical trials have shown that narrow-band ultraviolet B (UVB) can prove a useful adjunctive therapy for the treatment of moderate-to-severe atopic eczema when initiated in the presence of a topical corticosteroid.[32] However, a total of 20–30 treatments are necessary to achieve an effective level of control, and thus potential long-term adverse effects may include premature skin ageing and skin cancers.

Calcineurin inhibitors

Drugs of this class (e.g. tacrolimus and pimecrolimus) are known as non-steroidal immunomodulators and share a similar mechanism of action – transcriptional blockade of inflammatory cytokines from activated T-lymphocytes, through the inhibition of the phosphatase enzyme, calcineurin. In addition, they inhibit the release of inflammatory mediators from other inflammatory cells, including mast cells and basophils.[33,34] Thus, these agents represent a non-steroidal alternative to treating the inflammation associated with atopic eczema and are effective and well tolerated in both adults and children over the age of 2 years.[35–37] In contrast to corticosteroids, no suppressive effects on connective tissue cells have been observed, and thus these agents have low skin atrophogenic potential. Their principal side-effect is a local irritation at the application site, which is described principally as a burning sensation.

Ciclosporin

Ciclosporin is another calcineurin inhibitor which has potent immunosuppressive properties. However, it is inactive topically, and its use as an oral agent is limited by significant side-effects including raised serum creatinine, renal impairment, hypertension and relapse flares following discontinuation. Thus, these factors limit its use to short-term treatment periods in patients with severe, refractory atopic eczema.[38]

Tar preparations

Topical coal tar preparations have been used for the treatment of atopic eczema for many years, as a result of their anti-itch and anti-inflammatory effects on the skin. However, due to their relatively weak action, unpleasant odour, potential for staining and irritant effects on broken skin their use in the treatment of chronic eczema lesions is relatively limited.

Antibiotics

The use of antibiotics (e.g. erythromycin, flucloxacillin, azithromycin, clarithromycin, dicloxacilin and oxacillin) is advocated in patients with poorly controlled atopic eczema or in those displaying signs of clinical infection of scratched or broken skin, usually due to the bacterium *S. aureus*. A bacteriological skin swab may guide the clinician as to the nature of the pathogen and any antibiotic sensitivities which may be present.

Socioeconomic impact

Owing to its high prevalence, the management of atopic eczema exerts considerable pressure on limited public healthcare resources. Eczema-associated expenses incurred by hospitals, health authorities and individual families can be expected to increase as the frequency of the disease and cost of medication continues to rise. On the basis of prevalence estimates within the UK population, the annual personal cost, based on 1995 prices, to patients with atopic eczema has been estimated at £297 million. This is accompanied by costs to the health service of approximately £125 million, and an annual cost to society, in terms of lost schooling. The cost of lost working days has been estimated at £43 million annually.[39]

In the US, the annual cost of treating one patient with atopic eczema has been estimated at US$219, with costs escalating significantly with disease severity.[40] An Australian survey estimated the annual cost of treating a child with mild disease severity at Aus$1142, increasing up to Aus$6099 in those children with severe exacerbations.[40] For the parent, in addition to the personal financial cost of treatment, which exceeds that of asthma,[41,42] the management of atopic eczema in a child can also result in sleep deprivation, loss of employment and emotional burdens.

Key points

- Atopic eczema is a chronic skin condition generally associated with an abnormal production of IgE antibodies in response to common environmental allergens. Most common in children, it may persist into adulthood.
- The disease is characterised by patches of red, dry itchy skin, commonly localised to the head and limbs. Lichenification of the skin and skin infections may develop as a result of the excessive scratching of affected areas.
- Although there is usually a strong familial history of atopic disease, environmental factors, including socioeconomic status, family size, exposure to allergens and early childhood infection contribute heavily to disease manifestation.
- The increasing worldwide incidence of atopic eczema, particularly in developed countries, exerts significant pressure on healthcare resources.
- Current therapy is directed at the relief of eczema-related symptoms through the hydration of the skin and the reduction of localised inflammation.
- Topically applied corticosteroids represent the first-line therapy for atopic eczema, but prolonged use is associated with a number of local as well as systemic side-effects.
- Recently, alternative non-steroidal topical agents have been developed, which offer efficacy in the treatment of atopic eczema, with a lower potential for systemic side-effects.

References

1. Eichenfield L, Hanifin J, Beck L *et al*. Atopic dermatitis and asthma: parallels in the evolution of treatment. *Pediatrics* 2003; **111**: 608–16.
2. Johansson S, Hourihane J, Bousquet J *et al*. A revised nomenclature for allergy. An EAACI position statement from the EAACI nomenclature task force. *Allergy* 2001; **56**: 813–24.
3. Wollenberg A, Wetzel S, Burgdorf W, Haas J. Viral infections in atopic dermatitis: pathogenic aspects and clinical management. *J Allergy Clin Immunol* 2003; **112**: 667–74.
4. Leung D, Bieber T. Atopic dermatitis. *Lancet* 2003; **361**: 151–60.
5. Thestrup-Pedersen K. Clinical aspects of atopic dermatitis. *Clin Exp Dermatol* 2000; **25**: 535–43.
6. Hoare C, Li Wan Po A, Williams H. Systematic review of treatments for AE. *Health Technology Assessment* 2000; **4**: 13–15.
7. The AE/Dermatitis Syndrome. Allergic Diseases Resource Center 2003: http://www.worldallergy.org/professional/allergic_diseases_center/atopiceczema/index
8. Forrest S, Dunn K, Elliott K *et al*. Identifying genes predisposing to AE. *Am J Respir Crit Care Med* 1997; **156**: 1390–3.
9. Schultz Larsen F. Atopic dermatitis: a genetic-epidemiologic study in a population-based twin sample. *J Am Acad Dermatol* 1993; **28**: 719–23.
10. Hanifin J, Chan S. Biochemical and immunologic mechanisms in atopic dermatitis: new targets for emerging therapies. *J Am Acad Dermatol* 1999; **41**: 72–7.
11. Monti G, Tonetto P, Mostert M *et al*. *Staphylococcus aureus* skin colonization in infants with atopic dermatitis. *Dermatology* 1996; **193**: 83–7.
12. Tupker RA, Pinnagoda J, Coenraads PJ *et al*. Susceptibility to irritants: role of barrier function, skin dryness and history of atopic dermatitis. *Br J Dermatol* 1990; **123**: 199–205.
13. Laske N, Bunikowski R, Niggemann B. Extraordinarily high serum IgE levels and consequences for atopic phenotypes. *Ann Allergy Asthma Immunol* 2003; **91**: 202–4.
14. Hoffman DR, Specific IgE antibodies in atopic eczema. *J Allergy Clin Immunol* 1975; **55**: 256–67.
15. Ring J, Darsow U, Gfesser M *et al*. The 'atopy patch test' in evaluating the role of aeroallergens in AE. *Int Arch Allergy Immunol* 2001; **124**: 326–31.
16. Loffler H, Steffes A, Happle R, Effendy I. Allergy and irritation: an adverse association in patients with AE. *Int Arch Allergy Immunol* 1997; **113**: 379–83.
17. Hanifin J, Rajka G. Diagnostic features of atopic dermatitis. *Acta Derm Venereol Suppl (Stockh)* 1980; **92**: 44–7.
18. Williams H. Epidemiology of atopic dermatitis. *Clin Exp Dermatol* 2000; **25**: 522–9.
19. Schultz-Larsen F, Diepgen T, Svensson A. The occurrence of atopic dermatitis in north Europe: an international questionnaire study. *J Am Acad Dermatol* 1996; **34**: 760–4.
20. Schultz-Larsen F, Hanifin J. Epidemiology of atopic dermatitis. *Immunol Allergy Clin North Am* 2002; **22**: 1–24.
21. Williams H. Is the prevalence of atopic dermatitis increasing? *Clin Exp Dermatol* 1992; **17**: 385–91.
22. Williams H, Robertson C, Stewart A, *et al*. Worldwide variations in the prevalence of symptoms of atopic eczema in the International Study of Asthma and Allergies in Childhood. *J Allergy Clin Immunol* 1999; **103**: 125–38.
23. Fergusson D, Horwood L, Shannon F. Risk factors in childhood eczema. *J Epidemiol Community Health* 1982; **36**: 118–22.
24. Larsen F, Holm N, Henningsen K. Atopic dermatitis. A genetic-epidemiologic study in a population-based twin sample. *J Am Acad Dermatol* 1986; **15**: 487–94.
25. ISAAC. Worldwide variation in prevalence of symptoms of asthma, allergic rhinoconjunctivitis, and atopic eczema: ISAAC. The International Study of Asthma and Allergies in Childhood (ISAAC) Steering Committee. *Lancet* 1998; **351**: 1225–32.
26. Gdalevich M, Mimouni D, David M, Mimouni M. Breast-feeding and the onset of atopic dermatitis in childhood: a systematic review and meta-analysis of prospective studies. *J Am Acad Dermatol* 2001; **45**: 520–7.
27. Williams H, Strachan D, Hay R. Childhood eczema: disease of the advantaged? *BMJ* 1994; **308**: 1132–5.
28. McNally N, Phillips D, Williams H. The problem of atopic eczema: aetiological clues from the environment and lifestyles. *Soc Sci Med* 1998; **46**: 729–41.
29. Strachan D. Family size, infection and atopy: the first decade of the "hygiene hypothesis". *Thorax* 2000; **55**: S2–10.
30. Strachan D. Hay fever, hygiene, and household size. *BMJ* 1989; **299**: 1259–60.
31. Primary Care Dermatology Society & British Association of Dermatologists. Guidelines for the management of atopic eczema. *eGuidelines.co.uk* 2003; **19**.
32. Reynolds N, Franklin V, Gray J, Diffey B, Farr P. Narrow-band ultraviolet B and broad-band ultraviolet A phototherapy in adult atopic eczema: a randomised controlled trial. *Lancet* 2001; **357**: 2012–6.
33. Wollenberg A, Sharma S, von Bubnoff D, Geiger E, Haberstok J, Bieber T. Topical tacrolimus (FK506) leads to profound phenotypic and functional alterations of epidermal antigen-presenting dendritic cells in atopic dermatitis. *J Allergy Clin Immunol* 2001; **107**: 519–25.
34. Zuberbier T, Chong S, Grunow K, *et al*. The ascomycin macrolactam pimecrolimus (Elidel, SDZ ASM 981) is a potent inhibitor of mediator release from human dermal mast cells and peripheral blood basophils. *J Allergy Clin Immunol* 2001; **108**: 275–80.
35. Reitamo S, Rustin M, Ruzicka T, *et al*. Efficacy and safety of tacrolimus ointment compared with that of hydrocortisone butyrate ointment in adult patients with atopic dermatitis. *J Allergy Clin Immunol* 2002; **109**: 539–46.

36 Reitamo S, Van Leent E, Ho V, et al. Efficacy and safety of tacrolimus ointment compared with that of hydrocortisone acetate ointment in children with atopic dermatitis. *J Allergy Clin Immunol* 2002; **109**: 547–55.

37 Eichenfield L, Lucky A, Boguniewicz M, et al. Safety and efficacy of pimecrolimus (ASM 981) cream 1% in the treatment of mild and moderate atopic dermatitis in children and adolescents. *J Am Acad Dermatol* 2002; **46**: 495–504.

38 Sowden J, Berth-Jones J, Ross J, et al. Double-blind, controlled, crossover study of cyclosporin in adults with severe refractory atopic dermatitis. *Lancet* 1991; **338**: 137–40.

39 Herd R, Tidman M, Prescott R, Hunter J. The cost of atopic eczema. *Br J Dermatol* 1996; **135**: 20–3.

40 Weinmann S, Kamtsiuris P, Henke K, Wickman M, Jenner A, Wahn U. The costs of atopy and asthma in children: assessment of direct costs and their determinants in a birth cohort. *Pediatr Allergy Immunol* 2003; **14**: 18–26.

41 Kemp A. Atopic eczema: its social and financial costs. *J Paediatr Child Health* 1999; **35**: 229–31.

42 Su J, Kemp A, Varigos G, Nolan T. Atopic eczema: its impact on the family and financial cost. *Arch Dis Child* 1997; **76**: 159–62.

7. Benign prostatic hyperplasia

Dr Richard Clark
CSF Medical Communications Ltd

Summary

Benign prostatic hyperplasia (BPH) is a highly prevalent condition. Enlarged prostates are evident in as many as 50% of middle-aged males and nearly 90% of men in their eighties. BPH is associated with a number of significant and serious complications such as acute urinary retention, which may necessitate surgical intervention. Indeed, untreated acute urinary retention is associated with a significant mortality burden. BPH also impacts on a patient's quality of life and imposes a significant burden on public health services globally. However, with the advent of effective medical treatments for the condition – including α-adrenergic receptor antagonists and 5α-reductase inhibitors – the number of surgical interventions for BPH and its associated complications has fallen dramatically. The availability of these agents has also led to a shift in the responsibility for managing the condition – from urology specialists to general practitioners.

BPH is a benign enlargement of the prostate, occurring in 40–50% of men in their fifties, up to 70% in their sixties and 88% in their eighties.[1,2] Benign enlargement of the prostate can result in increased pressure on the urethra leading to obstruction of urinary flow.[1] Patients with BPH often present with lower urinary tract symptoms (LUTS) as a result of difficulties in voiding (e.g. hesitancy, straining, weak stream, dribbling, urgency and urge incontinence). However, the cause of these urinary symptoms varies, and whilst benign prostatic enlargement (BPE) may be the major cause, other aetiologies can also be involved. If left untreated, BPH and accompanying LUTS can progress in severity and become increasingly bothersome to the patient. Patients may also experience recurrent bladder infections, develop bladder calculi or acute urinary retention, and eventually may require prostate surgery.[3]

BPH is a specific histological term, commonly used to encompass BPE, bladder outflow obstruction (BOO) and the coexistence of LUTS.[4] Historically, older men with LUTS were described as suffering from prostatism or 'symptoms of benign prostatic hyperplasia', but the use of a

> The advent of therapeutic agents such as the α-AR antagonists and the 5α-reductase inhibitors has increased the proportion of men treated in primary care.

histological term is confusing in everyday clinical practice.[5] Prostatism implies a prostatic cause for symptoms, though little evidence exists for this, and there are no symptoms specific to BPH, or BOO, one of its complications.[5] Furthermore, BPH is evident in 70% of men over the age of 70 years, though only some patients with BPH develop BPE, with a minority developing BOO and voiding symptoms.[6] BPE indicates a clinically enlarged prostate, BOO a urodynamic obstruction with an unspecified cause, and benign prostatic obstruction (BPO) a urodynamic obstruction secondary to BPE. LUTS, BPE and BOO may occur on their own or in combination, with a combination of symptoms more likely to result in the requirement for invasive surgery.[7] In light of the above, it has been suggested that the terminology used in this therapeutic area should be more clearly defined to reflect clinical symptoms or aetiology (Table 1).[5] For example, LUTS should replace prostatism, and storage and voiding symptoms should replace irritative and obstructive symptoms, respectively.[5] This review will use specific clinical terms wherever possible in order to simplify and clarify the complexities in the field.

A pan-European survey of 80,774 males has demonstrated a linear increase in the incidence of LUTS, suggestive of BPH, from the ages of 46 to 80 years, with an overall prevalence of approximately 10% (Figure 1).[1] Moderate-to-severe LUTS symptoms were present in 15% of men aged 50–59, 27% aged 60–69, and 31% aged 70–79.[8] Other studies have suggested overall prevalence rates of clinical BPH of 9–20% in men aged 50–75 years in the Netherlands, and 41% with moderate-to-severe symptoms of LUTS in men aged over 50 years in the UK.[9,10] Historically, most men in the UK with LUTS were not actively treated by their GP; either they did not complain, accepting these symptoms as a natural consequence of ageing, or they were managed conservatively.[11] The advent of therapeutic agents such as the α-adrenergic receptor (AR) antagonists

Table 1. Abbreviations of prostate-specific terms.

BPH	Benign prostatic hyperplasia
LUTS	Lower urinary tract symptoms
BPE	Benign prostatic enlargement
BOO	Bladder outflow obstruction
BPO	Benign prostatic obstruction
TURP	Transurethral resection of the prostate
TUIP	Transurethral incision of the prostate
BNI	Bladder neck incision
RPP	Retropubic prostatectomy

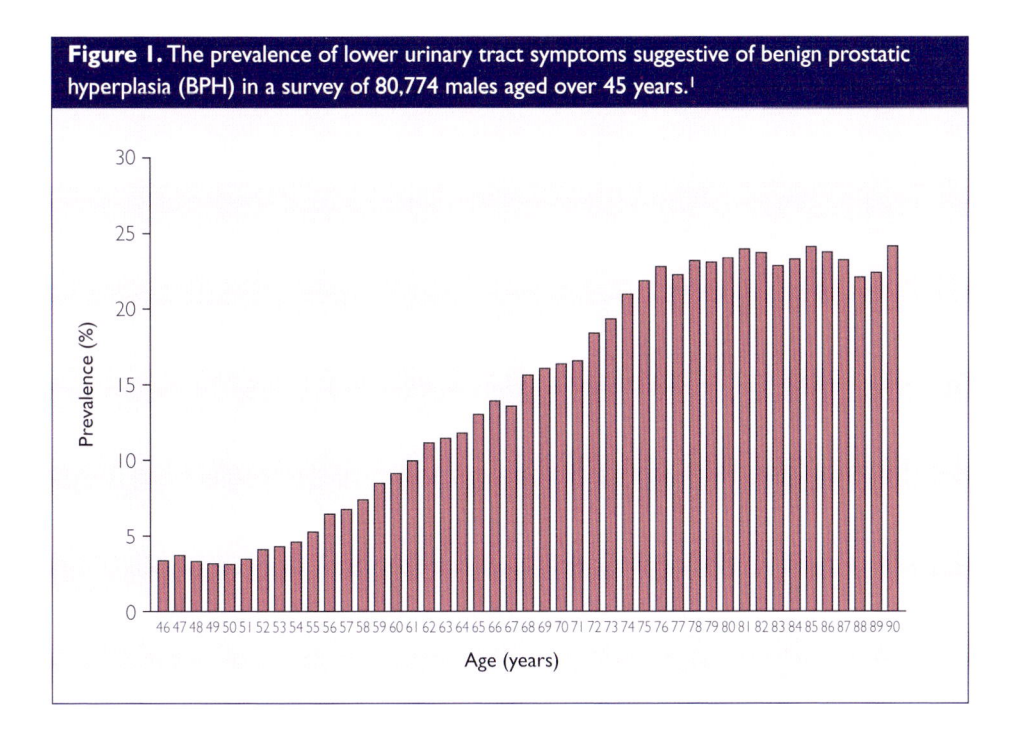

Figure 1. The prevalence of lower urinary tract symptoms suggestive of benign prostatic hyperplasia (BPH) in a survey of 80,774 males aged over 45 years.[1]

and the 5α-reductase inhibitors has increased the proportion of men treated in primary care in the UK but has not decreased the rate of surgical treatment for BPH, probably because of the low baseline rates of operative treatment.[11]

Impact of BPH

BPH has a huge impact on public health services worldwide. It accounts for approximately 2 million physician visits and 379,000 prostatectomies each year in the US, such that a 40-year-old man who lives to the age of 80 years would have a one-in-three chance of having a prostatectomy for BPH.[2] Annually in England and Wales, approximately 42,000 men undergo prostatectomy (including transurethral resection of the prostate [TURP], transurethral incision of the prostate [TUIP], alternatively known as bladder neck incision [BNI]; and open prostatectomy, also known as retropubic prostatectomy [RPP]). One-quarter of these patients present with acute retention of urine, which carries a two-fold greater risk of death and complications than for non-retentive patients undergoing this procedure.[11] Interestingly, the mortality rate from BPH has been declining, particularly in western countries such as the USA, Canada, Australia, New Zealand and Western Europe. A slower decline in mortality rates has been observed in Central and Eastern Europe.[2] In the UK, the age-adjusted rate of mortality

> A 40-year-old man who lives to the age of 80 years would have a one-in-three chance of having a prostatectomy for BPH.

from BPH fell from 16.5 per 100,000 in 1950–54 to 1.2 per 100,000 in 1985–89, probably due to improvements in surgical techniques, anaesthesia and improved medical management during the postoperative period.[2]

LUTS have a profound effect on patients' quality of life, as assessed by the Short Form-36 (SF-36) quality-of-life questionnaire.[12] Moderate-to-severe LUTS were found to be associated with small-to-moderate deficits in terms of anxious and depressed mood, and poorer role functioning related to the emotional problems arising from the illness. Severe LUTS were associated with significant fatigue and limitations on daily work and family activities, again related to the emotional problems contingent on the symptoms. Furthermore, feelings of anxiety or depression and low energy levels were greater in patients with severe LUTS than those with hypertension, diabetes, angina or gout. These results have been confirmed in a separate study that showed that the more severe the LUTS the lower the quality of life, as determined by an EQ-5D quality-of-life questionnaire, regardless of a diagnosis of BPH.[10] Furthermore, in a group of patients with LUTS suggestive of BPH, urgency, nocturia and hesitancy were the most bothersome symptoms, with the severity of the symptoms of incomplete bladder emptying and frequency of urination most strongly associated with a diminished sense of well-being.[13]

The management and treatment of BPH places a heavy burden on healthcare services, both in terms of direct costs (e.g. treatment costs, increased physician workload, increased risk of injury from nocturia-related falls) and indirect costs (e.g. loss of patient working hours).[14]

Pathophysiology and natural history

BPH is a chronic progressive condition, with LUTS and BPE becoming more common with increasing age.[15,16] A normal prostate weighs approximately 20 g at 21–30 years of age, and remains at this size unless BPH occurs.[16] The prevalence of pathological BPH is 8% by 40 years of age; however, 50% of males have pathological BPH when they are 51–60 years old, and the average weight of a prostate containing BPH at autopsy is 33 g.[17] The growth of the prostate usually begins before 30 years of age, with the early phase of BPH growth (men between 31 and 50 years) characterised by a doubling time of 4.5 years for prostate weight. In the mid-phase of BPH growth (men between 51 and 70 years) the doubling time is 10 years, though growth slows in patients over 70 years of age (with a BPH doubling time of over 100 years).[17] Although pathological changes in the prostate can begin from 30–40 years of age, symptoms such as LUTS rarely occur until men are aged 50 years or older.[11] In fact, the growth of the prostate gland does not always result in symptomatic problems as no strong relationship has been observed between the size of the prostate and obstructive symptoms.[11,15]

Although LUTS can be caused by BPE, other aetiologies include:
- age-related changes in bladder smooth muscle (detrusor muscle)
- idiopathic detrusor instability (phasic changes in bladder pressure found during filling, giving rise to symptoms of urgency and frequency)
- prostate cancer.[11]

BOO may also be caused by BPE, or other problems such as bladder neck dyssynergia, though the increase in outlet resistance can be overcome for some time by increased detrusor contraction, whereby the patient maintains his urinary flow under higher pressure (a condition termed 'silent prostatism').[11] If the obstruction continues, however, detrusor function is affected and urinary retention can occur. Acute urinary retention, in particular, can have devastating effects, with patients experiencing the sudden onset of painful, distressing symptoms requiring hospitalisation and the insertion of a catheter, frequently resulting in emergency surgery, with its attendant risk of morbidity and mortality.[3]

Risk factors

Risk factors for a diagnosis of clinical BPH (defined as frequent urination or difficulty urinating, together with an enlarged or swollen prostate or surgery for BPH) include elevated levels of free prostate-specific antigen (PSA), heart disease, and the use of β-blocker medications.[18] In contrast, current cigarette smoking and high levels of physical activity appeared to protect against the development of clinical BPH.[18]

Several factors are associated with the progression of BPH. These include:
- increased post-void residual urine
- reduced urinary flow rate
- increased urinary symptoms
- urodynamic evidence of obstruction.[16]

Three factors have been identified as associated with an increased risk of acute urinary retention or the need for prostate surgery:
- changes in the force of the urinary stream
- sensation of incomplete bladder emptying
- enlarged prostate on digital rectal examination.[3,19]

The presence of one, two or all three of these risk factors is associated with a 9, 16 and 37% increased risk, respectively, of acute urinary retention or prostate surgery.[3,19] Age is also an important independent risk factor. A man aged 70 years who has all three risk factors has an 11-fold greater risk of progressing to acute urinary retention or of having prostate surgery compared with a man aged 40 years with the same risk factors.[3]

Peak urinary flow rates decrease with advancing age, showing an average of 2 mL/second decrease with each passing decade (Figure 2).[20] This corresponds to an increase in prostate size of approximately 0.6 mL/year.[3] Men with enlarged prostates (>40 mL) are:
- three-times more likely to have LUTS
- twice as likely to be bothered by symptoms of LUTS
- twice as likely to experience interference with their normal daily activities.[21]

Even men with prostate volumes greater than 30 mL have three times the risk of suffering from acute urinary retention compared with those with smaller prostates.[21]

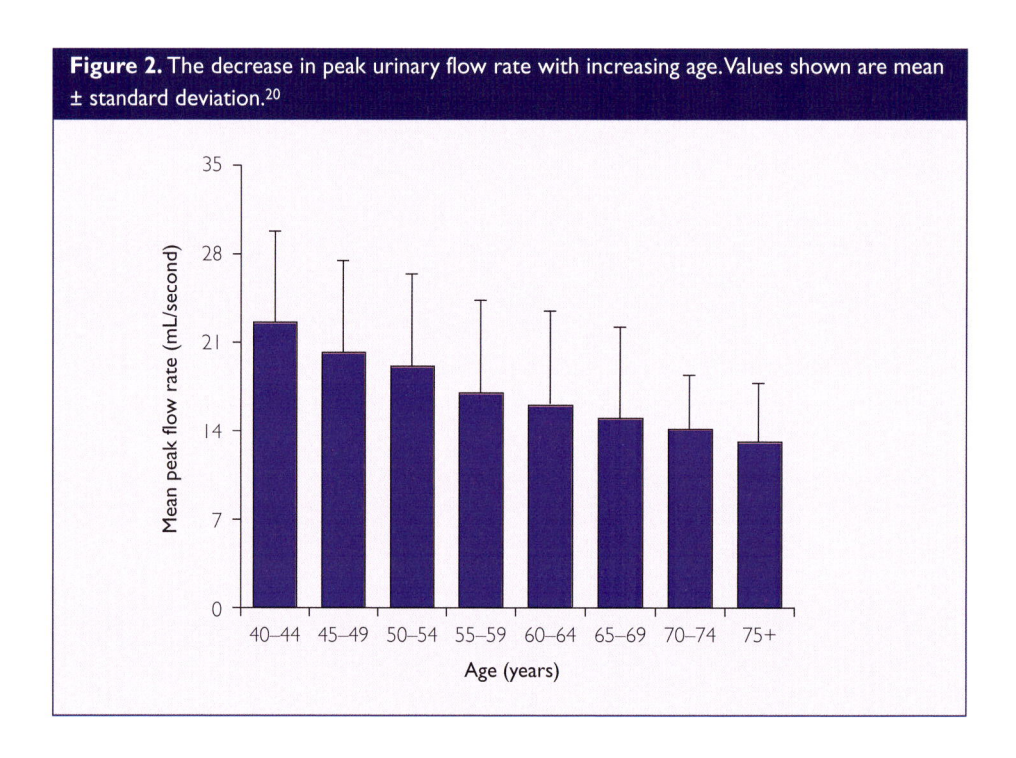

Peak urinary flow rates decrease with advancing age... this corresponds to an increase in prostate size.

Figure 2. The decrease in peak urinary flow rate with increasing age. Values shown are mean ± standard deviation.[20]

Symptoms

LUTS may have causes other than BPH, BPE or BOO, as discussed previously. LUTS are classified into voiding symptoms (formerly known as obstructive symptoms) and storage symptoms (formerly termed irritative symptoms).

The following voiding symptoms may occur:
- hesitancy (a sensation of delay in the onset of micturition from several seconds to several minutes)
- poor urinary stream and/or straining (a flow of less than 10 mL/second is suggestive of BOO)
- sensation of incomplete bladder emptying (may signal the presence of residual urine)
- terminal and post-micturition dribbling (flow ends abruptly at the end of normal voiding, or continues at a low level for some time)
- prolonged voiding time (BOO can reduce the force of the urine stream, resulting in prolonged voiding time)
- urinary retention (either acute or chronic retention may occur).[11]

The following storage symptoms may occur:
- frequency (normal daytime frequency is less than seven times per day)
- nocturia (being woken from sleep by the desire to void)
- urgency (the urgent desire to void, often accompanied by fear of impending leakage)
- urge incontinence (incontinence caused by severe detrusor instability, often caused by BOO or idiopathic detrusor instability)
- pain (though not a symptom of BPE, pain may accompany urinary retention and bladder conditions such as bladder stone and urinary tract infections, which may themselves be associated with BPE).[11]

Diagnosis

Most clinical diagnostic assessments target either BPE, LUTS, BOO, or detrusor dysfunction to identify patients with BPH and to exclude other underlying disease processes.[22] The assessments recommended for the diagnosis of BPH are outlined in Table 2,[22–24] and the International Prostate Symptom Score (IPSS) questionnaire, which is generally acknowledged as the best validated prostate diagnostic questionnaire, is shown in Table 3.[6] Whilst the measurement of PSA is recommended in the majority of guidelines to help rule out prostate cancer as the cause of LUTS, this remains a contentious issue amongst urologists.[22,23] Although opportunistic PSA screening is not recommended in the UK guidelines, in practice many

> Although opportunistic PSA screening is not recommended in the UK guidelines, in practice many GPs carry out PSA measurements before referral.

Table 2. Tests for the evaluation of benign prostatic hyperplasia.[22–24]

Assessment	Comments
Digital rectal examination	Mandatory test that helps to determine the size of the prostate and eliminate clinically evident prostate cancer.
Medical history/symptom score	Can describe and quantify symptoms (e.g. the International Prostate Symptom Score [IPSS]).
Prostate serum antigen (PSA)	Indicates the possible presence of prostate cancer and the size of the prostate.
Uroflowmetry	Maximum and average urinary flow rates should be interpreted with caution, allowing for age-related urodynamic changes.
Serum creatine measurement	To detect abnormalities in liver function, since long-standing bladder outlet obstruction can result in hydronephrosis or renal failure.
Imaging	Includes transrectal ultrasonography (TRUS), computed tomography, and magnetic resonance imaging.

GPs carry out PSA measurements before referral, predominantly due to concerns over litigation if prostate cancer is subsequently diagnosed.[11,25] However, there is no firm evidence to suggest that the presence of LUTS is predictive of localised prostate cancer, and there is a high likelihood of false positives and false negatives with this test.[22,25] All patients should receive counselling before PSA testing, and have a life expectancy of at least 10 years.[23]

Treatment options

When patients have been diagnosed with LUTS due to BOO or BPE, treatment can take the form of surveillance (watchful waiting), pharmacological treatment, or physical intervention (surgical or non-surgical). Immediate referral should be sought after an initial physical examination if the following complications are observed:
- urinary infection
- bladder stones
- haematuria
- chronic urinary retention
- upper-tract deterioration with the attendant risk of renal impairment.[6]

An algorithm for the management of patients with urinary symptoms in primary care is shown in Figure 3.[26]

Table 3. The International Prostate Symptom Score (IPSS) questionnaire. Adapted from Abrams, 1995.[6]

International Prostate Symptom Score (IPSS)

	Not at all	Less than 1 time in 5	Less than half the time	About half the time	More than half the time	Almost always
1. Over the past month, how often have you had a sensation of not emptying your bladder completely after you finished urinating?	0	1	2	3	4	5
2. Over the past month, how often have you had to urinate again less than two hours after you finished urinating?	0	1	2	3	4	5
3. Over the past month, how often have you found you stopped and started again several times when you urinated?	0	1	2	3	4	5
4. Over the past month, how often have you found it difficult to postpone urination?	0	1	2	3	4	5
5. Over the past month, how often have you had a weak urinary system?	0	1	2	3	4	5
6. Over the past month, how often have you had to push or strain to begin urination?	0	1	2	3	4	5

	None	1 time	2 times	3 times	4 times	5 or more times
7. Over the past month, how many times did you most typically get up to urinate from the time you went to bed at night until the time you got up in the morning?	0	1	2	3	4	5

Total IPSS Score

Quality of life due to urinary symtoms

	Delighted	Pleased	Mostly satisfied	Mixed[a]	Mostly dissatisfied	Unhappy	Terrible
1. If you were to spend the rest of your life with your urinary condition just the way it is now, how would you feel about that?							

Quality of life assessment index

[a] About equally satisfied and dissatisfied

Watchful waiting

Recent guidelines recommend watchful waiting for patients with mild symptoms (IPSS <7–8), with monitoring at 6- or 12-month intervals.[22–24] The variety of symptoms, their impact on the patient's daily activities, and the cost-effectiveness of this approach should also be considered.[24]

Figure 3. Management algorithm for urinary symptoms in primary care.[26]
DRE, digital rectal examination; IPSS, International Prostate Symptom Score; MSU, mid-stream urine; PSA, prostate-specific antigen; UTI, urinary tract infection.

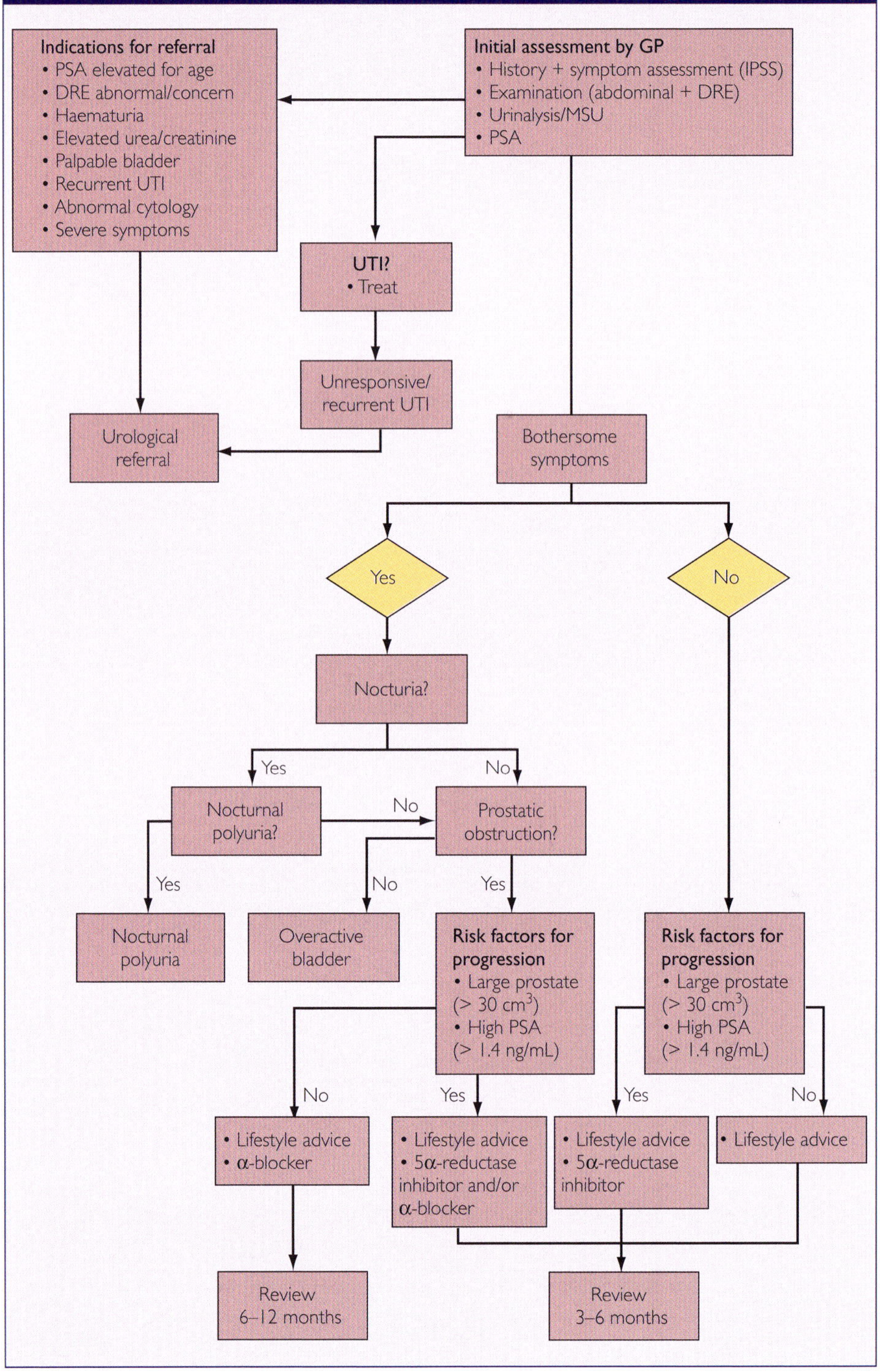

Indications for referral
- PSA elevated for age
- DRE abnormal/concern
- Haematuria
- Elevated urea/creatinine
- Palpable bladder
- Recurrent UTI
- Abnormal cytology
- Severe symptoms

Initial assessment by GP
- History + symptom assessment (IPSS)
- Examination (abdominal + DRE)
- Urinalysis/MSU
- PSA

UTI?
- Treat

Unresponsive/recurrent UTI → Urological referral

Bothersome symptoms → Yes / No

Yes → Nocturia?
- Yes → Nocturnal polyuria?
  - Yes → Nocturnal polyuria
  - No → Overactive bladder / Prostatic obstruction?
- No → Prostatic obstruction?
  - Yes → Risk factors for progression
    - Large prostate (> 30 cm³)
    - High PSA (> 1.4 ng/mL)
    - No → Lifestyle advice; α-blocker → Review 6–12 months
    - Yes → Lifestyle advice; 5α-reductase inhibitor and/or α-blocker → Review 3–6 months

No → Risk factors for progression
- Large prostate (> 30 cm³)
- High PSA (> 1.4 ng/mL)
- Yes → Lifestyle advice; 5α-reductase inhibitor → Review 3–6 months
- No → Lifestyle advice

Pharmacological treatments

Most guidelines recommend that patients with uncomplicated clinical BPH and moderate symptoms (IPSS 8–19) receive pharmacological intervention, though a few also advocate this approach for uncomplicated clinical BPH with moderate-to-severe symptoms (IPSS 8–35).[22–24] The α-AR antagonists (alfuzosin, doxazosin, indoramin, prazosin, tamsulosin and terazosin) and 5α-reductase inhibitors (finasteride and dutasteride) are commonly used. α-AR antagonists are used in patients with bothersome LUTS who do not have an absolute indication for surgery, regardless of prostate volume, whilst a 5α-reductase inhibitor may be beneficial in patients with bothersome LUTS and an enlarged prostate (>30 mL).[26]

α-AR antagonists:
- rapidly relax the smooth muscle of the prostate gland and bladder neck, improve urinary flow and reduce BOO, but do not affect the size of the prostate gland
- provide symptomatic improvements within 48 hours that can last up to 42 months
- can reduce symptom scores by 20–50%
- improve urinary flow rates by up to 20–30%.[24]

5α-reductase inhibitors:
- are slower acting than α-AR antagonists, with maximum effects observed after 6 months of treatment
- can reduce prostate size by 20–30%
- reduce symptom scores by approximately 15%
- cause moderate improvements in urinary flow rates.[24]

Interestingly, whilst the market for 5α-reductase inhibitors has remained stable since 1995, that of the α-AR antagonists is expanding rapidly worldwide.[27] Alternative treatments (e.g. phytotherapy) are generally not recommended, as their efficacy is unproven in well-designed, long-term trials.[22,23] One possible exception is Saw palmetto, which has demonstrated equivalent efficacy to finasteride for the reduction of LUTS in large numbers of patients, for up to 48 weeks.[28]

Surgery

Surgery is the main treatment option for patients who fail to respond to pharmacological therapy or who present with complicated BPH. The complications for which surgery is indicated are acute urinary retention, recurrent urinary tract infection, gross haematuria, bladder stones, renal insufficiency due to BPH, renal failure due to BOO, and large bladder diverticulum.[23] Surgery, which removes the enlarged part of the prostate and relieves the bladder obstruction, is often the best long-term solution in such patients.[23] The three surgical options are:

- TURP
- TUIP
- open prostatectomy.

Generally, TURP is the most frequently performed surgical technique, and it is suitable for patients with moderately enlarged prostates, provided the procedure lasts less than 1 hour.[23] TUIP is suitable for smaller prostates (25–30 mL), with no median lobe and a low risk of associated prostate cancer. Patients with severely enlarged prostate glands generally receive an open prostatectomy.[23] Laser surgery is not considered as a first-line surgical intervention, but may be useful in certain patient groups (e.g. those receiving anticoagulation medication or those not suitable for TURP).[23]

Other, less-invasive physical interventions are used less frequently than surgical techniques, as many are still considered to be investigational therapies (e.g. transrectal high-intensity focused ultrasound) or have high failure rates (e.g. transurethral needle ablation).[23] The most attractive non-surgical physical intervention is transurethral microwave thermotherapy, though this is probably best reserved for patients who prefer to avoid surgery or who are no longer responding to medication.[22,24] Furthermore, any physical interventions considered should ideally be compared with the 'gold standard' of TURP, be demonstrated in large numbers of patients, and show evidence of long-term efficacy.[22]

Key points

- BPH is a benign enlargement of the prostate occurring in 40–50% of men in their fifties, up to 70% of men in their sixties and 88% of men in their eighties.
- Patients with BPH often present with LUTS.
- Pathological changes in the prostate may be present from 30 to 40 years of age, though symptoms such as LUTS rarely occur until men are aged 50 years or older.
- If left untreated, BPH and accompanying LUTS may progress in severity, leading ultimately to prostate surgery.
- Treatment can take the form of surveillance (watchful waiting), pharmacological treatment, or physical intervention (surgical or non-surgical).
- α-AR antagonists are generally used in patients with bothersome LUTS without an absolute indication for surgery, regardless of prostate volume.
- Patients with bothersome LUTS and an enlarged prostate (>30 mL) may benefit from treatment with a 5α-reductase inhibitor.
- Surgery is the main treatment option for patients who fail to respond to pharmacological therapy or who present with complicated BPH.

References

1. Verhamme KM, Dieleman JP, Bleumink GS et al. Triumph Pan European Expert Panel. Incidence and prevalence of lower urinary tract symptoms suggestive of benign prostatic hyperplasia in primary care – the Triumph project. *Eur Urol* 2002; **42**: 323–8.
2. Napalkov P, Maisonneuve P, Boyle P. Worldwide patterns of prevalence and mortality from benign prostatic hyperplasia. *Urology* 1995; **46(Suppl A)**: 41–6.
3. Kirby RS. The natural history of benign prostatic hyperplasia: what have we learned in the last decade? *Urology* 2000; **56(Suppl 1)**: 3–6.
4. Abrams P. Benign prostatic hyperplasia has precise meaning. *BMJ* 2001; **322**:106.
5. Abrams P. New words for old: lower urinary tract symptoms for 'prostatism'. *BMJ* 1994; **308**: 929–30.
6. Abrams P. Fortnightly review: managing lower urinary tract symptoms in older men. *BMJ* 1995; **310**: 1113–17.
7. Ramsey EW. Benign prostatic hyperplasia: a review. *Can J Urol* 2000; **7**: 1135–43.
8. Norman RW, Nickel JC, Fish D, Pickett SN. 'Prostate-related symptoms' in Canadian men 50 years of age or older: prevalence and relationships among symptoms. *Br J Urol* 1994; **74**: 542–50.
9. Blanker MH, Groeneveld FP, Prins A, Bernsen RM, Bohnen AM, Bosch JL. Strong effects of definition and nonresponse bias on prevalence rates of clinical benign prostatic hyperplasia: the Krimpen study of male urogenital tract problems and general health status. *BJU Int* 2000; **85**: 665–71.
10. Trueman P, Hood SC, Nayak US, Mrazek MF. Prevalence of lower urinary tract symptoms and self-reported diagnosed 'benign prostatic hyperplasia', and their effect on quality of life in a community-based survey of men in the UK. *BJU Int* 1999; **83**: 410–15.
11. Neal DE, Neal RR, Donovan J. Benign prostatic hyperplasia. http://hcna.radcliffe-oxford.com/urinframe.html (accessed May 2003).
12. Welch G, Weinger K, Barry MJ. Quality-of-life impact of lower urinary tract symptom severity: results from the Health Professionals Follow-up Study. *Urology* 2002; **59**: 245–50.
13. Eckhardt MD, van Venrooij GE, van Melick HH, Boon TA. Prevalence and bothersomeness of lower urinary tract symptoms in benign prostatic hyperplasia and their impact on well-being. *J Urol* 2001; **166**: 563–8.
14. Anderson JB, Roehrborn CG, Schalken JA, Emberton M. The progression of benign prostatic hyperplasia: examining the evidence and determining the risk. *Eur Urol* 2001; **39**: 390–9.
15. Jacobsen SJ, Girman CJ, Lieber MM. Natural history of benign prostatic hyperplasia. *Urology* 2001; **58(Suppl 1)**: 5–16.
16. Djavan B, Nickel JC, de la Rosette J, Abrams P. The urologist view of BPH progression: results of an international survey. *Eur Urol* 2002; **41**: 490–6.
17. Berry SJ, Coffey DS, Walsh PC, Ewing LL. The development of human benign prostatic hyperplasia with age. *J Urol* 1984; **132**: 474–9.
18. Meigs JB, Mohr B, Barry MJ, Collins MM, McKinlay JB. Risk factors for clinical benign prostatic hyperplasia in a community-based population of healthy aging men. *J Clin Epidemiol* 2001; **54**: 935–44.
19. Arrighi HM, Guess HA, Metter EJ, Fozard JL. Symptoms and signs of prostatism as risk factors for prostatectomy. *Prostate* 1990; **16**: 253–61.
20. Girman CJ, Panser LA, Chute CG et al. Natural history of prostatism: urinary flow rates in a community-based study. *J Urol* 1993; **150**: 887–92.
21. Girman CJ, Jacobsen SJ, Rhodes T, Guess HA, Roberts RO, Lieber MM. Association of health-related quality of life and benign prostatic enlargement. *Eur Urol* 1999; **35**: 277–84.
22. de la Rosette JJ, van der Schoot DK, Debruyne FM. Recent developments in guidelines on benign prostatic hyperplasia. *Curr Opin Urol* 2002; **12**: 3–6.
23. Roehrborn CG, Bartsch G, Kirby R et al. Guidelines for the diagnosis and treatment of benign prostatic hyperplasia: a comparative, international overview. *Urology* 2001; **58**: 642–50.
24. de la Rosette JJ, Alivizatos G, Madersbacher S et al. European Association of Urology. EAU Guidelines on benign prostatic hyperplasia (BPH). *Eur Urol* 2001; **40**: 256–63.
25. Prodigy Guidance. Prostate – benign hyperplasia. January 2003. http://www.prodigy.nhs.uk
26. Speakman MJ, Kirby RS, Joyce A, Abrams P, Pocock R. The guidelines for the primary care management of male lower urinary tract symptoms. *BJU Int* 2004; **93**: 985–90.
27. Höfner K. Alpha(1)-blocker therapy in the nineties: focus on the disease. *Prostate Cancer Prostatic Dis* 1999; **2(Suppl 4)**: S9–S15.
28. Saw palmetto and prostatic hypertrophy. *Bandolier*. http://www.jr2.ox.ac.uk/bandolier/band73/b73-2.html (accessed May 2003).

Acknowledgements

Figure 1 is adapted from Verhamme *et al.*, 2002.[1]
Figure 2 is adapted from Girman *et al.*, 1993.[20]
Figure 3 is adapted from Speakman *et al.*, 2004.[26]

8. Cholera

Dr Duncan West
CSF Medical Communications Ltd

Summary

Cholera accounts for more than 120,000 deaths each year, with fatality rates as high as 40% of infected individuals in certain affected regions, with children being at particular risk. The causative pathogen is *Vibrio cholerae* which produces a potent enterotoxin that leads to acute diarrhoea by disrupting ion transport in intestinal epithelial cells. Epidemics of cholera are almost exclusively caused by the O1 and O139 serogroups, with the O1 variant being the most predominant globally. Acute diarrhoea can persist for several days, and in severe cases can cause death as a consequence of severe dehydration. Poor hygiene and sanitation are the major causes of the spread of infection, and, consequently, cholera remains endemic in areas of the world with limited access to safe and clean water supplies. The risk of infection can be minimised by following appropriate hygiene and sanitary measures. However, in those individuals visiting areas of cholera endemicity, vaccination is recommended against the disease. Currently, the World Health Organization recommend the oral inactivated whole-cell/cholera toxin B subunit vaccine (or Dukoral®) for prophylaxis of cholera.

Introduction

Cholera and other diarrhoeal diseases caused by enterotoxigenic bacteria are a major cause of illness and death in many parts of the world. Cholera has existed for many centuries and during this time has claimed the lives of millions of people. Even today, with recent medical advances, it is estimated that the disease is responsible for about 120,000 deaths each year.[1]

Cholera is an acute enteric infection caused by the bacterium *Vibrio cholerae* and morbidity is mediated by the potent enterotoxin that it produces. Infected individuals suffer acute diarrhoea of several days duration and in extreme cases cholera can be one of the most rapidly progressing fatal infectious diseases, bringing about death by dehydration in as little as 6–8 hours after the onset of symptoms.[1] Humans are the only known natural host for the bacterium, and the disease is spread by faecal contamination of water and food. Consequently, poor sanitation is largely to blame for the endemicity and epidemicity of the disease. With proper treatment and sanitation less than 1% of cases should prove fatal, but in affected regions fatality rates as high as 40% have been reported.[1]

There is an inverse relationship between age and cholera risk that is thought to reflect a protective immunity that is acquired through previous disease or pathogen exposure (inapparent infection). As a result, it is predominantly children who are at greatest risk of infection in regions where the disease is endemic, although people of all ages are susceptible.[2] The protective immunity conferred by cholera infection is a physiological response that has formed the foundation for the development of cholera vaccines, a strategy that until recently had proved largely ineffective.

The pathogen: *Vibrio cholerae*

The infectious agent responsible for cholera was first described in 1854 by Filipo Pacini who noted the unusual appearance of a curved bacterium, *Vibrio cholerae*, in the gastrointestinal tracts of infected patients.[3] However, it was not until 1883 that Robert Koch demonstrated a causative link between the bacterium and the disease.[3]

V. cholerae is a motile, curved, Gram-negative, water-borne bacillus of the family Vibrionaceae that lives in coastal waters throughout the world.[4,5] Like many bacterial pathogens, infection occurs as a result of the ingestion of contaminated food and/or water. *V. cholerae* is a well defined species with over 200 serogroups identified on the basis of the composition of the major polysaccharide surface antigen of the cell wall – the so called 'O' antigen.[5,6] However, the species is by no means homogeneous in terms of its pathogenic potential.[4] Epidemics have almost exclusively been caused by *V. cholerae* of the O1 and O139 serogroups, with O1 being the predominant variant worldwide.[1,4–6] The remaining serogroups are considered to be either non-pathogenic or occasional pathogens. The O1 subgroup can be further classified into three antigenic serotypes – Inaba, Ogawa and the much rarer Hikojima. In addition, the O1 subgroup may also be divided into two biotypes – El Tor and Classical – and various combinations of sero- and biotype can be found (i.e. Classical and El Tor strains which are either Inaba or Ogawa).[1,4–6] The O139 serogroup shares many characteristics with El Tor O1 strains possessing all the virulence determinants but displaying a mutation in the genes encoding the O antigen.[7] In addition the O139 strain also produces a polysaccharide capsule and has an increased capacity for both toxin production and for bacterial proliferation.[8]

V. cholerae has the ability to persist in infected regions for months, if not years, due to its ability to enter a dormant, but viable, state until it is activated by environmental triggers such as an increase in temperature or a decrease in salinity. The bacterium is characteristically water-borne and can also bind to chitin, a component of crustacean shells, and can also colonise the surfaces of algae, phytoplankton and the roots of aquatic plants.[5] As a result, *V. cholerae* can survive for 2–14 days in food and for many weeks in living shellfish.[10]

V. cholerae infection begins with the ingestion of contaminated food and/or water which enables the bacterium to colonise and adhere to the mucosal lining of the small intestine where it produces a potent enterotoxin that disrupts ion transport in intestinal epithelial cells. The subsequent loss of water and electrolytes in turn leads to the severe diarrhoea that is characteristic of cholera.[4]

Epidemiology

One of the most important and characteristic features of cholera is its ability to occur in explosive outbreaks. Cholera epidemics usually arise as a result of the introduction of *V. cholerae* to non-endemic areas where the majority of the population is not immune.[11] The morbidity and mortality observed with cholera can be profound. During an outbreak in West Africa in 1970, there were over 150,000 cases of cholera and in excess of 20,000 associated deaths in the first year alone.[12] Epidemics are often unpredictable, but in various countries there does seem to be a seasonal relationship. In Bangladesh, cholera becomes most prevalent in winter, whereas in South America cholera peaks during summer months. In tropical jungle regions it is the cool dry season that is most commonly associated with cholera epidemics.[5]

Outbreaks of cholera become endemic when a large proportion of the population is immune or semi-immune. With cholera, protective immunity is acquired as a result of previous pathogenic exposure – therefore the incidence of cholera is greatest in young children and decreases with age.

Since the turn of the nineteenth century, there have been seven recorded pandemics. In each of these, the disease originated from Asia and spread to other continents where a large number of countries were affected for many years.[4] In all but the most recent pandemic the disease arose from the Indian subcontinent, usually from the Ganges delta, and was probably caused by the Classical O1 strain. The latest pandemic, however, was caused by the El Tor biotype of the O1 strain and emerged from Indonesia in 1961 and has since spread across the globe, reaching West Africa in 1970 and South America in 1991. By the end of 1996, the pandemic had spread to

21 countries in Latin America resulting in over 1 million cases of cholera and more than 12,000 deaths.[6] This pandemic has proved to be the most extensive outbreak of cholera on record, both in terms of its geographical spread and its duration, and continues to be a problem in affected regions.[4]

A more recent outbreak of cholera, although not a pandemic as initially feared, emerged from India and Bangladesh in 1992. This outbreak was unusual in that although the clinical symptoms were typical of cholera, it was not caused by the O1 strains responsible for the previous seven pandemics but by the previously unrecognised and more virulent O139 strain.[4,6] The lack of cross-immunity between the O139 and O1 strains led to major epidemics in India, Bangladesh and across South-East Asia, totally displacing existing O1-associated cholera.[13,14] However, by 1994 O1 had replaced O139 as the leading cause of cholera leading many observers to conclude that this was a transient event. Such conclusions appeared premature as O139 reappeared in 1996.[15] The latest epidemiological data suggests that O139 currently accounts for 17% of laboratory-confirmed cholera cases in Asian countries where the disease is endemic.[16]

According to the WHO, 58 countries reported 184,311 cases of cholera in 2001, which resulted in 2,728 deaths (Figure 1).[16] African countries accounted for 94% of the global cholera cases (Table 1). This represents an increase of one-third over the previous year's total and highlights the sustained prevalence of the disease. However, the actual figures are likely to

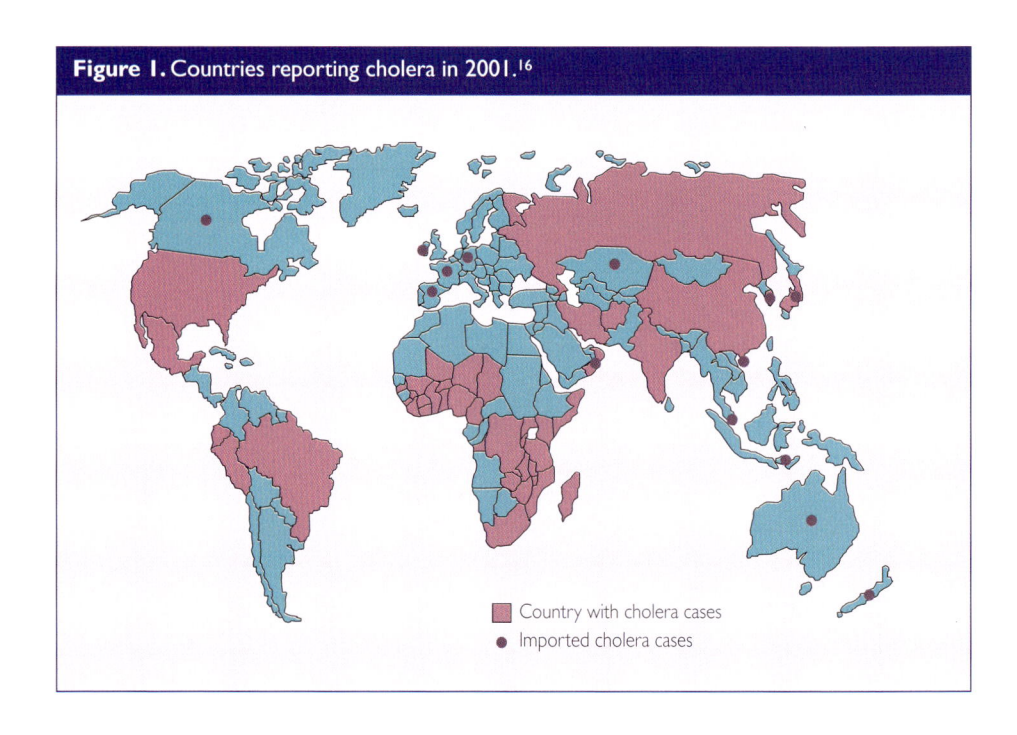

> According to the WHO, 58 countries reported 184,311 cases of cholera in 2001, which resulted in 2,728 deaths. The WHO estimates that reported cases represent just 5–10% of actual cases occurring worldwide.

Figure 1. Countries reporting cholera in 2001.[16]

- Country with cholera cases
- Imported cholera cases

Table 1. Global cases of cholera and associated deaths reported to WHO, 2001.[16]

Continent	Number of cases	No of deaths	Fatality rate (%)	Proportion of global cases (%)
Africa	173,359	2,590	1.5	94
Americas	535	0	0	0.3
Asia	10,340	138	1.3	5.6
Europe	58	0	0	0.03
Oceania	19	0	0	0.01
World total	184,311	2,728	1.5	100

be much higher due to under-reporting prompted by political and economic pressures together with limitations in the surveillance and reporting of cholera cases.[1,6,16] In 1991, for example, there were an estimated 235,000 cases of cholera during an outbreak in Bangladesh, yet none of these were officially reported.[17] As a result, the WHO estimates that reported cases represent just 5–10% of actual cases occurring worldwide.

Despite great efforts being made by many countries to manage and control the spread of the disease, cholera is on the rise again and the global burden of the disease does not appear to be relenting. Hygienic water supplies are essential for the control of cholera transmission and this explains why cholera is so prevalent in developing countries. Inadequate sanitation and healthcare can have disastrous effects as highlighted by an outbreak among Rwandan refugees in Zaire where in one refugee camp the fatality rate was 48%.[18,19] Global events such as war, political unrest, climatic change and natural catastrophes all lead to increased human migration which often results in large numbers of people being crowded in confined areas under poor sanitary conditions.[1] This forms the ideal environment for the rapid spread of cholera.

It is not just the indigenous population that is at risk of infection. Travellers to affected countries are also at risk. The risk for European and North American travellers has been estimated at 0.2 cases per 100,000.[6,20] The total number of cases in Europe, North America, Australia, New Zealand and Japan is stable at about 100 cases per year, the majority of which are imported from other countries.[6] However, there is reason to believe that these are underestimates. As the incubation period is very short, it is likely that many infected subjects suffer abroad and recover fully before returning home.[6] In addition, the disease may not be as severe in travellers as its severity is often related to a patient's general physical condition and their immune status. Consequently, infected travellers may not seek medical advice and therefore the infection is not reported.[6] Clearly, those travellers that visit developing countries and endemic regions are at greatest risk. Surveillance of US Embassy personnel during the cholera outbreak in Peru during 1991–93 showed that the incidence of cholera among these workers was 44 cases per 100,000 per month of exposure.[21] Likewise backpackers may be at greater risk, not just because they may journey to endemic regions, but because these regions may be remote and offer no medical services.

Whilst the human impact of cholera is substantial, so is the economic impact of the disease. In Peru, which witnessed a major cholera outbreak in the early 1990s, the losses, due to reduced productivity, failing food exports and decreased tourism, were estimated at US$495 million in 1 year alone, or almost 1% of the nation's gross domestic product.[22]

Pathophysiology

V. cholerae infection begins with the ingestion of contaminated food and/or water and, after passage through the acidic environment of the stomach, the bacterium colonises and adheres to the mucosal lining of the small intestine. The adherent vibrios then produce a potent enterotoxin, simply termed cholera toxin (CT), which disrupts ion transport in intestinal epithelial cells. The subsequent loss of water and electrolytes in turn leads to the severe diarrhoea that is characteristic of cholera.[4]

V. cholerae is extremely virulent. Clinical studies in human volunteers estimate that approximately 10^{11} vibrios are required to induce cholera.[23] However, when administered with a pH buffer to neutralise gastric acid in the stomach, the number required falls to 10^6. Further studies suggest that as few as 100–1000 vibrios are necessary to cause cholera, although such inocula are associated with a reduced severity of the disease.[24] Although gastric acidity clearly plays a role in determining susceptibility to infection, other mostly unidentified host factors are thought to be important.[4] One such factor is blood type, with individuals of blood group O demonstrating more severe disease than those of other blood types.[25–28]

All pathogenic *Vibrio* strains carry a set of virulence genes that are necessary for the development of the disease. These include genes which encode CT, a colonisation factor, toxin co-regulated pilus (TCP), and a regulatory protein, ToxR, which co-regulates the expression of both CT and TCP.[29] Therefore, cholera pathogenesis depends on the synergistic effect of a number of pathogenic gene products.

The critical role of CT in the pathogenesis of the disease is illustrated by the observation that ingestion of 25 µg of purified toxin caused severe diarrhoea (~20 litres) in human volunteers.[30] However, vibrios genetically modified so that they were unable to produce the toxin were also capable of inducing diarrhoea, although much milder in severity.[31] Therefore, although CT is responsible for the profuse diarrhoea witnessed in infected patients, additional factors appear to be involved.

So what is the mechanism of action of CT and how does it cause such profound symptoms? After ingestion of *V. cholerae*, the bacterium colonises the small intestine and releases CT which binds to ganglioside G_{M1} receptors on the epithelial cell surface.[32] CT consists of a single biologically active A subunit, comprised of two physically coupled polypeptide chains (A_1 and A_2), and five identical B subunits that serve to bind the toxin to the G_{M1} receptors on the cell surface.[4,32] Upon binding, the toxin's A subunit is transferred across the epithelial cell membrane, probably via endocytosis, and is proteolytically cleaved by the acidic environment of the endosome to liberate its constituent A_1 and A_2 peptides.[4] The intracellular target of the A_1 peptides is the enzyme adenylate cyclase, which mediates the transformation of ATP to cAMP, an important signalling molecule involved in a variety of cellular processes. Adenylate cyclase is regulated by GTP-binding regulatory proteins (G proteins), in particular the protein G_S, which serves to couple cell surface receptors to effector proteins in the cell membrane. G_S can switch between two states: active when GTP is bound, and inactive when GDP is bound. In its inactive state G_S exists as a trimeric complex of α, β, and γ subunits. However, activation of the protein by exchange of GDP for GTP causes the α-subunit to dissociate from the complex and bind to and activate membrane-bound adenylate cyclase. This activation persists until the intrinsic GTPase activity of the α-subunit converts it back to its inactive state. It is this last step that is targeted by CT since the A_1 peptide has the ability to inhibit the hydrolysis of GTP to GDP, maintaining the α-subunit permanently in its active state (Figure 2).[33–35] Sustained activation of adenylate cyclase results in a 100-fold increase in cAMP that in turn activates cAMP-dependent protein kinases that phosphorylate key cellular components.[32] This leads to increased chloride ion (Cl⁻) secretion from intestinal crypt cells, perhaps by direct phosphorylation of Cl⁻ channels, and decreased NaCl-coupled absorption by intestinal villi.[36] The resulting net movement of electrolytes into the gut lumen results in a transepithelial osmotic gradient which promotes the flow of water into the lumen. Under normal conditions this water would be reabsorbed by the distal small intestine and colon but fluid is produced on such a scale that this physiological mechanism is overwhelmed resulting in the severe diarrhoea that characterises cholera.[4,32]

The three-dimensional crystal structure of CT has recently been determined and appears to closely resemble that of the heat-labile enterotoxin (LT) produced by enterotoxigenic *Escherichia coli* (ETEC).[37,38]

Figure 2. Mode of action of cholera toxin (CT). After binding to the cell membrane via G_{M1} receptors on the cell surface, the A subunit of CT enters the cell where it is proteolytically cleaved to yield the active A_1 peptide which targets the α-subunit of the G_s protein that regulates the membrane bound adenylate cyclase (AC). The A_1 peptide maintains the α-subunit in its active state by preventing the hydrolysis of GTP to GDP. This results in a sustained activation of adenylate cyclase which leads to a 100-fold increase in the signalling molecule cAMP. cAMP-dependent phosphorylation of key cellular components leads to the disruption of ion transport and the loss of water from the cell.[4]

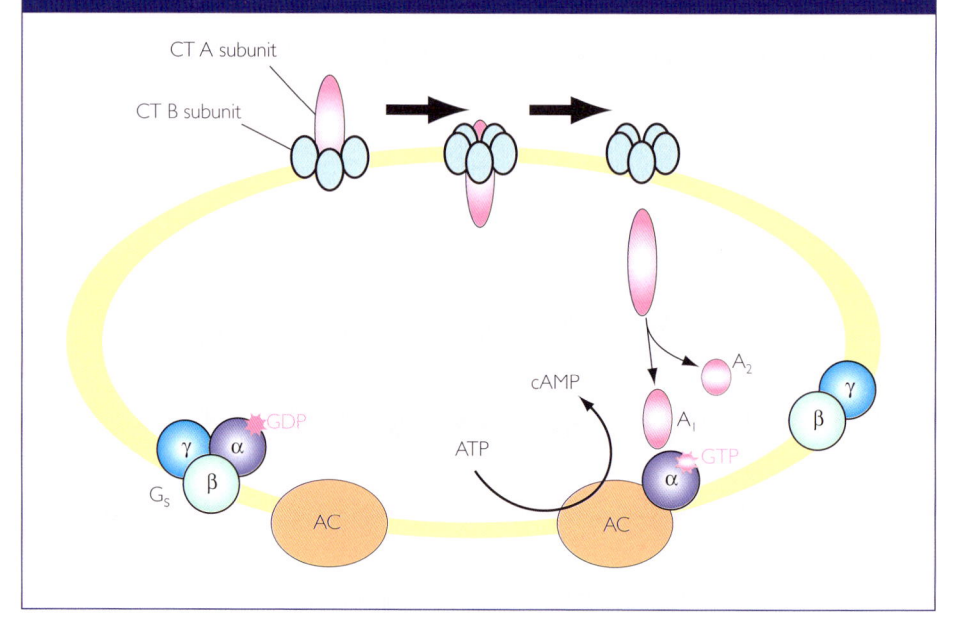

Analysis of the primary structure of these two toxins reveals that they share approximately 80% sequence homology.[37] In addition, the A_1 peptide has structural homology with the catalytic region of *Pseudomonas aeruginosa* exotoxin A and diphtheria toxin.[38] It is not surprising, therefore, that clinical studies have shown that oral cholera vaccine comprising purified CT also offers protection against ETEC infection.[39,40]

As stated previously, additional factors are thought to contribute to the pathogenesis of cholera. The observation that CT-deficient *V. cholerae* strains maintain the ability to cause mild-to-moderate diarrhoea has prompted a search for additional pathogenic agents. This has lead to the identification of a second toxin, termed Zot, which increases the permeability of the intestinal mucosa by affecting the structure of intercellular tight junctions.[41] It is hypothesised that this may lead to a loss of water and electrolytes into the gut lumen and contribute to the diarrhoeal effects associated with cholera.[41] However, the precise role of Zot and other putative pathogenic factors remains to be determined.

Diagnosis and treatment

Most people infected with *V. cholerae* present with mild diarrhoea or may even be asymptomatic.[6] However, the disease can progress at an alarming rate and is one of the most rapidly fatal infections known.[6] The incubation period of cholera can range from a matter of hours to five days, dependent on the inoculum size.[5,24] As discussed above, as few as 100–1000 vibrios may cause mild disease but around 1 million are required to reliably induce classical cholera.[23,24]

In severe cases, patients experience profuse watery diarrhoea, perhaps up to 1 litre per hour, resulting in a loss of body weight of more than 10% within the first 24 hours.[6] Such drastic fluid loss can lead to tachycardia, hypotension and vascular collapse.[4,5,42] Initially, stools are brown with faecal matter but they soon turn colourless and flecked with mucus, the so-called rice water appearance. Peripheral pulses may be absent and it may not be possible to measure blood pressure. In addition the patient may become lethargic with sunken eyes and poor skin turgor. Painful muscle cramps are not uncommon. Left untreated, cholera has a 50% fatality rate, but suitable treatment can reduce this to 1% or less.[6]

However, only a minority of people infected with *V. cholerae* go on to develop the severe form of the disease. It has been estimated that 11% of patients infected with the Classical O1 strain develop severe cholera, compared with 2% with the El Tor strain.[43] An additional 15% and 5% of infections respectively result in moderate illness (i.e. not requiring hospitalisation).

The key to the successful treatment of patients with cholera is rapid rehydration. The WHO has published guidelines on the assessment and treatment of infected patients (Table 2).[44] Immediate intravenous administration of Ringer's lactate or normal saline together with an oral rehydration solution (ORS) is recommended for those patients with severe dehydration. For those patients with mild or moderate dehydration ORS alone is considered sufficient. Antibiotics have been shown to shorten the duration of cholera-associated diarrhoea, with tetracycline or doxycycline being the reported drugs of choice.[4,45,46] In addition, by killing the bacterium, antibiotic therapy may help prevent the spread of the disease.[6] However, the WHO does not advocate antibiotic therapy for mass prophylaxis and only recommends such treatment for severe cases of cholera.[1]

Table 2. Rehydration therapy for patients with cholera as recommended by the WHO. ORS, oral rehydration solution.[44]

Assessment	No dehydration	Mildly dehydrated	Severe dehydration
General condition	Well, alert	Restless, irritable	Lethargic or unconscious
Eyes	Normal	Sunken	Very sunken and dry
Tears	Present	Absent	Absent
Mouth and tongue	Moist	Dry	Very dry
Thirst	Drinks normally, not thirsty	Thirsty, drinks eagerly	Drinks poorly or not able to drink
Skin pinch	Goes back quickly	Goes back slowly	Goes back very slowly
Recommended treatment	ORS to be given at home	Give ORS, monitor over 4 hours and reassess	Give i.v. fluid immediately plus ORS when able. Reassess after 3 hours.

Disease prevention

Organisations such as the WHO advise that the risk from cholera can be minimised by taking simple precautions to avoid potentially contaminated food or drink when in susceptible regions of the world.[47] However, no matter how careful one is, it is impossible to guarantee absolute protection. For example, carefully prepared food may become unwittingly contaminated by flies. Therefore, prophylactic measures may be necessary.[6,48]

The use of antibiotics prophylactically is debatable, especially since antibiotic resistance is high in those regions where cholera is most prevalent.[49–51] Therefore, the standard approach has been to vaccinate those individuals at risk of infection.[6] Parenteral, whole-cell cholera vaccines have been used since the late nineteenth century, but with limited success. This is partly due to the fact that *V. cholerae* remains in the gut lumen and does not invade intestinal tissue. As a result it is not serum antibodies but gastrointestinal antibodies, particularly the secretory IgA antibodies produced locally by the intestinal mucosa, that are the major contributors to immunoprotection.[2,52] Parenteral vaccines do not effectively stimulate an intestinal immune response and consequently offer limited immunoprotection that is of short duration.[2,4,53,54] As a result, these vaccines are no longer recommended by the WHO.[1]

However, oral cholera vaccines have proven to offer better and more prolonged protection by virtue of their ability to stimulate an intestinal immune response. Currently two types of oral vaccine are marketed internationally: (1) a live attenuated vaccine containing a genetically modified classical *V. cholerae* strain (CVD 103-HgR) and (2) a vaccine comprising inactivated whole-cell *V. cholerae* strains (Classical and El Tor) plus purified recombinant cholera toxin B subunit (Dukoral™). However, only the latter vaccine is currently licensed in the UK. In addition, the WHO have concluded that Dukoral is the only vaccine to have demonstrated convincing protection in field conditions and remains the only vaccine to be recommended by them.[6]

Key points

- Cholera remains a major cause of disease around the world accounting for an estimated 120,000 deaths per year.
- The disease is caused by the bacterium *Vibrio cholerae* that causes severe diarrhoea in infected individuals and can lead to tachycardia, hypotension and vascular collapse.
- Cholera is one of the most rapidly fatal infectious diseases.
- *Vibrio cholerae* of the O1 and O139 serogroups have been solely responsible for all recorded cholera outbreaks.
- The disease is mediated by a potent toxin produced by the bacterium which disrupts ion transport in intestinal epithelial cells. The subsequent loss of water and electrolytes leads to the severe diarrhoea that is characteristic of the disease.
- The mechanism of action of cholera toxin involves the sustained activation of adenylate cyclase resulting in a 100-fold increase in cytosolic cAMP levels.
- Cholera infection results from the ingestion of contaminated water and/or food and therefore can be avoided by following strict hygiene and sanitary guidelines.
- Oral inactivated whole-cell/cholera toxin B subunit vaccine (Dukoral) offers an effective prophylactic intervention and is currently the only vaccine recommended by the WHO.

References

1 WHO. Cholera vaccines. WHO position paper. *Wkly Epidemiol Rec* 2001; **76**: 117–24.
2 Holmgren J, Svennerholm AM. Cholera and the immune response. *Prog Allergy* 1983; **33**: 106–19.
3 Pollitzer R. *Cholera*. Geneva: World Health Organization, 1959.
4 Kaper JB, Morris JG, Jr., Levine MM. Cholera. *Clin Microbiol Rev* 1995; **8**: 48–86.
5 Sanchez JL, Taylor DN. Cholera. *Lancet* 1997; **349**: 1825–30.
6 Steffen R, Acar J, Walker E, Zuckerman J. Cholera: assessing the risk to travellers and identifying protection. *Trav Med Infect Dis* 2003; **1**: 80–88.
7 Hall RH, Khambaty FM, Kothary M, Keasler SP. Non-O1 Vibrio cholerae. *Lancet* 1993; **342**: 430.
8 Morris JG. *Vibrio cholerae* O139 Bengal. In: Wachsmuth IK, Blake PA, Olsvik O, eds. Vibrio cholerae *and cholera: molecular to global perspectives*. Washington D.C.: American Society for Microbiology, 1994:95–115.
9 Kolvin JL, Roberts D. Studies on the growth of *Vibrio cholerae* biotype El Tor and biotype classical in foods. *J Hyg (Lond)* 1982; **89**: 243–52.
10 Colwell RR, Huq A. Vibrios in the environment: viable but nonculturable *Vibrio cholerae*. In: Wachsmuth IK, Blake PA, Olsvik O, eds. Vibrio cholerae *and cholera: molecular to global perspectives*. Washington D.C.: American Society for Microbiology, 1994:117–33.
11 Shears P. Cholera. *Ann Trop Med Parasitol* 1994; **88**: 109–22.
12 Goodgame RW, Greenough WB. Cholera in Africa: a message for the West. *Ann Intern Med* 1975; **82**: 101–6.
13 Sack RB, Albert MJ, Siddique AK. Emergence of *Vibrio cholerae* O139. *Curr Clin Top Infect Dis* 1996; **16**: 172–93.
14 Nair GB, Ramamurthy T, Bhattacharya SK et al. Spread of *Vibrio cholerae* O139 Bengal in India. *J Infect Dis* 1994; **169**: 1029–34.
15 Sinha S, Chakraborty R, De K et al. Escalating association of *Vibrio cholerae* O139 with cholera outbreaks in India. *J Clin Microbiol* 2002; **40**: 2635–7.
16 WHO. Cholera, 2001. *Wkly Epidemiol Rec* 2002; **77**: 257–68.
17 WHO. Cholera in 1991. *Wkly Epidemiol Rec* 1992; **67**: 253–60.
18 Siddique AK, Salam A, Islam MS et al. Why treatment centres failed to prevent cholera deaths among Rwandan refugees in Goma, Zaire. *Lancet* 1995; **345**: 359–61.
19 Public health impact of Rwandan refugee crisis: what happened in Goma, Zaire, in July, 1994? Goma Epidemiology Group. *Lancet* 1995; **345**: 339–44.
20 Wittlinger F, Steffen R, Watanabe H, Handszuh H. Risk of cholera among western and Japanese travelers. *J Travel Med* 1995; **2**: 154–58.
21 Taylor DN, Rizzo J, Meza R, Perez J, Watts D. Cholera among Americans living in Peru. *Clin Infect Dis* 1996; **22**: 1108–9.
22 The economic impact of the cholera epidemic, Peru, 1991. *Epidemiol Bull* 1992; **13**: 9–11.
23 Cash RA, Music SI, Libonati JP et al. Response of man to infection with *Vibrio cholerae*. I. Clinical, serologic, and bacteriologic responses to a known inoculum. *J Infect Dis* 1974; **129**: 45–52.
24 Levine MM, Black RE, Clements ML et al. Volunteer studies in development of vaccines against cholera and enterotoxigenic *Escherichia coli*: a review. In: Holme T, Holmgren J, Merson MH, Mollby R, eds. *Acute enteric infections in children. New prospects for treatment and prevention*. Amsterdam: Elsevier/North-Holland Biomedical Press, 1981:443–59.
25 Glass RI, Holmgren J, Haley CE et al. Predisposition for cholera of individuals with O blood group. Possible evolutionary significance. *Am J Epidemiol* 1985; **121**: 791–6.
26 Levine MM, Nalin DR, Rennels MB et al. Genetic susceptibility to cholera. *Ann Hum Biol* 1979; **6**: 369–74.
27 Tacket CO, Losonsky G, Nataro JP et al. Extension of the volunteer challenge model to study South American cholera in a population of volunteers predominantly with blood group antigen O. *Trans R Soc Trop Med Hyg* 1995; **89**: 75–7.
28 Clemens JD, Sack DA, Harris JR et al. ABO blood groups and cholera: new observations on specificity of risk and modification of vaccine efficacy. *J Infect Dis* 1989; **159**: 770–3.
29 Faruque SM, Albert MJ, Mekalanos JJ. Epidemiology, genetics, and ecology of toxigenic *Vibrio cholerae*. *Microbiol Mol Biol Rev* 1998; **62**: 1301–14.
30 Levine MM, Kaper JB, Black RE, Clements ML. New knowledge on pathogenesis of bacterial enteric infections as applied to vaccine development. *Microbiol Rev* 1983; **47**: 510–50.
31 Levine MM, Kaper JB, Herrington D et al. Volunteer studies of deletion mutants of *Vibrio cholerae* O1 prepared by recombinant techniques. *Infect Immunol* 1988; **56**: 161–7.
32 Raufman JP. Cholera. *Am J Med* 1998; **104**: 386–94.
33 Cassel D, Selinger Z. Mechanism of adenylate cyclase activation by cholera toxin: inhibition of GTP hydrolysis at the regulatory site. *Proc Natl Acad Sci USA* 1977; **74**: 3307–11.
34 Cassel D, Pfeuffer T. Mechanism of cholera toxin action: covalent modification of the guanyl nucleotide-binding protein of the adenylate cyclase system. *Proc Natl Acad Sci USA* 1978; **75**: 2669–73.
35 Moss J, Vaughan M. Activation of adenylate cyclase by choleragen. *Annu Rev Biochem* 1979; **48**: 581–600.
36 Field M. Secretion of electrolytes and water by mammalian small intestine. In: Johnson LR, ed. *Physiology of the gastrointestinal tract*. New York: Raven Press, 1981:963–82.
37 Zhang RG, Scott DL, Westbrook ML et al. The three-dimensional crystal structure of cholera toxin. *J Mol Biol* 1995; **251**: 563–73.
38 Sixma TK, Pronk SE, Kalk KH et al. Crystal structure of a cholera toxin-related heat-labile enterotoxin from *E. coli*. *Nature* 1991; **351**: 371–7.
39 Clemens JD, Sack DA, Harris JR et al. Cross-protection by B subunit-whole cell cholera vaccine against diarrhea associated with heat-labile toxin-producing enterotoxigenic *Escherichia coli*: results of a large-scale field trial. *J Infect Dis* 1988; **158**: 372–7.
40 Peltola H, Siitonen A, Kyronseppa H et al. Prevention of travellers' diarrhoea by oral B-subunit/whole-cell cholera vaccine. *Lancet* 1991; **338**: 1285–9.

41 Fasano A, Baudry B, Pumplin DW *et al*. *Vibrio cholerae* produces a second enterotoxin, which affects intestinal tight junctions. *Proc Natl Acad Sci USA* 1991; **88**: 5242–6.

42 Morris JG, Jr., Black RE. Cholera and other vibrioses in the United States. *N Engl J Med* 1985; **312**: 343–50.

43 Gangarosa EJ, Mosley WH. Epidemiology and surveillance of cholera. In: Barua D, Burrows W, eds. *Cholera*. Philadelphia: Saunders, 1974:381–403.

44 WHO. Management of the patient with cholera. WHO/CDD/SER/91.15 REV.1. www.who.int/emc, 1991.

45 Swerdlow DL, Ries AA. Cholera in the Americas. Guidelines for the clinician. *JAMA* 1992; **267**: 1495–9.

46 Seas C, DuPont HL, Valdez LM, Gotuzzo E. Practical guidelines for the treatment of cholera. *Drugs* 1996; **51**: 966–73.

47 WHO. *International Travel and Health*. WHO, 2003.

48 Fotedar R. Vector potential of houseflies (*Musca domestica*) in the transmission of *Vibrio cholerae* in India. *Acta Trop* 2001; **78**: 31–4.

49 Albert MJ, Siddique AK, Islam MS *et al*. Large outbreak of clinical cholera due to *Vibrio cholerae* non-O1 in Bangladesh. *Lancet* 1993; **341**: 704.

50 Finch MJ, Morris JG, Jr., Kaviti J, Kagwanja W, Levine MM. Epidemiology of antimicrobial resistant cholera in Kenya and East Africa. *Am J Trop Med Hyg* 1988; **39**: 484–90.

51 Ramamurthy T, Pal A, Bhattacharya MK *et al*. Serovar, biotype, phage type, toxigenicity & antibiotic susceptibility patterns of *Vibrio cholerae* isolated during two consecutive cholera seasons (1989–90) in Calcutta. *Indian J Med Res* 1992; **95**: 125–9.

52 Quiding M, Nordstrom I, Kilander A *et al*. Intestinal immune responses in humans. Oral cholera vaccination induces strong intestinal antibody responses and interferon-gamma production and evokes local immunological memory. *J Clin Invest* 1991; **88**: 143–8.

53 Bhadra RK, Dasgupta U, Das J. Cholera vaccine: developmental strategies and problems. *Indian J Biochem Biophys* 1994; **31**: 441–8.

54 Kaper JB. *Vibrio cholerae* vaccines. *Rev Infect Dis* 1989; **11 (Suppl 3)**: S568–73.

Acknowledgements

Figure 1 is adapted from the World Health Organization, 2002.[16]

9. Chronic pain

Dr Eleanor Bull
CSF Medical Communications Ltd

Summary

Chronic, or persistent, pain affects millions of people worldwide and represents the most common symptom for which patients seek medical help. Whilst acute pain serves a protective function, when pain is chronic it becomes a disease process in itself and may lead to a decline in functional status and diminished quality of life. A psychological as well as a physical impairment, chronic pain not only affects individual patients but also disrupts the lives of their families. Understanding and effectively managing chronic pain is a priority in primary care and medical research into the condition is ongoing. However, the subjective nature of chronic pain can make diagnosis and the selection of an appropriate treatment approach difficult. Despite stigmatisation, the opioids, specifically morphine, remain at the forefront of chronic pain management, although constipation, respiratory depression and the development of tolerance may limit their use. The development of transdermal routes of administration may reduce side-effects and resolve some compliance issues for this highly costly and debilitating condition.

Introduction

Pain is defined as an unpleasant sensory and emotional experience associated with actual or potential tissue damage.[1] Many aspects of pain continue to elude both scientists and physicians, and the understanding and effective management of pain represents a significant challenge in primary care, not least because of the subjective nature of the condition. In recognition of the scale of the problem, in 2000, the US government launched the Decade of Pain Control and Research.

Whilst acute pain has an important protective physiological function, when pain manifests chronically, it becomes a disease in its own right and can have a devastating effect on the lives of patients and their families.[2]

Chronic pain is defined by the International Association for the Study of Pain (IASP) as "pain that persists beyond normal tissue healing time, which is assumed to be 3 months". The aetiology of chronic pain is multifactorial

> Chronic pain is defined as pain that persists beyond normal tissue healing time, which is assumed to be 3 months.

and may be as a result of underlying disease (e.g. cancer, osteoarthritis, multiple sclerosis), nerve damage or physical injury. If left untreated, chronic pain can lead to helplessness, depression, isolation and family breakdown.[2]

Chronic pain is a major public health problem in terms of patient suffering and lost productivity and is one of the most common reasons why people seek medical attention. Patients presenting with pain are estimated to access health services up to five-times more frequently than the general population.[3] Although the effective management of chronic pain has become an increasingly critical healthcare issue, expertise in treating chronic pain is scarce and specialist pain services struggle to meet demand.[2] Guidelines issued by the Royal College of Anaesthetists and the Pain Society in 2003, addressed the shortcomings in existing pain management strategies and aimed to improve the quality of care available to patients.[1]

Epidemiology

Our understanding of the epidemiology of chronic pain remains limited, in part due to a lack of good, community-based epidemiology studies conducted with large sample sizes and clear case definitions.[3] What is clear, however, is that chronic pain is widespread throughout the general population. A review of 15 epidemiological studies performed in developed countries found that the prevalence of chronic pain within the adult population ranged between 2 and 40%, with a median value of 15%.[4] However, the incidence of pain varies widely across different geographical regions and ethnic groups.[5,6] Moreover, there is evidence to indicate gender differences in presentation of pain, with women reporting more severe, more frequent and longer-lasting pain than men.[7] The age of the population can also dictate the type of pain experienced. For example, in the elderly, pain in the joints, the back, legs and feet is most common, with visceral pain and headache reported less frequently.[8]

The extrapolation of currently published data suggests that between 2 and 6 million people in the UK would describe themselves as having persistent, severe pain that is not associated with cancer.[9] Approximately 7% of the UK population suffers chronic pain at any one time and up to one-quarter of the population experiences bouts of musculoskeletal pain.[2] Back pain tends to be the most common presentation of chronic pain. For example, in 1993, over 16 million people in the UK experienced low-back pain, of whom, 1.6 million attended hospital and 24,000 underwent corrective surgery.[10]

Since pain is a hugely subjective phenomenon, patient questionnaires represent one of the most effective methods of estimating its prevalence. In a self-evaluation study conducted in the Grampian region of Scotland, 3605 individuals enrolled in 29 general practices were surveyed by a postal self-completion questionnaire.[3] Of these, 50.4% reported chronic pain, equivalent to 46.5% of the general population after standardisation of the sample to the age and sex distribution of the total population. Back pain and arthritis accounted for one-third of all complaints and age, sex, housing tenure and employment status were all identified as important predictors of pain. In a similar study of 4611 subjects, 14.1% reported significant chronic pain whilst 6.3% reported severe chronic pain.[11] A 4-year follow-up study of 2184 of these subjects found that 79% of those patients reporting chronic pain at baseline were still suffering after 4 years, testament to the low recovery rate associated with the condition.[12]

Pathophysiology

Nociception – the perception of noxious stimuli – involves a complex interaction of peripheral and central nervous system structures, extending from the skin, the viscera and the musculoskeletal tissues, to the cerebral cortex. Under normal conditions, the acute response to pain fulfils an important protective function. By signalling whether a stimulus is noxious, or harmful, acute pain conditions the individual to avoid potentially dangerous situations or stimulates protective recuperative behaviour.[13]

Chronic pain fulfils no physiological purpose, arises spontaneously and impinges profoundly on health and general well-being.[13] The differentiation between acute, subchronic and chronic pain is illustrated in Table 1.[13] The pathophysiology of chronic pain shows alterations of normal physiological pain pathways, giving rise to hyperalgesia or allodynia.[14] Hyperalgesia, an increase in the sensitivity to pain elicited by a noxious stimulus, may reflect the sensitisation of peripheral nociceptive nerve terminals and the central facilitation of synaptic transmission. Allodynia refers to pain evoked by a normally innocuous stimulus.

Nociception

Both visceral and somatic pain are associated with electrical activity in the small diameter primary afferent fibres of the peripheral nerves whose nerve endings innervate the skin and viscera, and which may be activated by mechanical, thermal or chemical stimuli of noxious intensity.[15] These fibres can be myelinated (A fibres) or non-myelinated (C fibres) and, as a result, have rapid and slow conduction velocities, respectively. In general, A fibres transmit sharp localised pain and C fibres transmit dull, burning pain sensations. These nociceptive afferent neurones have their cell bodies

> Pain is associated with electrical activity in the small diameter primary afferent fibres of the peripheral nerves that may be activated by mechanical, thermal or chemical stimuli.

Table 1. Pathophysiological classification of some major features of pain.[13]

Type	Duration	Temporal features	Major characteristics	Adaptive value	Adaptive response	Examples
Acute	Seconds	Instantaneous	Proportional to cause	High Preventative	Withdrawal Escape	Contact with hot surface
Subchronic	Hours to days	Resolves upon recovery	Primary and secondary Hyperalgesia Allodynia Spontaneous	Protective Recovery	Quiescence Avoidance of contact with injured tissue	Inflamed wound
Chronic	Months to years	Persistent Long-term disease Exceeds resolution of tissue damage	Primary and secondary Hyperalgesia Allodynia Spontaneous Affective component	None Maladaptive	Psychological and cognitive	Arthritis CNS injury Cancer

CNS, central nervous system.

located in the dorsal root ganglia and terminate in the grey matter of the dorsal horn of the spinal cord.

Neuropathic pain

Neuropathic pain is defined by the IASP as "initiated or caused by a primary lesion or dysfunction in the nervous system". Such nerve damage may be caused by infection, trauma, metabolic abnormalities, chemotherapy, surgery, radiation, neurotoxins or nerve compression.[16] Neuropathic pain may have a peripheral or central origin and may arise spontaneously or be evoked by a particular stimulus. Typically, neuropathic pain is burning or shooting and can be either intermittent or continuous.[15,17] The mechanism behind it is poorly understood, but spontaneous activity in damaged sensory neurones may be implicated. Post-herpetic neuralgia and painful diabetic neuropathy are amongst the most common types of neuropathic pain.[16]

> Neuropathic pain is "initiated or caused by a primary lesion or dysfunction in the nervous system".

Transmitters involved in the pain response

The two most important systems mediating nociception are the N-methyl-D-aspartate (NMDA) and opioid receptor systems. Other transmitters that feature strongly in pain transmission include nitric oxide, the tachykinins – substance P and neurokinin A – serotonin and noradrenaline.[13,18,19]

Glutamate

Glutamate is an excitatory amino acid neurotransmitter and the endogenous activator of NMDA receptors. Glutamate and glutamate receptors are located in the areas of the brain, spinal cord and periphery that are involved in pain sensation and transmission.[20] The activation of glutamate receptors in some brain areas (e.g. thalamus, trigeminal nucleus) seems to be pronociceptive, or pain-inducing, whereas the activation of glutamate receptors in other brain areas (e.g. periaqueductal grey, ventrolateral medulla) seems to be antinociceptive, or analgesic.[20] The opioid system interacts with the glutamate system by either inhibiting or potentiating NMDA receptor-mediated events.[14]

Opioid peptides

Of the opioid peptides, met-enkephalin and β-endorphin in particular, play an important role in the modulation of pain transmission. Opioids, whether endogenous or exogenous (e.g. morphine-like analgesics), act on one of three subtypes of opioid receptors, μ, δ and κ. Opioid receptors are located at specific locations within the brain, including the periaqueductal grey (μ receptor), the rostral ventral medulla (μ/δ receptors), the substantia nigra (μ receptor) and within the spinal dorsal horn (μ/δ/κ receptors). The opioid receptors are coupled to G-proteins and the cellular actions of the opioids are mainly inhibitory.[21] The discovery of endogenous opioid receptors and ligands provided a compelling scientific rationale for their therapeutic application. Gene knockout studies in animals have demonstrated considerable variability in opioid receptor affinity, demonstrating a genetic basis for the variability in the response to opioid analgesics observed in patients, a phenomenon known as 'opioid sensitivity'.[22,23]

Risk factors for chronic pain

A wide range of disease conditions may predispose an individual to chronic pain. Of those cases of chronic pain presenting to the GP, around 20% are due to malignancy, whilst non-malignant pain is most commonly linked to the limbs, joints and back.[24] The most prominent causes of chronic pain include:
- cancer
- diabetic neuropathy
- post-herpetic neuralgia
- low-back pain
- fibromyalgia

- arthritis (rheumatoid and osteoarthritis)
- nerve damage
- advanced progressive disease (e.g. multiple sclerosis, HIV infection or AIDS)
- chronic headache
- inherited conditions (e.g. sickle cell disease, haemophilia).

Diagnosis

The diagnosis and classification of pain can be extremely difficult for the physician. In most chronic pain conditions, no organic cause can be discerned and diagnosis must be made solely from the subjective symptoms reported by the patient. There are few objective signs which the doctor can use to judge the severity of reported pain.[25] Doctors should be sympathetic to the patient and attempt to elucidate the most probable cause of the pain in order to determine the most appropriate management strategy.

The most important method of pain assessment is to listen to the patient. By getting patients to describe their pain in terms of its precise nature, the circumstances under which it occurs and how it makes them feel, the physician will develop a clearer understanding of the situation.[10] Table 2 details a comprehensive approach to interviewing a patient.[25]

When dealing with chronic pain in particular, patients should be encouraged to use diaries to record the nature and frequency of their pain over extended periods of time. This may limit the errors and bias associated with recall-based self-reports and result in a richer dataset.[26] In their diaries, patients should specify the intensity of the pain (none, mild, moderate or severe) and the effectiveness of their pain relief (none, slight, moderate, good or complete).[25] The use of paper diaries may be confounded by the poor quality of data collected and non-compliance of patients. As such, electronic systems, if available, are preferable.[26]

Pain scales represent a reliable means of evaluating pain. The most commonly used is the visual analogue scale (VAS), a scale segmented into portions and anchored at each end by verbal descriptors (e.g. 'no pain' and 'worst imaginable pain').[26] However, this approach does not eliminate bias as the categories are open to interpretation by the individual patient.[26]

Pain management

In response to the shortcomings in pain management resources at the time, in 2003 the Royal College of Anaesthetists, in collaboration with the Pain Society, published a number of recommendations pertaining to the management of chronic pain. These included:

Table 2. The diagnosis of pain – pain history.[25]

Site of pain	Where do you feel the pain?
	Does it go anywhere else?
	Is it numb where you feel the pain?
Character of pain	What sort of pain is it?
	(e.g. burning/shooting/stabbing/dull)
History of pain	How long have you had this pain?
	How did it start?
	Did it come out of the blue or was it triggered by something?
Relieving factors	Does anything make it better?
	(e.g. position/drugs/distraction/alcohol)
Accentuating factors	Does anything make it worse?
	(e.g. position/exercise/weather)
Pattern	Is there any pattern to the pain?
	Is it worse at any particular time of day?
Sleep disturbances	Do you get off to sleep with no trouble?
	Does the pain keep you awake?
	Does the pain wake you up?
Activities	What does the pain stop you doing which you would otherwise do?
Previous treatments	What methods have been tried already?
	Did they help the pain?

- the provision of core services for chronic pain management in all district general hospitals and most specialist hospitals
- the provision of specialised services for pain management on a regional basis
- the provision of a fixed number of patient consultations with specialists in pain management, adequate support staff, accommodation, facilities and equipment
- close liaison between pain management services and other healthcare groups in order to provide an individualised, interdisciplinary approach
- special arrangements for vulnerable groups (elderly, children, non-verbal, physically and mentally disabled).[1]

A chronic pain relief strategy should aim to:
- alleviate pain
- alleviate psychological and behavioural dysfunction and distress
- reduce disability and restore function
- rationalise use of medication
- reduce utilisation of healthcare services
- attend to social, family and occupational issues
- educate nursing, medical staff and other healthcare professionals.[1]

Pharmacological interventions

The vast majority of patients suffering from chronic pain are managed with medication, although drug treatment tends to be more effective if used as part of an overall management strategy.[17]

The World Health Organization's (WHO) pain treatment ladder is widely regarded as the 'gold standard' for pain management (Figure 1).[27,28] This ladder advocates the step-wise addition of increasingly potent drugs to an individual's treatment regimen until the patient is free of pain. In general, pain relief is given 'by the clock' at recognised treatment times, rather than 'on demand', although this may vary for individual patients. In those circumstances in which the patient is administering pain relief on an 'as needed' basis, the speed of onset of relief is crucial. The duration of effect may be prolonged by the use of sustained-release oral formulations and subcutaneous or intravenous infusions.

Opioid analgesics

Opioids act as agonists at endogenous opioid receptors (found throughout the central and peripheral nervous systems) and elicit the characteristic actions of endogenous morphine-like ligands (e.g. β-endorphin, met-enkephalin).[9] Despite stigmatisation as drugs of abuse, opioids (e.g. morphine, buprenorphine, dextropropoxyphene, fentanyl) remain at the forefront of chronic pain management, with morphine representing the benchmark against which other opioids are compared. International confidence has seen the development of opioid pain management guidelines from many countries and national organisations (Table 3).[29–35] More than 20 different opioids are available in the UK and most are delivered orally, although transdermal preparations are available (e.g. fentanyl).[9] Opioids are not suitable for all patients and may not be effective against all types of

> Opioids remain at the forefront of chronic pain management, with morphine representing the benchmark against which other opioids are compared.

Figure 1. The World Health Organization's analgesic ladder.[27,28]

Step 1
Non-opioid
+/– adjuvant

Step 2
'Mild opioid' for mild–moderate pain
+/– non-opioid
+/– adjuvant

Step 3
'Strong opioid' for severe pain
+/– non-opioid
+/– adjuvant

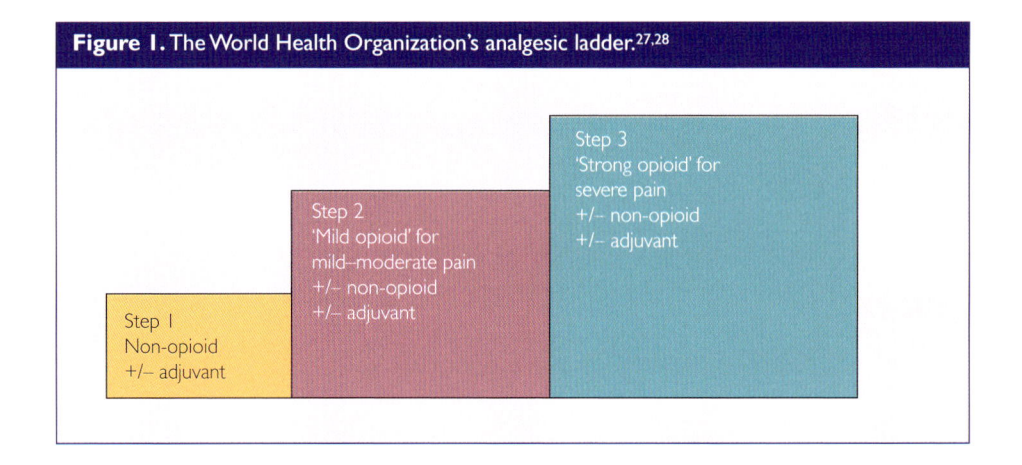

Table 3. Opioid pain management guidelines from different countries.[29–35]

Country	Reference
America	Tennant and Uelmen, 1983.[29]
	Portenoy, 1996.[30]
Australia	Graziotti and Goucke, 1997.[31]
Canada	Hagen et al., 1995.[32]
France (Limoges recommendations)	Perrot et al., 1999.[33]
Europe (Amsterdam)	Kalso et al., 2003.[34]
New Zealand	Merry et al., 1992.[35]

chronic pain. Since the clinical response to opioids can be variable, switching patients between different opioids, or 'opioid rotation', may represent a viable treatment approach.[9]

The opioids are associated with a number of side-effects, including nausea, vomiting, itching and somnolence, most of which occur within the first few days and decrease over time.[9] Constipation is particularly common and tends to persist for the duration of treatment, although the incidence may be reduced by transdermal delivery.[9] Potentially, more serious problems include respiratory depression, hormonal effects and hypotension, although these can be minimised through the implementation of an appropriate dosage regimen, reached through careful and gradual dose-titration.[9,36,37] Tolerance, where a given dose produces a diminished effect, can be associated with long-term opioid treatment and may necessitate dose-escalation in order to maintain adequate pain relief.[38]

Non-steroidal anti-inflammatory drugs (NSAIDs)

As anti-inflammatory compounds, the NSAIDs (e.g. aspirin, ibuprofen) are most commonly used to relieve those types of pain associated with chronic inflammation, including rheumatoid and osteoarthritis. The NSAIDs exert their analgesic effects by inhibiting cyclo-oxygenase-1 and -2 (COX-1 and -2), the enzymes that produce the prostanoid mediators of the inflammatory response. However, use of these agents may be restricted by the peptic ulceration and gastrointestinal bleeding associated with the non-selective inhibition of the COX-1 isoenzyme. The development of the COX-2-selective compounds (e.g. celecoxib, etoricoxib, rofecoxib, valdecoxib) collectively known as the coxibs, has limited the extent of gastrotoxicity associated with non-selective COX-1 inhibition, without compromising anti-inflammatory potency. These agents, therefore, may improve the risk–benefit ratio of NSAID therapy.[39] However, the coxibs do not provide protection against ischaemic cardiovascular events and are not recommended in those patients at high risk of cardiovascular disease.[37] The National Institute for Clinical Excellence (NICE) recommended in 2001 that coxibs should not be used routinely in the management of patients with rheumatoid or osteoarthritis.[37]

Corticosteroids

The corticosteroids (e.g. dexamethasone) may be particularly effective in relieving the pressure associated with compression neuropathy, thereby reducing pain.[37] The same principle applies to the relief of nerve compression pain and headaches associated with intracranial pressure. The side-effects associated with long-term use of steroidal compounds can be serious and include gastrointestinal perforation, osteoporosis, skin thinning, insomnia and diabetes.

Antidepressants

Although an unlicensed indication, the tricyclic antidepressants (e.g. amitriptyline) are frequently used to relieve neuropathic pain, by enhancing the descending inhibitory pathways leading from the brain to the spinal cord.[37,40] Pain relief is achieved at half the dosage used to treat depression and it may take several weeks of therapy before an antinociceptive effect is observed. Side-effects may include sedation, dry mouth, postural hypotension, seizures, arrhythmias, glaucoma, urine retention and constipation.

Anticonvulsants

The anticonvulsant drugs (e.g. carbamazepine, gabapentin, lamotrigine) may be used to relieve the pain associated with trigeminal neuralgia and diabetic neuropathy. Although the mechanism of action of these drugs in this regard is not well understood, it is thought to involve ion channels at the level of the spinal cord. If taken during the acute stages of trigeminal neuralgia, these compounds may reduce the frequency and severity of attacks.[37] Side-effects include drowsiness, confusion, dizziness, tremor, ataxia and hepatic dysfunction.

Cannabinoids

Much of the recent debate regarding the decriminalisation of cannabis has centred on the analgesic potential of its active constituent, Δ^9-

tetrahydrocannabinol (Δ^9-THC), which acts on cannabinoid receptors in the central and peripheral nervous system.[41] It has been postulated that cannabinoids may provide effective pain relief in those patients with diseases such as multiple sclerosis and resistant neuropathic pain.[42,43] Sativex®, a sublingual spray, is currently in phase 3 clinical trials for the relief of pain associated with multiple sclerosis.

Topical capsaicin

Capsaicin, the compound in chilli peppers responsible for their hot taste, can be used to provide topical pain relief from post-herpetic neuralgia and painful diabetic neuropathy under the supervision of a consultant.[37] Following an initial burning sensation upon application, capsaicin induces a refractory period in which sensitivity is reduced, possibly due to the depletion of substance P from afferent C-fibres.[44]

Management of cancer pain

Guidelines issued by the Scottish Intercollegiate Guidelines Network (SIGN) state that the effective management of cancer pain should be driven by the needs of the individual patients, who should be encouraged to take an active role in their own pain control.[28] Analgesia for continuous pain should be prescribed on a regular basis, not as required.[28] Pain relief should be optimised in accordance with the treatment principles outlined in the WHO analgesic ladder and orally administered morphine is usually the first choice of therapy for moderate-to-severe cancer pain.[45]

Non-pharmacological interventions

Although drug therapy remains the cornerstone of most pain management strategies, there is evidence to suggest that the implementation of alternative treatment approaches, either in addition to, or in place of, drug therapy, may be of therapeutic benefit to a proportion of patients. Some techniques are listed below:
- neurosurgical treatment (only appropriate in those circumstances in which there is clear evidence of nerve damage [e.g. severe sciatica])
- transcutaneous electrical nerve stimulation (TENS)
- cognitive behaviour therapy (CBT)
- palliative radiotherapy
- massage
- exercise therapy
- relaxation techniques
- acupuncture.[10,15,17,46]

Socioeconomic impact

Chronic pain represents one of the major reasons for healthcare visits and as such, places an enormous burden on healthcare resources.[27] As one of the main causes of absence from work, chronic pain impacts significantly on the taxpayer, in terms of social security payments and unemployment.[1] In the UK, approximately 12.5% of unemployed people cite back pain as the reason for their unemployment.[3]

Chronic pain is one of the most costly conditions for which an economic analysis has been carried out in the UK.[47] In 1998, the estimated direct cost of back pain, in terms of healthcare costs, was estimated as £1632 million. A breakdown of these costs in terms of healthcare resource utilisation is illustrated in Figure 2. Since a large proportion of these costs is derived from the private sector (35%) much of this cost will have been financed by patients and their families.[47] Overall, the cost of informal care and the production losses related to back pain in the UK in 1998 were in the region of £10,668 million.[47]

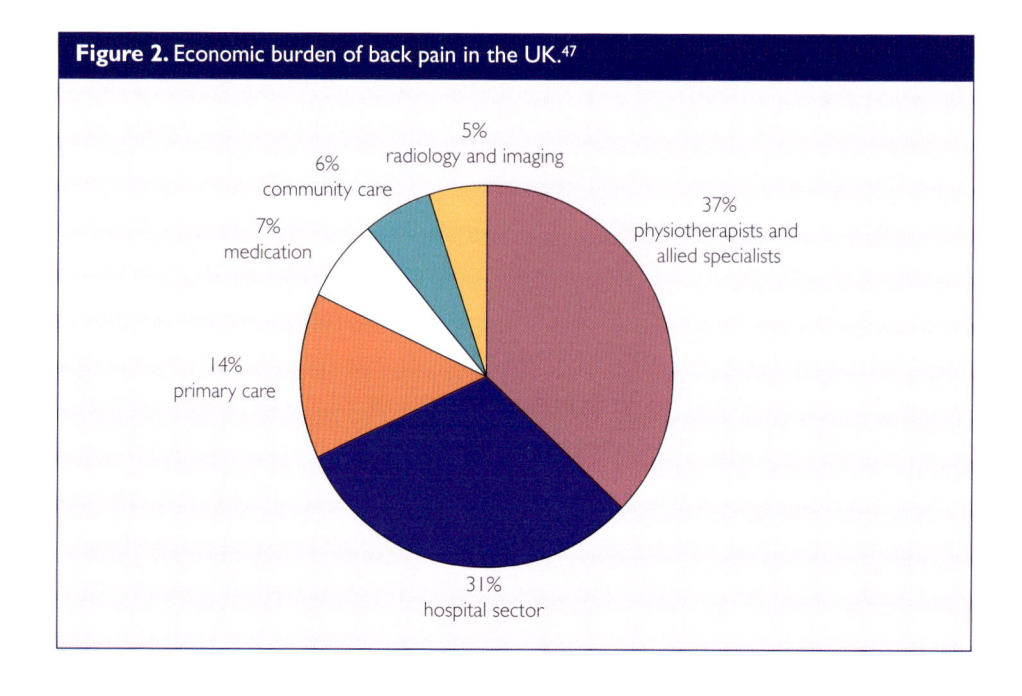

> Chronic pain is one of the most costly conditions for which an economic analysis has been carried out in the UK.

Figure 2. Economic burden of back pain in the UK.[47]

- 5% radiology and imaging
- 6% community care
- 7% medication
- 14% primary care
- 31% hospital sector
- 37% physiotherapists and allied specialists

Key points

- Chronic pain is described as "pain that persists beyond normal tissue healing time, taken, in the absence of other criteria, to be 3 months."

- A disease in its own right, chronic pain impacts heavily on well-being and productivity. Patients may experience depression and diminished self-esteem, as well as financial difficulties associated with an inability to work.

- Owing to its subjective nature and complexity, the management of chronic pain represents a significant challenge to the physician, and a multidisciplinary approach is recommended.

- The scale of the problem is immense, with millions of the UK population estimated to have been affected by chronic pain.

- Chronic pain is multifactorial and may result from underlying disease (e.g. cancer, multiple sclerosis), nerve damage or physical trauma. Low-back pain is amongst the most common causes of chronic pain in the UK.

- The pathophysiology of chronic pain is not well understood but may involve the development of hyperalgesia and allodynia – abnormal responses to noxious and innocuous stimuli, respectively.

- The management of pain is largely pharmacological, with opioid analgesics and NSAIDs remaining the cornerstone of the therapeutic approach.

- The World Health Organization's therapeutic ladder provides a rational basis for the progressive management of pain.

References

1. The Royal College of Anaesthetists and the Pain Society. *Pain Management Services: Good Practice*. London, 2003.
2. Clinical Standards Advisory Group. *Services for patients with pain: a summary of the CSAG report on services for NHS patients with acute and chronic pain*. Oxford, 2000.
3. Elliott A, Smith B, Penny K, Smith W, Chambers W. The epidemiology of chronic pain in the community. *Lancet* 1999; **354**: 1248–52.
4. Verhaak P, Kerssens J, Dekker J, Sorbi M, Bensing J. Prevalence of chronic benign pain disorder among adults: a review of the literature. *Pain* 1998; **77**: 231–9.
5. Gureje O, Von Korff M, Simon G, Gater R. Persistent pain and well-being: a World Health Organization Study in Primary Care. *JAMA* 1998; **280**: 147–51.
6. Green C, Anderson K, Baker T et al. The unequal burden of pain: confronting racial and ethnic disparities in pain. *Pain Med* 2003; **4**: 277–94.
7. Dao T, LeResche L. Gender differences in pain. *J Orofac Pain* 2000; **14**: 184–95.
8. Helme R, Gibson S. The epidemiology of pain in elderly people. *Clin Geriatr Med* 2001; **17**: 417–31.
9. The Pain Society, the Royal College of Anaesthetists, the Royal College of General Practitioners and the Royal College of Psychiatrists. *Recommendations for the appropriate use of opioids for persistent non-cancer pain: a consensus statement*. London: The Pain Society, 2004.
10. Priest T, Hoggart B. Chronic pain: mechanisms and treatment. *Curr Opin Pharmacol* 2002; **2**: 310–15.
11. Smith B, Elliott A, Chambers W et al. The impact of chronic pain in the community. *Fam Pract* 2001; **18**: 292–9.
12. Elliott A, Smith B, Hannaford P, Smith W, Chambers W. The course of chronic pain in the community: results of a 4-year follow-up study. *Pain* 2002; **99**: 299–307.
13. Millan M. The induction of pain: an integrative review. *Prog Neurobiol* 1999; **59**: 1–164.
14. Riedel W, Neeck G. Nociception, pain, and antinociception: current concepts. *Z Rheumatol* 2001; **60**: 404–15.
15. Hall E, Sykes N. Analgesia for patients with advanced disease: I. *Postgrad Med J* 2004; **80**: 148–54.
16. Dworkin R. An overview of neuropathic pain: syndromes, symptoms, signs, and several mechanisms. *Clin J Pain* 2002; **18**: 343–9.
17. Goucke C. The management of persistent pain. *Med J Aust* 2003; **178**: 444–7.
18. Besson J. The neurobiology of pain. *Lancet* 1999; **353**: 1610–5.
19. Pleuvry B, Lauretti G. Biochemical aspects of chronic pain and its relationship to treatment. *Pharmacol Ther* 1996; **71**: 313–24.
20. Fundytus M. Glutamate receptors and nociception: implications for the drug treatment of pain. *CNS Drugs* 2001; **15**: 29–58.
21. Bovill J. Mechanisms of actions of opioids and non-steroidal anti-inflammatory drugs. *Eur J Anaesthesiol Suppl* 1997; **15**: 9–15.
22. Pasternak G. The pharmacology of mu analgesics: from patients to genes. *Neuroscientist* 2001; **7**: 220–31.
23. Mogil J. The genetic mediation of individual differences in sensitivity to pain and its inhibition. *Proc Natl Acad Sci USA* 1999; **96**: 7744–51.
24. Smith B, Hopton J, Chambers W. Chronic pain in primary care. *Fam Pract* 1999; **16**: 475–82.
25. McQuay H. Relief of chronic non-malignant pain. In: Morris P, Malt R, eds. *Oxford Textbook of Surgery*. Oxford University Press, 1994.
26. Gendreau M, Hufford M, Stone A. Measuring clinical pain in chronic widespread pain: selected methodological issues. *Best Pract Res Clin Rheumatol* 2003; **17**: 575–92.
27. World Health Organization. *The World Health Report 2001: pain and well-being*.
28. Scottish Intercollegiate Guidelines Network. *Control of pain in patients with cancer: publication number 44*. Edinburgh, 2000.
29. Tennant F, Uelmen G. Narcotic maintenance for chronic pain. Medical and legal guidelines. *Postgrad Med* 1983; **73**: 81–94.
30. Portenoy R. Opioid therapy for chronic nonmalignant pain: a review of the critical issues. *J Pain Symptom Manage* 1996; **11**: 203–17.
31. Graziotti P, Goucke C. The use of oral opioids in patients with chronic non-cancer pain. Management strategies. *Med J Aust* 1997; **167**: 30–4.
32. Hagen N, Flynne P, Hays H, MacDonald N. Guidelines for managing chronic non-malignant pain. Opioids and other agents. College of Physicians and Surgeons of Alberta. *Can Fam Physician* 1995; **41**: 49–53.
33. Perrot S, Bannwarth B, Bertin P et al. Use of morphine in nonmalignant joint pain: the Limoges recommendations. The French Society for Rheumatology. *Rev Rhum Engl Ed* 1999; **66**: 571–6.
34. Kalso E, Allan L, Dellemijn P et al. Recommendations for using opioids in chronic non-cancer pain. *Eur J Pain* 2003; **7**: 381–6.
35. Merry A, Schug S, Richards E, Large R. Opioids in chronic pain of non-malignant origin: state of the debate in New Zealand. *Eur J Pain* 1992; **13**: 2.
36. McQuay H. Opioids in pain management. *Lancet* 1999; **353**: 2229–32.
37. *British National Formulary (BNF) 47*. London: the British Medical Association and the Royal Pharmaceutical Society of Great Britain, 2004.
38. Inturrisi CE. Clinical pharmacology of opioids for pain. *Clin J Pain* 2002; **18**: S3–13.
39. Markenson J. The demographics of chronic pain management. *J Pain Symptom Manage* 2002; **24**: S10–17.
40. Reisner L. Antidepressants for chronic neuropathic pain. *Curr Pain Headache Rep* 2003; **7**: 24–33.
41. Croxford J. Therapeutic potential of cannabinoids in CNS disease. *CNS Drugs* 2003; **17**: 179–202.
42. Pertwee R. Cannabinoids and multiple sclerosis. *Pharmacol Ther* 2002; **95**: 165–74.
43. Finn D, Chapman V. Cannabinoids as analgesic agents: evidence from *in vivo* studies. *Curr Neuropharm* 2004; **2**: 75–89.

44 Mason L, Moore R, Derry S, Edwards J, McQuay H. Systematic review of topical capsaicin for the treatment of chronic pain. *BMJ* 2004; **328**: 991.
45 Hanks G, Conno F, Cherny N *et al.* Morphine and alternative opioids in cancer pain: the EAPC recommendations. *Br J Cancer* 2001; **84**: 587–93.
46 Hall E, Sykes N. Analgesia for patients with advanced disease: 2. *Postgrad Med J* 2004; **80**: 190–5.
47 Maniadakis N, Gray A. The economic burden of back pain in the UK. *Pain* 2000; **84**: 95–103.

Acknowledgements

Figure 1 is adapted from the World Health Organization and the Scottish Intercollegiate Guidelines Network.[27,28] Figure 2 is adapted from Maniadakis and Gray, 2000.[47]

10. COPD

Dr Susan Chambers and Dr Scott Chambers
CSF Medical Communications Ltd

Summary

Chronic obstructive pulmonary disease (COPD) is a potentially fatal, slowly progressive disease of the airways, characterised by airflow obstruction that is not fully reversible. This is in contrast to the situation in asthma, where airflow obstruction is reversible. COPD encompasses a number of conditions that are now recognised as being different aspects of the same problem. These include: emphysema, chronic bronchitis, asthmatic bronchitis, chronic obstructive airways disease and chronic airflow limitation. COPD is a major cause of death, and has a significant impact on patients' quality of life. However, it tends to be underdiagnosed and undertreated. There is no cure, and treatment is aimed mainly at controlling symptoms.

Pathophysiology of COPD

COPD is caused by two main mechanisms: chronic inflammation of the small airways and gradual destruction of the alveoli.[1] Chronic inflammation results in fibrosis, which in turn leads to narrowing of the airways. The inflammation observed in COPD is different from that seen in asthma, and is driven by neutrophils.[2] Various protease enzymes released by neutrophils damage the elasticity and support of the alveoli. Furthermore, terminal bronchioles collapse or are blocked by mucus plugs, and as a result their alveoli die. COPD is also associated with excessive mucus production, causing the airways to become clogged, and spasm of the muscles surrounding the airways. Air becomes trapped in the distal airways, causing hyperinflation. This reduces tidal volume and increases dead space and, in combination with narrowed airways and reduced gas exchange from loss of alveoli, leads to respiratory failure. Hypoxia increases pulmonary vascular resistance, causing pulmonary hypertension and, ultimately, right-heart failure. COPD is a gradually progressive condition, and the majority of damage is not amenable to drug treatment.

Symptoms

The main symptoms of COPD include chronic cough and/or wheezing, a tight chest, shortness of breath, difficulty in breathing, increased sputum production, and frequent clearing of the throat.[3] Other possible symptoms are shown in Table 1. A typical course of COPD might begin after a person has been smoking for 10 years, during which time the symptoms are not usually noticeable.[4] The patient then develops a productive, chronic cough. After 40 years of age, the patient may experience shortness of breath, which gets worse with time. The signs and symptoms of COPD vary over time with the severity of the disease, but most patients will show a gradual deterioration over the course of 4–5 years.

Different stages of COPD are recognised according to the severity of symptoms and the extent of airflow obstruction. The latter is measured as the volume of air that the patient can exhale in the first second of forced expiration (the forced expiratory volume in 1 second or FEV_1) using the technique of spirometry. The FEV_1 cut-off points used to classify the different stages of COPD are used for simplicity – they have not been clinically validated. The British and American (BTS and ATS) Thoracic Societies currently recognise three stages of the disease (Stages 1, 2 and 3, or mild, moderate and severe, respectively);[5,6] but the recently updated Global Initiative for Chronic Obstructive Lung Disease (GOLD) classifies the disease into five stages (Table 2).[7]

Table 1. Possible symptoms of chronic obstructive pulmonary disease.

- Shortness of breath
- Chronic cough and/or wheezing
- Tight chest
- Breathing difficulty
- Increased sputum production
- An increase in the thickness or stickiness of sputum
- A change in sputum colour to yellow or green
- Blood in the sputum
- Frequent clearing of the throat
- A general feeling of ill health
- Ankle swelling
- Forgetfulness, confusion, slurring of speech and drowsiness
- Sleeping difficulty
- An unexplained increase or decrease in weight
- Fatigue and lack of energy
- Lack of sexual drive
- Increasing morning headaches, dizzy spells, restlessness

Table 2. The different stages of chronic obstructive pulmonary disease (COPD) and their characteristics as set out by the Global Initiative for Chronic Lung Disease (GOLD).[7]

Stage of disease	Spirometry and symptom characteristics
Stage 0: at risk	• Normal spirometry • Chronic symptoms (cough, sputum production)
Stage 1: mild COPD	• FEV_1/FVC <70% • FEV_1 ≥80% of predicted • ± chronic symptoms (cough, sputum production)
Stage 2: moderate COPD	• FEV_1/FVC <70% • FEV_1 50–80% of predicted • ± chronic symptoms (cough, sputum production)
Stage 3: severe COPD	• FEV_1/FVC <70% • FEV_1 30–50% of predicted • ± chronic symptoms (cough, sputum production)
Stage 4: very severe COPD	• FEV_1/FVC <70% • FEV_1 <30% of predicted or <50% of predicted plus chronic respiratory failure • ± chronic symptoms (cough, sputum production)

FEV_1, forced expiratory volume in 1 second; FVC, forced vital capacity.

Impact of COPD

COPD is a major cause of death. In the USA, it was the fourth leading cause of death in 1998, accounting for more than 112,000 deaths.[8] In the UK each year there are over 30,000 deaths attributed to COPD.[9] In 1999, a total of 32,155 deaths were reported. COPD exacerbations account for one in eight of all hospital admissions in the UK. Besides AIDS, COPD is the only cause of death that is increasing.[10,11]

COPD also has a significant impact on patients' quality of life. A recent survey performed in the USA showed that millions of sufferers experience shortness of breath so severe that it interferes with even the most basic daily activities: of the nearly 600 COPD sufferers interviewed, almost half experienced shortness of breath whilst washing and dressing or doing light housework, a third experienced shortness of breath whilst talking, a third had difficulty breathing when lying down or sitting still, and one-in-four said their condition had made them an invalid.[12]

Nearly 900,000 people in the UK are diagnosed as having COPD, and half as many again are believed to go undiagnosed.[9] In the USA, 16 million patients were diagnosed with COPD in 1994, but as many as 16 million people were thought to be undiagnosed.[13] Identifying patients with COPD

Identifying patients with COPD and giving appropriate treatment is vital to improve quality of life and reduce the mortality rate associated with the disease.

and giving appropriate treatment is therefore vital to improve quality of life and reduce the mortality rate associated with the disease.

Aetiology

The main cause of COPD is tobacco smoking – it accounts for 80–90% of all cases of COPD, and a smoker is 10-times more likely to die of the disease than a non-smoker.[14] Smoking causes irreversible structural changes to the lungs and accelerates the decline in lung function normally seen with increasing age. If a patient with COPD stops smoking, however, the rate of decline in lung function returns to that of a non-smoker (Figure 1).[15] Thus, early detection of COPD is important if sufferers are to be encouraged to stop smoking.

Other risk factors for COPD include middle/old age, genetic factors (including deficiency of the antiprotease enzyme α_1-antitrypsin), passive smoking, exposure to air pollution at work, and a history of childhood respiratory infections.[15–20] Lifelong heavy smokers who are over 40 years of age and patients who are exposed to respiratory irritants (e.g. fumes and dust) during the course of their work are at greatest risk of developing COPD.

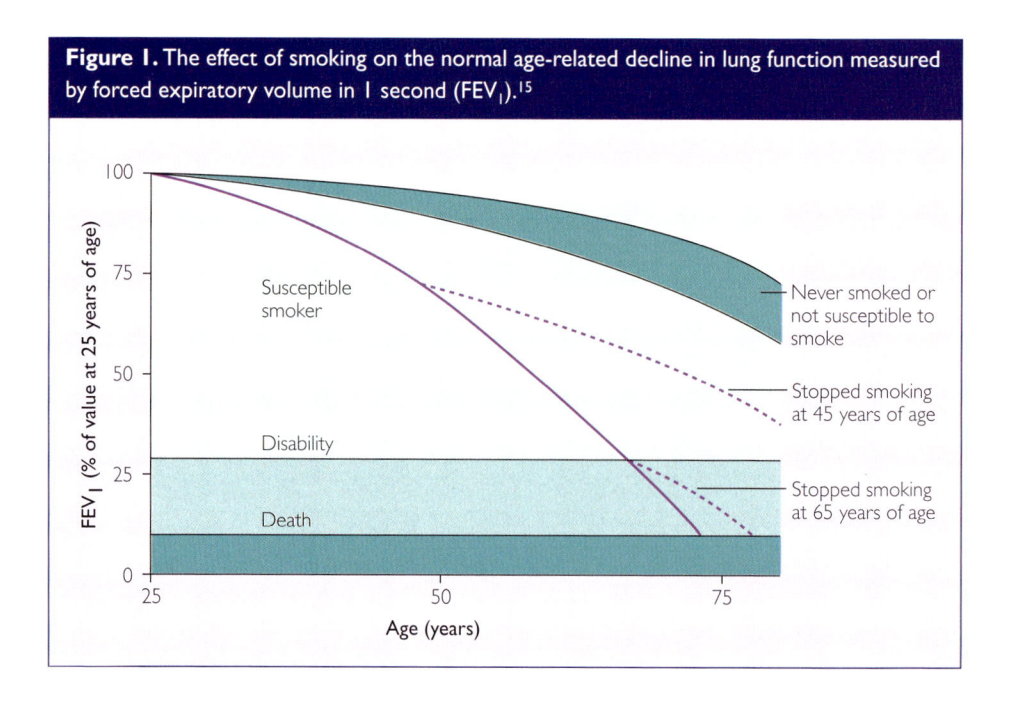

Figure 1. The effect of smoking on the normal age-related decline in lung function measured by forced expiratory volume in 1 second (FEV_1).[15]

Diagnosis

The presence of COPD is usually apparent from symptoms associated with this disease, such as breathlessness and wheezing. However, for a definite diagnosis to be made, it is necessary to prove the presence of airflow limitation that is not fully reversible. This can be achieved through lung function tests. The main problem is distinguishing COPD from asthma, particularly chronic asthma in patients who smoke. However, it is important to differentiate between the two diseases as they require different treatments. In the first instance, a patient's history can help. COPD is suggested by:

- onset in mid-life
- slowly progressive symptoms
- history of smoking
- chronic cough and sputum
- breathlessness on exertion

whereas a patient's history for asthma is markedly different:

- onset early in life
- symptoms vary from day to day
- symptoms at night/early morning
- allergy, rhinitis or eczema also present
- family history of asthma.

For example, patients whose symptoms started before 40 years of age are more likely to be asthmatic, particularly if they are non-smokers. Serial peak-flow monitoring may also help to distinguish between the two conditions, or, alternatively, bronchodilator and/or corticosteroid reversibility tests can be performed (Table 3).[6] Many patients being assessed for COPD are already receiving inhaled corticosteroids, with a presumptive diagnosis of asthma. In these patients, a trial withdrawal of the inhaled corticosteroids is indicated to see whether their condition deteriorates. If it does deteriorate, they probably have asthma; if it does not, they are likely to have COPD and do not need the corticosteroids.

Spirometry is the key diagnostic technique for patients with suspected COPD. This is a sensitive technique that assesses lung function by measuring a patient's airflow. Patients with COPD will show largely irreversible airflow obstruction presenting as an FEV_1 value of less than 80% of the predicted value for a person of the same sex, age and height, and a FEV_1/forced vital capacity (FVC) ratio of less than 70% of the predicted value. Spirometry is the gold standard for diagnosing and assessing COPD, yet research shows that it is underused, mainly because of

Table 3. Distinguishing chronic obstructive pulmonary disease (COPD) from asthma (see *www.brit-thoracic.org.uk*).

Investigation	COPD	Asthma
FEV_1	Always reduced and airflow limitation not reversible	Variable and airflow limitation largely reversible
Daily variations in peak expiratory flow rate	Minimal	'Morning dip' and day-to-day variation
Objective response to bronchodilator therapy[a]	Partial at best	Partial/complete
Objective response to corticosteroid trial[a]	Partial response in 10–20% of patients	Good response in majority of patients

[a]A positive response is an increase in FEV_1 that is both >200 mL and a 15% increase from baseline. FEV_1, forced expiratory volume in 1 second.

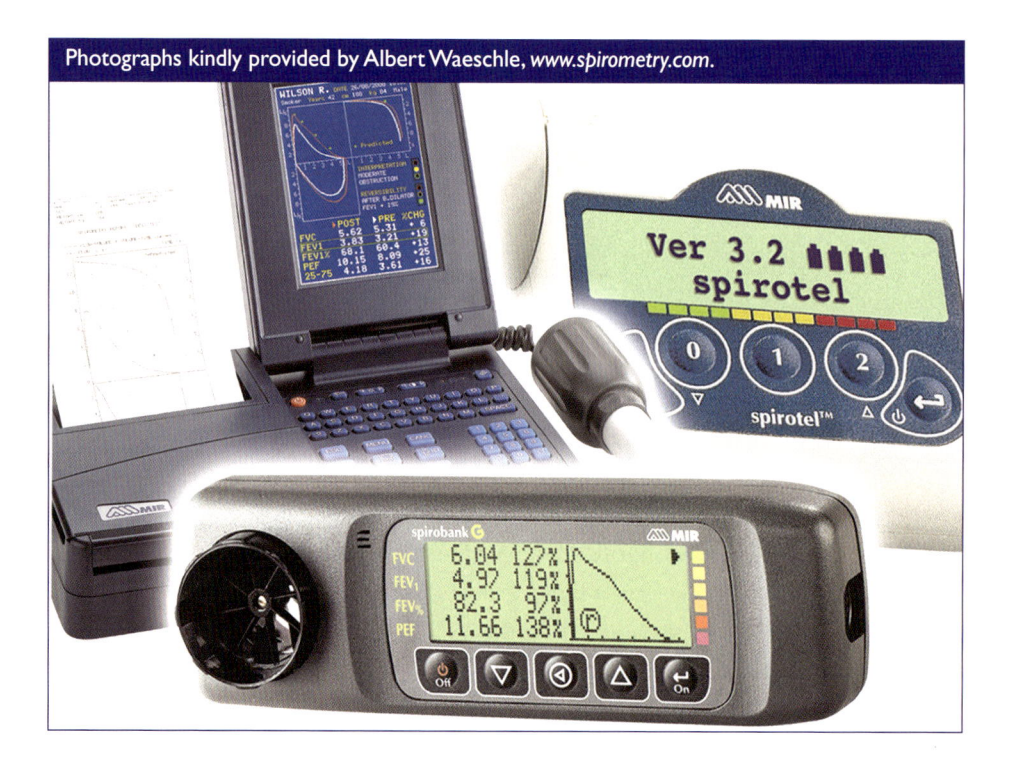

Photographs kindly provided by Albert Waeschle, *www.spirometry.com*.

lack of confidence among health professionals in conducting the test and in interpreting the results.[21] The BTS COPD consortium has produced a booklet of information on performing spirometry and interpreting the results.[a]

Other tests that may aid in the diagnosis of COPD include a chest radiograph, a full blood count and electrocardiogram (ECG). For example, a chest radiograph cannot be used to diagnose COPD, but is a useful screening tool to exclude other pathologies such as lung cancer. A full blood count will identify anaemia and polycythaemia, a condition commonly associated with more advanced COPD, whilst an ECG provides useful information relating to the presence of ischaemic heart disease.

An algorithm for the diagnosis of COPD is illustrated in Figure 2.[22]

Treatment of COPD

GOLD initiative

Over 40 national guidelines for the management of COPD have been developed worldwide by local respiratory societies, including the European Respiratory Society, the ATS and the BTS.[5,6,23] These guidelines are all based on a consensus of local key opinion leaders. GOLD is a programme aimed at developing global recommendations for the management of COPD. It is supported by the World Health Organization (WHO) and the US National Heart, Lung and Blood Institute. The first step in the GOLD programme was to prepare a global consensus report on the management of COPD. The report was developed by a worldwide expert panel and is evidence based. It provides up-to-date information about COPD and specific recommendations on the most appropriate management and prevention strategies.[7] The GOLD guidelines were recently updated in 2003, and further information about the GOLD initiative can be found at *www.goldcopd.com*.

National Institute for Clinical Excellence guidelines

The National Institute for Clinical Excellence (NICE) in the UK recently published guidelines on the diagnosis and management of COPD in primary and secondary care.[22] These guidelines address issues relating to the management of COPD from a British perspective, and set out a number of key priorities with the aim of raising the standard of care of COPD patients within the UK NHS.

---

[a]This booklet can be accessed via *www.brit-thoracic.org.uk/pdf/COPDSpirometryInPractice.pdf*

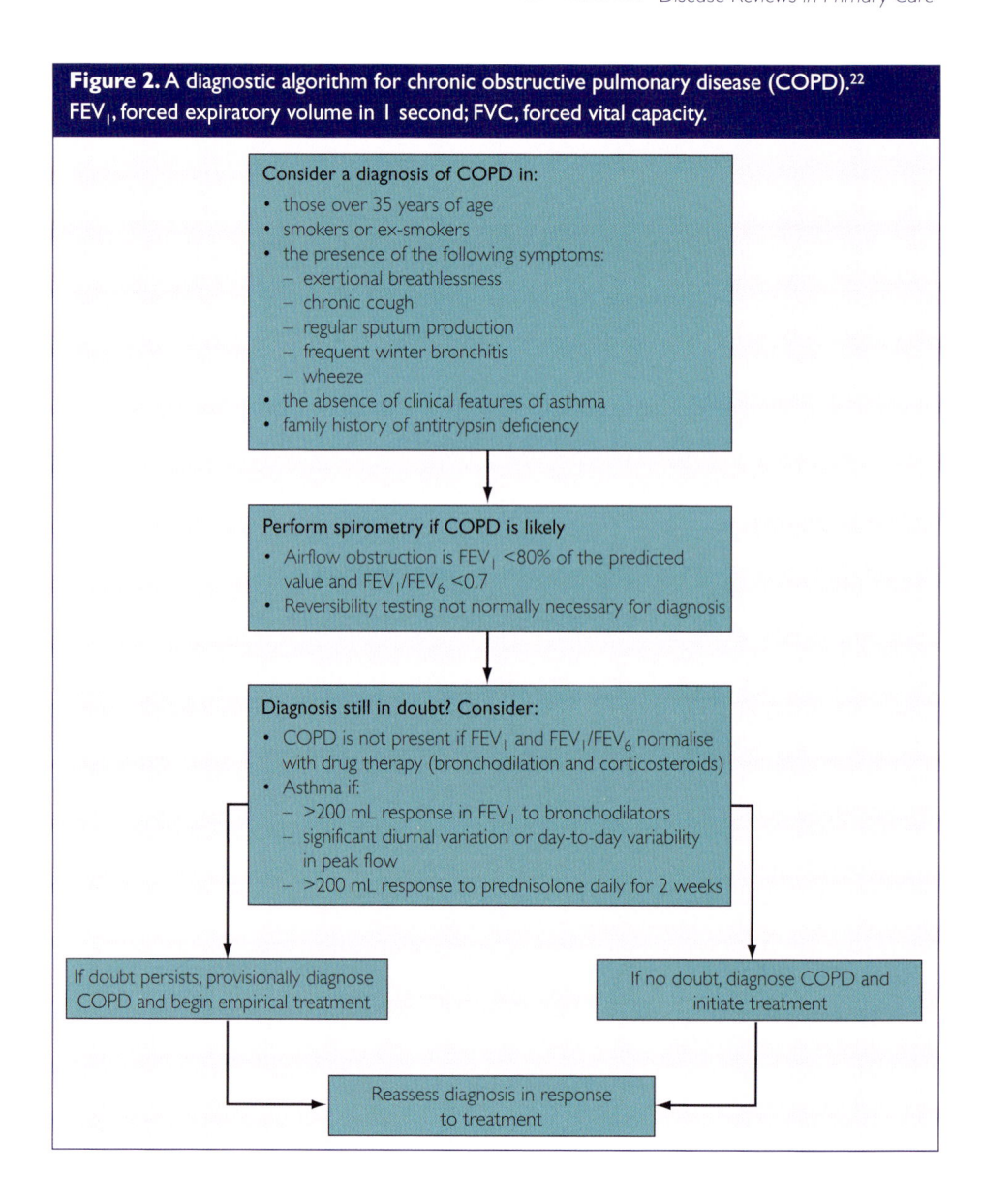

Figure 2. A diagnostic algorithm for chronic obstructive pulmonary disease (COPD).[22] FEV_1, forced expiratory volume in 1 second; FVC, forced vital capacity.

Consider a diagnosis of COPD in:
- those over 35 years of age
- smokers or ex-smokers
- the presence of the following symptoms:
  - exertional breathlessness
  - chronic cough
  - regular sputum production
  - frequent winter bronchitis
  - wheeze
- the absence of clinical features of asthma
- family history of antitrypsin deficiency

Perform spirometry if COPD is likely
- Airflow obstruction is FEV_1 <80% of the predicted value and FEV_1/FEV_6 <0.7
- Reversibility testing not normally necessary for diagnosis

Diagnosis still in doubt? Consider:
- COPD is not present if FEV_1 and FEV_1/FEV_6 normalise with drug therapy (bronchodilation and corticosteroids)
- Asthma if:
  - >200 mL response in FEV_1 to bronchodilators
  - significant diurnal variation or day-to-day variability in peak flow
  - >200 mL response to prednisolone daily for 2 weeks

If doubt persists, provisionally diagnose COPD and begin empirical treatment

If no doubt, diagnose COPD and initiate treatment

Reassess diagnosis in response to treatment

In terms of the FEV_1 cut-off points for different stages of airway obstruction, the NICE guidelines are closely aligned to the updated GOLD guidelines (Table 2), although there is some variation in the terminology employed. Thus, in the NICE guidance, an FEV_1 of 50–80% of the predicted value constitutes mild obstruction, 30–40% is moderate obstruction and less than 30% severe obstruction.

NICE have outlined the following major priorities to improve the standards of care in COPD:
- effective diagnosis on the basis of a history, confirmed via spirometry if COPD seems likely (the NICE guidance emphasises that reversibility

testing is not a necessary part of the diagnostic work-up or as a tool to determine an initial treatment plan [Figure 2])
- smoking cessation programmes
- effective inhaled pharmacological interventions (with effectiveness determined by symptoms, impact on routine daily activities, exercise capacity, in addition to lung function tests)
- availability of pulmonary rehabilitation
- non-invasive ventilation during COPD exacerbations
- effective prevention of exacerbations through the appropriate use of inhaled corticosteroids, bronchodilators and vaccination
- effective management of exacerbations via self-management advice, appropriate use of oral steroids and antibiotics and the use of hospital-at-home or assisted discharge schemes
- multidisciplinary working.

Aims of treatment

COPD is progressive and irreversible. There is no cure, so treatment is essentially palliative. An effective plan for the management of COPD has four main components: assess and monitor the disease, reduce risk factors, manage the disease and manage any exacerbations. Thus, the main aims in the management of the disease are to:
- provide optimum symptom control
- prevent disease progression
- improve the patient's quality of life
- improve exercise tolerance
- prevent and treat complications
- prevent and treat exacerbations
- reduce mortality.[7]

Lifestyle changes

One of the most effective interventions to retard the progression of COPD is for a smoker to stop smoking.[14,15,24,25] The NICE guidelines urge support for patients with regard to smoking cessation at every opportunity available, including the use of pharmacotherapy as part of the cessation programme.[22] Such interventions help to slow the decline in lung function (Figure 1).[15] Other beneficial lifestyle changes include:
- avoiding dust, excessive air pollution, cigarette smoke and work-related fumes
- avoiding excessive heat, cold or high altitudes
- avoiding contact with people who have colds or influenza

> One of the most effective interventions to retard the progression of COPD is for a smoker to stop smoking.

- immunisation against influenza and pneumococcal pneumonia
- coughing in such a way as to clear the lungs of mucus within two or three coughs
- drinking plenty of fluid to help thin the mucus in the airways
- eating a healthy diet
- regular exercise to improve physical endurance
- regular monitoring of the disease.

Pharmacological treatment

Because COPD is progressive, pharmacological treatment should be increased in a step-wise manner according to the severity of the disease. Regular treatment should be maintained at the same level for long periods of time unless significant side-effects occur or the disease progresses. The step-down approach used for the chronic treatment of asthma is *not* suitable for COPD.[7]

Bronchodilators are the mainstay of pharmacological therapy for COPD. They provide relief from breathlessness, improve exercise tolerance and allow the lungs to work more efficiently.[26,27] They can be taken as needed, or on a regular basis. The choice is between:

- inhaled short-acting β_2-agonists such as fenoterol, salbutamol and terbutaline
- inhaled long-acting β_2-agonists (formoterol [eformoterol] and salmeterol)
- inhaled anticholinergics (ipratropium bromide, oxitropium bromide and tiotropium bromide).

Long-acting inhaled agents are preferable to short-acting oral agents because adverse events are less likely to occur with inhaled than with oral agents.[28] Inhaled anticholinergics are more effective than short-acting inhaled β_2-agonists.[29,30] Evidence for the efficacy of long-acting inhaled β_2-agonists in COPD is inconclusive, though they do provide additive bronchodilatory effects when given in combination with inhaled anticholinergics.[31,32] In view of this additive effect, the GOLD guidelines recommend a combination of bronchodilators from different classes rather than an increased dose of a single bronchodilator. This approach has the added benefit of reducing the risk of side-effects.[31–33] Some concern has been expressed about the regular use of short-acting β_2-agonists in COPD but the evidence is not strong enough to advise against their use.[34] There has also been disagreement as to whether older patients with COPD respond as well to these drugs as younger patients.[34–38]

Slow-release oral theophylline preparations are also used as bronchodilators. However, their use is in decline because of the poor side-effect profile, which generally outweighs any efficacy benefits. Thus, theophylline should be used only in patients with more severe COPD where other treatments have failed to provide adequate symptom control.[6]

Inhaled or oral corticosteroids are also commonly prescribed for COPD, but their use is controversial since they do not reduce the inflammatory response in COPD and do not prevent progression of the disease.[39,40] The GOLD guidelines advise against the long-term use of corticosteroids in COPD. However, there is some evidence that inhaled corticosteroids are useful in patients with severe COPD who have frequent exacerbations.[7] In view of this, the GOLD guidelines recommend the short-term use of inhaled steroids for acute exacerbations. NICE has clarified the role of inhaled corticosteroids in moderate-to-severe COPD further.[22] Their recommendations propose the addition of corticosteroids into the treatment plan if a patient's FEV_1 is 50% or less than the predicted value and if they have had two or more exacerbations in the preceding 12 months.[22]

Vaccination against influenza is recommended for all patients with COPD, as is vaccination against pneumococcal infection.[41]

Finally, antibiotics are recommended at the first sign of a respiratory infection for any patient with COPD (i.e. if two or more of the following signs are present: increased breathlessness, increased sputum volume, purulent sputum).[42]

Additional treatment options

Additional treatment options for COPD are:
- pulmonary rehabilitation, which can improve exercise tolerance
- supplemental oxygen for later stages of the disease
- surgical removal of large air spaces in the lungs (bullectomy)
- surgical removal of areas of the lungs showing major damage (lung volume reduction surgery) in carefully selected cases
- lung transplantation, which has proved effective in patients with end-stage COPD
- mechanical respiratory assistance – this may be required for end-stage disease.

Pulmonary rehabilitation programmes are becoming increasingly recognised as an effective part of COPD management. The primary objective of such programmes is to improve patients' exercise tolerance, thereby improving the quality of life. Disabling breathlessness in patients with COPD is a primary cause of physical deconditioning, which in turn leads to worsening breathlessness and an inability to cope with the disease. Worsening breathlessness can be accompanied by panic and anxiety, which can also lead to an increase in hospital admissions. This vicious cycle of spiralling decline in lung function can be reversed to some extent by pulmonary rehabilitation. Such programmes usually comprise a mixture of education, lower- and upper-extremity training, breathing retraining and chest physiotherapy and are usually aimed at patients with moderate-to-severe COPD. NICE recommend that pulmonary rehabilitation is made available to all patients who are functionally disabled by COPD, although it is not suitable for those patients who are unable to walk, or who have unstable angina or a recent myocardial infarction.[22]

Long-term oxygen therapy should be reserved for severe cases, in whom it can improve prognosis. Such therapy requires specialist assessment of the patient's arterial blood gases as it can lead to serious carbon dioxide retention and should be considered if the patient's arterial blood oxygen level is less than 7.3 kPa and FEV_1 is less than 1.5 L.[6]

GOLD recommendations for the treatment of COPD are summarised in Table 4 whilst the treatment recommendations from the NICE guidelines are presented in Table 5.[22]

Treatment of acute exacerbations

Patients with severe COPD are likely to experience frequent exacerbations, which may require hospital admission. Acute exacerbations present as a worsening of the previous stable situation which is beyond normal day-to-day variation and is acute in onset.[22] The main symptoms are:
- increased wheezing
- increased difficulty in breathing
- increased sputum volume
- increased sputum purulence
- chest tightness
- fluid retention.

Exacerbations not requiring hospitalisation should be managed with an increased frequency of bronchodilator therapy (possibly via a nebuliser), the use of antibiotics in the presence of purulent symptoms and the use of oral prednisilone unless contra-indicated.[22]

Although some patients with acute exacerbations will require hospitalisation, many can be managed at home. The basic strategy for treating an acute exacerbation of COPD at home is shown in Table 6.

Table 4. Global Initiative for Chronic Lung Disease (GOLD) guidelines for the management of stable chronic obstructive pulmonary disease (COPD).[7]

Stage of disease	Recommended intervention
Stage 0: at risk	• Avoidance of risk factors • Influenza vaccination
Stage 1: mild COPD	• Avoidance of risk factors • Influenza vaccination • Add short-acting bronchodilator[a] as needed
Stage 2: moderate COPD	• Avoidance of risk factors • Influenza vaccination • Add short-acting bronchodilator[a] as needed • Add regular treatment with long-acting bronchodilators[a] • Add rehabilitation
Stage 3: severe COPD	• Avoidance of risk factors • Influenza vaccination • Add short-acting bronchodilator[a] as needed • Add regular treatment with long-acting bronchodilators[a] • Add rehabilitation • Add inhaled corticosteroids if repeated exacerbations
Stage 4: very severe COPD	• Avoidance of risk factors • Influenza vaccination • Add short-acting bronchodilator[a] as needed • Add regular treatment with long-acting bronchodilators[a] • Add rehabilitation • Add inhaled corticosteroids if repeated exacerbations • Add long-term oxygen if chronic respiratory failure. • Consider surgical intervention

[a]β_2-agonist or anticholinergic.

Socioeconomic impact of COPD

As we have seen in the earlier sections of this overview, COPD can profoundly impair patients' quality of life and reduce their overall health status. In many cases of moderate-to-severe disease, patients' symptoms preclude them from working and from many routine daily activities. As their disease progresses and their lung function deteriorates further patients become even more dependent on family and carers. In severe disease, patients may become house-bound, socially isolated and depressed, leading to even greater consumption of social and health service resources.[43]

As the course of COPD progresses, disease exacerbations occur with increasing frequency, often necessitating hospital admission for their management. As a consequence, COPD exacerbations are a major contributor to the already overwhelming economic burden that is associated

Table 5. Management of stable chronic obstructive pulmonary disease (COPD) according to the guidelines of the National Institute for Clinical Excellence.[22]

	Management intervention recommendations
Smoking	• Support to stop at every opportunity • Combine support with pharmacotherapy within cessation programme
Breathlessness and exercise limitation	• Use short-acting bronchodilator[a] as needed • If still symptomatic, combine short-acting β_2-agonist and short-acting anticholinergic • If still symptomatic, use a long-acting bronchodilator[a] In moderate/severe COPD: • If still symptomatic consider a trial of a combination of a long-acting bronchodilator and an inhaled corticosteroid. Discontinue in the absence of benefit after 4 weeks • If still symptomatic consider adding theophylline NB: in all cases, stop therapy if it is ineffective after 4 weeks • Offer pulmonary rehabilitation to those who consider themselves functionally disabled • Consider referral for surgery
Exacerbations	• Offer annual influenza and pneumoccocal vaccination • Give self-management advice • Optimise bronchodilator therapy with one or more long-acting bronchodilators[a] • Add inhaled corticosteroids if FEV_1 ≤50% and there have been two or more exacerbations in the preceding 12 months (usually with long-acting bronchodilators[a])
Respiratory failure	• Assess for oxygen therapy • Consider referral for long-term non-invasive ventilation
Cor pulmonale	• Need for oxygen therapy • Use diuretics
Abnormal BMI	• Refer for dietary advice • If BMI is low, initiate dietary supplements
Chronic productive cough	• Consider trial of mucolytic therapy and continue if there is symptomatic improvement
Anxiety and depression	• Be aware of anxiety and depression; screen in the most physically disabled patients • Treat with conventional pharmacotherapy
Palliative care	• Opiates for the palliation of breathlessness in end-stage COPD unresponsive to other medical therapy • Use benzodiazepines, tricyclic antidepressants, major tranquillisers and oxygen where appropriate • Involve multidisciplinary palliative-care teams

[a]β_2-agonist or anticholinergic.
BMI, body mass index; FEV_1, forced expiratory volume in 1 second.

with the condition. Moreover, the burden of COPD hospitalisations is on the increase, with admission rates increasing by 50% from 1991 to 2000.[44] Emergency admissions due to COPD are thought to account for one-in-eight of all hospital admissions.

Direct costs of COPD are very high. A recent analysis estimated that the NHS spends £818 million annually (at 1996/1997 prices) to manage COPD in the UK.[43,45] For the year 2000–2001, across the UK there were

Table 6. Management of an acute exacerbation of chronic obstructive pulmonary disease at home.

- Add or increase the dose of bronchodilator
- Consider theophylline if other treatments fail to control symptoms
- Give an antibiotic if the patient shows at least two of the following:
  - increased breathlessness
  - increased sputum volume
  - purulent sputum
- Consider oral corticosteroids if:
  - the patient has previously responded to these drugs
  - the airflow obstruction fails to respond to an increase in the dose of bronchodilator
  - this is the first presentation of airflow obstruction

308,355 emergency admissions for COPD involving an average hospital stay of 7.87 days.[46–49] Assuming a cost of £242 per bed day, this means that COPD hospitalisations alone cost the NHS £587,135,802 over this period.[46–49] Whilst pharmacological interventions which can reduce the incidence of acute exacerbations will inevitably increase the direct costs in terms of drug acquisition, they have the potential to bring about substantial savings with regard to hospital admission, as well as providing symptomatic and quality of life improvements for the patients.

Costs to society in terms of lost productivity are also significant. In 1994 to 1995, 24 million working days were lost, with an estimated loss in productivity of about £2.7 billion.[43]

Finally, social and economic inequity persists in COPD. The majority of sufferers of COPD are amongst the least affluent of the population, principally living in urban conurbations. As an illustration of this inequity, men from unskilled, manual occupations are 14-times more likely to be COPD sufferers than those from higher social classes.[43]

Key points

- COPD is a potentially fatal, progressive disease of the airways, characterised by airflow obstruction that is not fully reversible. This contrasts with asthma where the airflow limitation is reversible, though in the later stages of asthma airflow restriction becomes less reversible because of structural changes in the airways.

- The main symptoms of COPD are a chronic cough and/or wheezing, a tight chest, shortness of breath, difficulty breathing, increased sputum production and frequent clearing of the throat.

- COPD causes more deaths than any other respiratory disease. Early diagnosis and treatment are key to reducing the number of deaths and to improving patients' quality of life.

- The main cause of COPD is tobacco smoking. Other risk factors include middle/old age, genetic factors and exposure to air pollution.

- The main problem in diagnosing COPD is differentiation from asthma. The patient's history can help with this.

- Spirometry is the key technique for diagnosing COPD. This technique assesses a patient's lung function by measuring the patient's airflow.

- One of the most effective measures to stop the progression of COPD is for a smoker to stop smoking.

- The most commonly prescribed pharmacological treatments for COPD are inhaled bronchodilators. The choice is between anticholinergics and β_2-agonists, or a combination of both. These provide symptom relief but do not stop progression of the disease.

- Acute exacerbations of COPD may require hospitalisation, though many patients can be managed at home with appropriate treatment. Exacerbations are a major component of the high cost associated with managing COPD.

References

1. Barnes PJ. New treatments for COPD. *Nat Rev Drug Discov* 2002; **1(6)**: 437–46.
2. Barnes PJ. Mechanisms in COPD: differences from asthma. *Chest* 2000; **117**: 10–14S.
3. National Institutes of Health. *COPD Questions and Answers* (publication no. 95–2020). www.nih.gov Bethesda: National Institutes of Health, 1995; 4–7.
4. Pearson MG, Calverley PMA. Clinical and laboratory assessment. In: Calverley PMA, Pride NB, eds. *Chronic Obstructive Pulmonary Disease*. London: Chapman & Hall, 1994.
5. American Thoracic Society. Standards for the diagnosis and care of patients with chronic obstructive pulmonary disease. *Am J Respir Crit Care Med* 1995; **152**: S77–120.
6. British Thoracic Society. Guidelines for the management of chronic obstructive pulmonary disease. *Thorax* 1997; **52(Suppl 5)**: S1–28. www.brit-thoracic.org.uk/pdf/COPDtext.pdf
7. Pauwels RA, Buist AS, Ma P, Jenkins CR, Hurd SS. Global strategy for the diagnosis, management, and prevention of chronic obstructive pulmonary disease: National Heart, Lung, and Blood Institute and World Health Organization Global Initiative for Chronic Obstructive Lung Disease (GOLD): executive summary. *Respir Care* 2001; **46**: 798–825.
8. National Center for Health Statistics. *Report of Final Morbidity Statistics, 1970–1998*. Hyattsville, Maryland: National Center for Health Statistics, 1998.
9. The British Thoracic Society. The BTS COPD consortium. www.brit-thoracic.org.uk/copd/copd_guidelines.html
10. Lopez AD, Murray CC. The global burden of disease, 1990–2020. *Nature Med* 1998; **4**: 1241–3.
11. World Health Organization. The World Health Report 2000. *Health Systems: Improving Performance*. Geneva: WHO, 2000.
12. Confronting COPD in America. www.lungusa.org/press/lung_dis/asn_copd21601.html
13. Petty TL. A national strategy for COPD. *J Resp Dis* 1997; **18**: 365–9.
14. Doll R, Peto R, Wheatley K, Gray R, Sutherland J. Mortality in relation to smoking: 40 years observations on male British doctors. *BMJ* 1994; **309**: 901–10.
15. Fletcher C, Peto R. The natural history of chronic airflow obstruction. *BMJ* 1977; **1**: 1645–8.
16. Janus ED, Phillips NT, Carroll RW. Smoking, lung function and α_1-antitrypsin deficiency. *Lancet* 1985; **1**: 152–4.
17. Korn RJ, Dockery DW, Speizer FE, Ware JH, Ferris BG. Occupational exposures and chronic respiratory symptoms. A population-based study. *Am Rev Respir Dis* 1987; **136**: 296–304.
18. Oxman AD, Muir DCF, Shannon HS *et al*. Occupational dust exposure and chronic obstructive pulmonary disease. A systematic overview of the evidence. *Am Rev Respir Dis* 1993; **148**: 38–48.
19. Tashkin DP, Detek R, Simmons M *et al*. The UCLA population study of chronic obstructive respiratory disease: impact of air pollution and smoking on annual change in FEV_1. *Am J Respir Crit Care Med* 1994; **149**: 1209–17.
20. Erhabor GE, Kolawole OA. Chronic obstructive pulmonary disease: a ten-year review of clinical features in OAUTHC, Ile-Ife. *Niger J Med* 2002; **11**: 101–4.
21. Bellamy D, Buchanan A, Coutts I, Hart L, Pearson M, Rudolf M, on behalf of the COPD Consortium. Impact of BTS COPD guidelines. www.brit-thoracic.org.uk/pdf/COPDImpact.pdf
22. National Institute for Clinical Excellence (NICE). Chronic obstructive pulmonary disease. Management of chronic obstructive pulmonary disease in adults in primary and secondary care. Quick reference guide. www.nice.org.uk
23. Siafakas NM, Vermiere P, Pride NB *et al*. Optimal assessment and management of chronic obstructive pulmonary disease (COPD). *Eur Respir J* 1995; **8**: 1398–420.
24. Traver GA, Clinc MG, Burrows B. Predictors of mortality in COPD. *Am Rev Respir Dis* 1979; **119**: 895–902.
25. Anthonisen N, Connett J, Kiley J *et al*. Effects of smoking intervention and the use of an inhaled anticholinergic bronchodilator on the rate of decline of FEV_1: the Lung Health Study. *JAMA* 1994; **272**: 1497–505.
26. Gross NJ, Skorodin MS. Anti-cholinergic, anti-muscarinic bronchodilators. *Am Rev Respir Dis* 1984; **139**: 1185–91.
27. Gross NJ, Co E, Skorodin MS. Cholinergic bronchomotor tone in COPD: estimates of its amount in comparison with that in normal subjects. *Chest* 1989; **96**: 984–7.
28. Shim CS, Williams MH. Bronchodilator response to oral aminophylline and terbutaline versus aerosol albuterol in patients with chronic obstructive pulmonary disease. *Am J Med* 1983; **75**: 697–701.
29. Braun SR, McKenzie WN, Copeland C *et al*. A comparison of the effect of ipratropium and albuterol in the treatment of chronic airways disease. *Arch Intern Med* 1989; **149**: 544–7.
30. The Combivent Inhalation Aerosol Study. Combination of ipratropium and albuterol is more effective than either agent alone. *Chest* 1994; **105**: 1411–9.
31. Appleton S, Smith B, Veale A, Bara A. Long-acting β_2-agonists for chronic obstructive pulmonary disease. *Cochrane Database Syst Rev* 2000; **2**: CD001104.
32. Van Noord JA, de Munck DR, Bantje TA *et al*. Long-term treatment of chronic obstructive pulmonary disease with salmeterol and the additive effect of ipratropium. *Eur Respir J* 2000; **15**: 878–85.
33. Combivent Inhalation Study Group. Routine nebulized ipratropium and albuterol together are better than either alone in COPD. *Chest* 1997; **112**: 1514–21.
34. Van Schayck CP, Dompeling E, van Herwaarden CLA *et al*. Bronchodilator treatment in moderate asthma or chronic bronchitis: continuous or on demand. A randomised controlled study. *BMJ* 1991; **303**: 1426–31.
35. Corris PA, Neville E, Nariman S, Gibson GJ. Dose-response study of inhaled salbutamol powder in chronic airflow obstruction. *Thorax* 1983; **39**: 292–6.
36. Guyatt GH, Townsend M, Nogradi S *et al*. Acute response to bronchodilator. An imperfect guide for bronchodilator therapy in chronic airflow limitation. *Arch Intern Med* 1988; **148**: 1949–52.
37. Berger R, Smith D. Effect of inhaled metaproterenol on exercise performance in patients with stable fixed airway obstruction. *Am Rev Respir Dis* 1988; **138**: 626–9.

38. Nisar M, Earis JE, Pearson MG, Calverley PMA. Acute bronchodilator trials in chronic obstructive pulmonary disease. *Am Rev Respir Dis* 1992; **146**: 555–9.
39. Barnes PJ. Inhaled corticosteroids are not helpful in chronic obstructive pulmonary disease. *Am J Respir Crit Care Med* 2000; **161**: 342–4.
40. Calverley PM. Inhaled corticosteroids are beneficial in chronic obstructive pulmonary disease. *Am J Respir Crit Care Med* 2000; **161**: 341–2.
41. Immunisation Against Infectious Disease 1996. 'The Green Book'. *http://www.doh.gov.uk/greenbook*
42. Anthonisen NR, Manfreda J, Warren CPW *et al*. Antibiotic therapy in exacerbations of chronic obstructive pulmonary disease. *Ann Intern Med* 1987; **106**: 196–204.
43. The Respiratory Alliance. *Bridging the Gap. Commissioning and Delivering High Quality Integrated Respiratory Healthcare*. A report from the Respiratory Alliance, 2003.
44. Lung and Asthma Information Agency. *Trends in Emergency Hospital Admissions for Lung Disease*. London: Lung and Asthma Information Agency, 2001.
45. Guest JF. The annual cost of chronic obstructive pulmonary disease to the UK's National Health Service. *Dis Management Outcomes* 1999; **5**: 93-100.
46. Department of Health, Social Services and Public Safety, Northern Ireland.
47. *Hospital Episode Statistics*. Department of Health, England.
48. *Health Solutions Wales*. National Health Service, Wales.
49. Information and Statistics Division, Common Services Agency. National Health Service, Scotland.

Acknowledgements

Figure 1 is adapted from Fletcher and Peto, 1977.[15]
Figure 2 is adapted from the National Institute for Clinical Excellence.[22]

11. Coronary heart disease

Dr Richard Clark
CSF Medical Communications Ltd

Summary

Coronary heart disease (CHD) is the greatest cause of mortality in the UK and, in the vast majority of cases of CHD, death is due to a myocardial infarction (MI). MI accounts for more than 120,000 deaths per year in the UK (one death in five). MI typically results from coronary occlusion, marked by sudden chest pain, shortness of breath, nausea, sweating and sometimes loss of consciousness, and which can lead to death. MI is a clinical presentation of CHD, but the underlying pathophysiological problem is atherosclerosis. Rupture of atherosclerotic plaques can trigger MI. It is essential to diagnose and treat MI rapidly to limit infarct size and prevent or manage complications. Long-term clinical management for secondary prevention post-MI should include dietary modification, cardiac rehabilitation and pharmacological intervention.

Scope

As CHD represents such a broad disease process, in this review we will focus specifically on its principal clinical manifestation, MI, and the pathophysiological processes that lead to this event. We will also discuss current diagnostic procedures and treatment both at the time of an index MI and in the long-term secondary prevention of future events.

Prevalence and impact

Cardiovascular disease (CVD) is amongst the most prevalent global causes of mortality, accounting for over 15 million deaths every year.[1] In the UK in 2000:
- CVD was the main cause of death accounting for more than 245,000 deaths per annum, representing 45% of the total mortality
- the principal manifestations of CVD – CHD and stroke – were responsible for approximately half and one-quarter of all deaths from CVD, respectively

> Each year, over 270,000 people in the UK have an MI, which is fatal in about 50% of cases.

- CHD alone was the most common cause of death, and nearly all deaths from CHD are caused by an MI – commonly called a heart attack over 270,000 people had an MI
- MI accounted for more than 120,000 deaths (one death in five), whilst strokes accounted for one-in-ten deaths.[2]

In addition to these extremely high fatality rates, MI also accounts for an enormous burden of CVD morbidity (Table 1).[2–6] This is likely to increase in the future due to an ageing population and the rapidly increasing prevalence of diabetes, which is itself a risk factor for CHD/MI. These epidemiological data highlight the huge burden of CHD/MI and the management challenge facing medical practitioners. For example, the burden of MI is such that:

- 25% of patients die in the period immediately following an MI
- 10% of survivors of an MI will die within the first year and 5% per year thereafter
- 18% of male and 35% of female survivors will have a recurrent MI within 6 years
- there is a 5-year rate of stroke in MI survivors of 8.1%.[7–10]

However, it must be remembered that many of the common risk factors for MI and CHD are modifiable, either by lifestyle interventions or by pharmacotherapy. For example, high blood lipid levels and high blood pressure can be reduced, smoking can be stopped, exercise levels can be increased and healthier diets adopted. A gradual but steady reduction in mortality from CHD has occurred in the UK since the 1970s, as some of these risk factors have been addressed (Figure 1).[11] In fact, the last 10 years have seen a reduction of 40% in mortality from CHD in adults under 65 years of age.[11]

Table 1. The incidence of new patients per year presenting with vascular disease in the UK population and in a theoretical general practice list of 2000 patients.[2–6]

Condition	Prevalence in the UK	Incidence per 2000 patients
Myocardial infarction[2]	274,000	9.2
Unstable angina/non-ST elevation MI[3]	180,000	6.0
Stroke[4,5]	155,000	5.2
Peripheral artery disease[6]	23,920	0.8

MI, myocardial infarction.

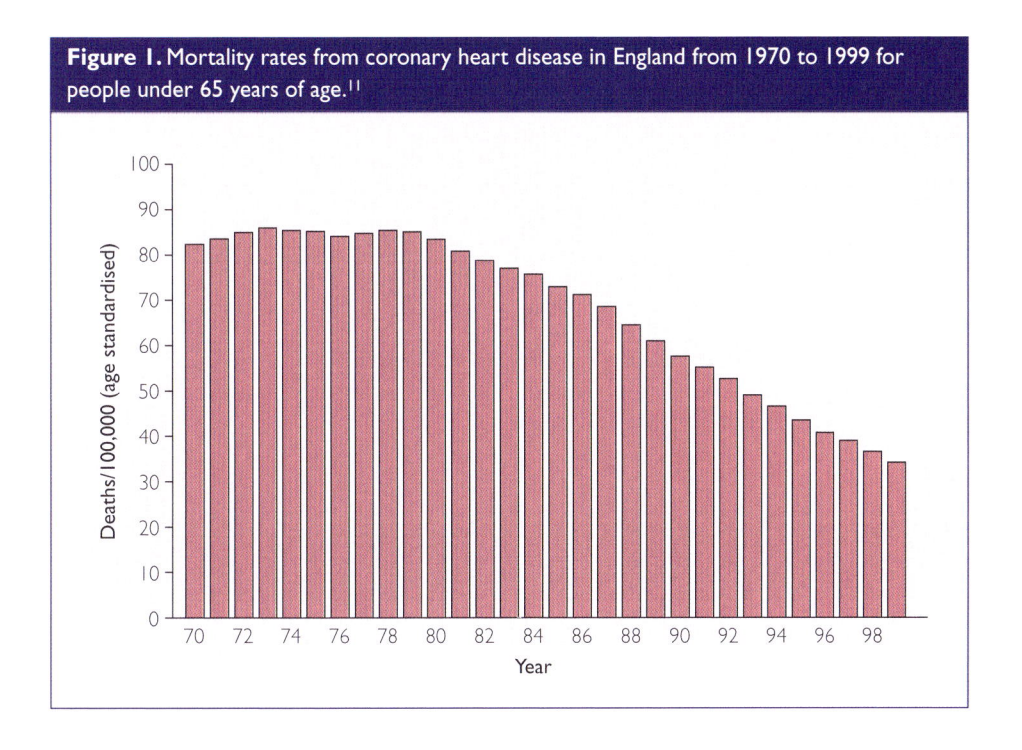

Figure 1. Mortality rates from coronary heart disease in England from 1970 to 1999 for people under 65 years of age.[11]

Clinical presentation of MI

MI can be defined as an infarction of the myocardium that results typically from coronary artery occlusion, that may be marked by sudden chest pain, shortness of breath, nausea, sweating and sometimes loss of consciousness, and which can lead to death. MI should be clearly differentiated from angina. Angina is an indication that part of the myocardium is at times not receiving enough oxygen (e.g. during exercise, when the heart has to work harder). In contrast, MI occurs when blood flow to the heart is suddenly cut off, causing permanent damage to the myocardium. Typically, chest pain associated with MI lasts longer and is more severe than angina, and does not dissipate with rest or with sublingual nitroglycerin medication.[12] In addition, whilst angina is typically a chronic syndrome, MI (by definition) is an acute manifestation of CHD, and, consequently, is often termed acute MI. Some patients, particularly older women, can have silent MI (no symptoms) or atypical chest discomfort, which may go unrecognised.[12] Furthermore, approximately one-third of all MIs go unrecognised.[13] As will be discussed in Pathophysiology of Atherosclerosis, Atherothrombosis and MI, the majority of atherothrombotic events probably do not lead to coronary symptoms (i.e. clinical symptoms of an MI). However, MI is characterised by electrocardiogram (ECG) changes and can be classified into:

- Q-wave infarcts or ST-segment elevation MI (STEMI)
- non-Q-wave infarcts or non-ST-segment elevation MI (NSTEMI).[14]

STEMI is the classical presentation of MI.[12] In STEMI the ECG changes gradually 'evolve' in a sequence, starting with tall, hyperacute T waves and ST-segment elevation, with Q waves appearing over the next few hours or days, the ST segments returning to normal and the T waves becoming inverted (Figure 2).[14] It is usual for a permanent abnormality of the ECG to persist following an MI, and this may take the form of 'pathological' Q waves, though T waves may also remain permanently inverted.[12,14]

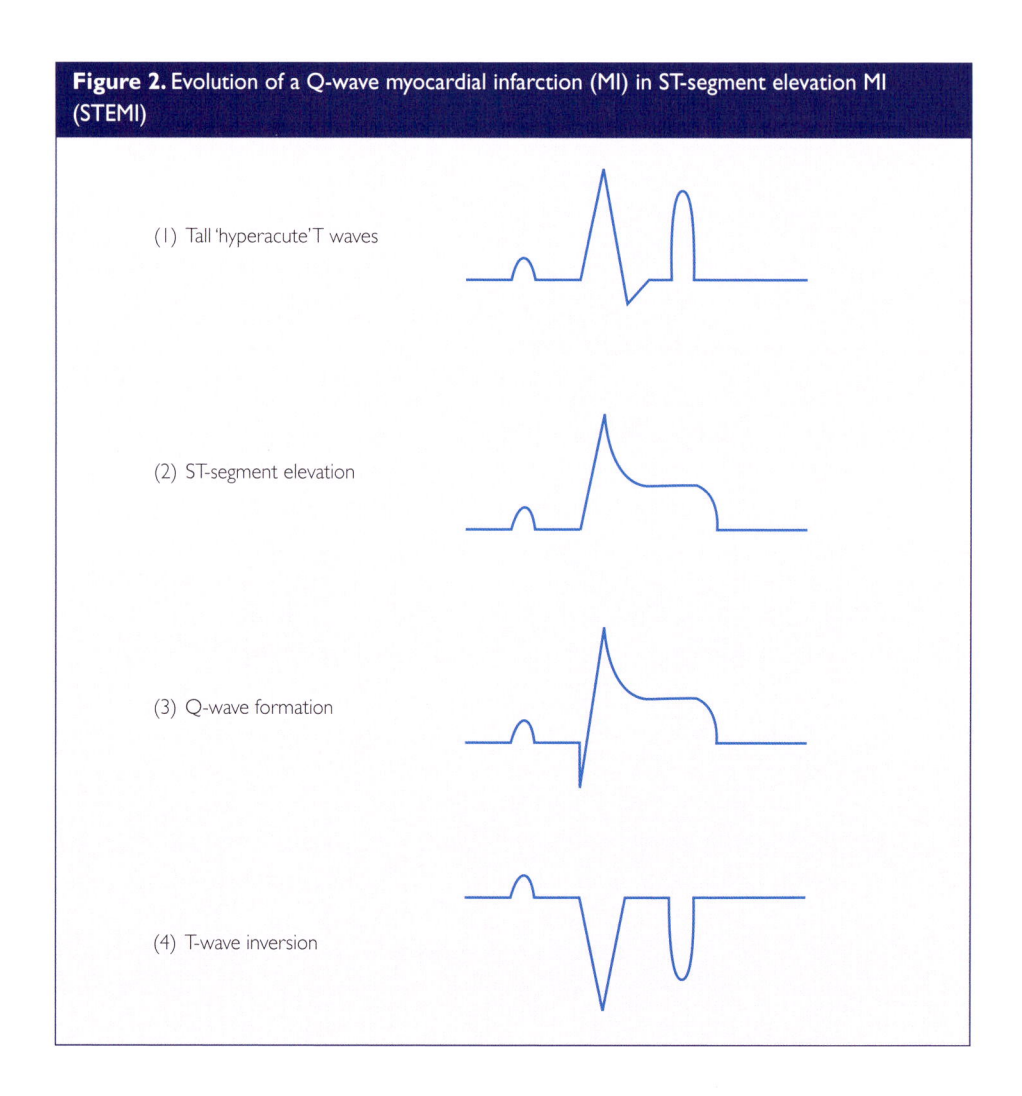

Figure 2. Evolution of a Q-wave myocardial infarction (MI) in ST-segment elevation MI (STEMI)

(1) Tall 'hyperacute' T waves

(2) ST-segment elevation

(3) Q-wave formation

(4) T-wave inversion

Pathophysiology of atherosclerosis, atherothrombosis and MI

MI is a clinical presentation of an underlying problem, namely atherosclerosis. Underlying CHD is usually caused by the progression of a stable atherosclerotic plaque, though a minority of patients may have no obvious angiographic lesion.[15]

Atherosclerosis is a long-term process that causes structural changes in the intimal and medial walls of major arteries, initially resulting in endothelial abnormalities and, ultimately, atherosclerotic plaques. The progression from atherosclerosis to atherothrombosis (atherosclerosis with a superimposed thrombus) usually occurs due to the rupture of the fibrous cap of the plaque or superficial erosion of the endothelial layer.[16] The composition of the plaque rather than the severity of stenosis may be the most important determinant of plaque disruption and subsequent thrombosis.[17] In general, vulnerable or high-risk plaques are characterised by the following features:

- a thin, fibrous cap with disorganised collagen
- a large atheromatous lipid core containing high concentrations of cholesteryl esters
- infiltration by large numbers of macrophages and other inflammatory cells such as T-lymphocytes
- a scarcity of smooth muscle cells
- a high concentration of tissue factor.[16–18]

In contrast, stable plaques are characterised by a small lipid core covered by a thick fibrous cap.

Passive plaque rupture tends to occur more frequently at the shoulders of a plaque, possibly as a consequence of physical forces, blood flow or even due to the high concentrations of macrophages located in these areas. The abundant activated macrophage population within a vulnerable atheroma may be involved in plaque destabilisation through the secretion of proteolytic enzymes, particularly matrix metalloproteinases, which degrade the extracellular matrix components of the fibrous cap.[17] A variety of local, mechanical and haemodynamic forces subject plaques to constant stresses that may trigger disruption of vulnerable plaques (Figure 3).[19] Changes in blood flow due to arterial stenosis, hypertension, dyslipidaemia and irritants in tobacco smoke can also accelerate the process of plaque vulnerability and rupture.[20]

The rupture or erosion of the plaque results in the abrupt exposure of thrombogenic plaque components (e.g. the lipid core, collagen,

> MI is a clinical presentation of an underlying problem, namely atherosclerosis.

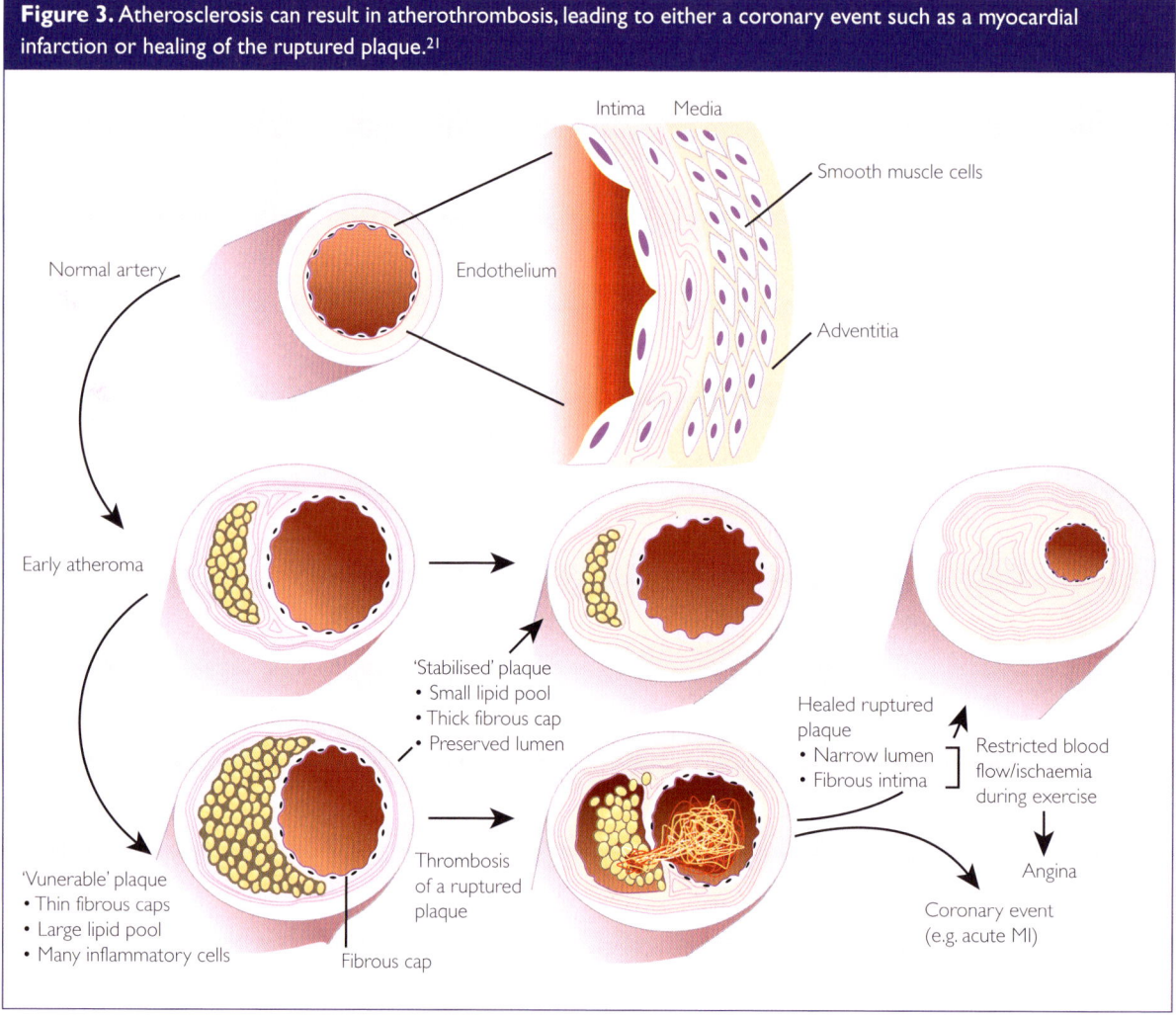

Figure 3. Atherosclerosis can result in atherothrombosis, leading to either a coronary event such as a myocardial infarction or healing of the ruptured plaque.[21]

macrophages and tissue factor) to circulating blood. Although disrupted coronary plaques are frequently found in the arteries of patients who have died of MI, plaque rupture or erosion does not always result in a lumen-occluding thrombus and a subsequent clinical coronary event.[16,19] In fact, most plaque disruptions probably do not cause any coronary symptoms.[21] When the prevailing fibrinolytic mechanisms outweigh the procoagulant pathways this leads to the formation of a limited mural thrombus rather than an occlusive and sustained blood clot.[21] However, though resorption of the mural thrombus can occur, the healing process can lead to fibrous tissue formation, thickening the fibrous cap and causing further expansion of the intima in an inwards direction. It is also possible to stabilise vulnerable plaques to yield a more stable plaque with a thick fibrous cap and preserved lumen diameter (Figure 3). Plaque stabilisation may be achieved through lipid-lowering therapies (e.g. statins), dietary and lifestyle changes, cessation of smoking and angiotensin-converting enzyme (ACE) inhibition.[19]

Risk factors

The major modifiable risk factors for CHD (and thus MI) are:
- dyslipidaemia
- hypertension
- tobacco smoking
- diabetes mellitus.[14]

Non-modifiable risk factors for MI are:
- increased age
- male gender
- family history of CHD.[14]

Diagnosis

MI must be diagnosed quickly and effectively, and it is recommended that patients with suspected MI are transferred as soon as possible to a hospital emergency department.[22,23] A clinical history, physical examination and a 12-lead ECG should be performed and assessed rapidly, and blood samples taken for cardiac enzyme assay. A physical examination may exclude differential diagnoses such as pleuritis, pericarditis or pneumothorax, as well as revealing evidence of ventricular failure and haemodynamic instability.[24] Cardiac markers commonly measured in suspected cases of MI are troponins I and T, creatine kinase (CK) or its isoenzyme CK-MB, aspartate transaminase (AST) and lactate dehydrogenase (LDH). However, changes in cardiac enzyme levels may not be detectable for several hours after an MI, so they have little role to play in the initial diagnosis of an MI.[14] However, they can be useful in the retrospective differentiation between NSTEMI and unstable angina.

Clinical management

Key interventions

Interventions that patients with an MI should receive, unless contra-indicated, can be divided into pre-hospital treatment, hospital treatment and continuing care. Pre-hospital interventions should include:
- cardiopulmonary resuscitation and defibrillation in the event of a cardiac arrest
- oxygen

- pain relief (e.g. intravenous diamorphine or morphine, with co-administered anti-emetic)
- aspirin, at least 300 mg
- immediate transfer to hospital.[25]

Hospital interventions should include:
- aspirin, at least 300 mg, if not given already
- oxygen
- pain relief (e.g. intravenous diamorphine or morphine, with anti-emetic) thrombolytic therapy given without delay (i.e. within 1 hour of the onset of symptoms if possible)
- β-blockers
- ACE inhibitors
- insulin-glucose infusion for people with diabetes.[25]

Continuing care interventions should include:
- patient education (advice about smoking cessation, physical activity levels and diet)
- low-dose aspirin (75 mg/day)
- continued β-blocker therapy
- advice and treatment to maintain blood pressure below 140/85 mmHg
- lipid-lowering pharmacological treatment and omega-3 acid ethyl esters supplementation
- the control of glucose levels in diabetic patients
- the assessment of the potential benefit from coronary revascularisation
- arranging systematic individualised rehabilitation and secondary prevention.[25]

Treatment

Initial/hospital treatment

Treatment of MI prior to and during admission to the emergency department is aimed at keeping infarct size to a minimum and preventing or managing complications. To this end, myocardial reperfusion should be started as soon as possible. Current treatment strategies address the component parts of coronary arterial thrombi – platelets, coagulation proteins and fibrin. Aspirin (or clopidogrel if aspirin is not tolerated) acts as an inhibitor of platelet aggregation. Anticoagulants or thrombolytics (e.g. heparin or warfarin) can inhibit thrombus formation, and fibrinolytics (e.g. streptokinase or recombinant tissue plasminogen activator) may be used to dissolve a thrombus.[26]

Primary angioplasty or coronary artery bypass graft procedures can be used to restore blood flow mechanically to the myocardium, particularly if thrombolysis is contra-indicated or when other reperfusion strategies have failed.[26,27]

Treatment in the community

All patients who have had an MI and do not have heart failure should receive long-term treatment with a β-blocker and an antiplatelet drug (i.e. aspirin or clopidogrel), a statin and an ACE inhibitor, except where contra-indicated.[28] A β-blocker reduces the workload on the heart whilst aspirin at low doses reduces the risk of blood clotting. ACE inhibitors lower blood pressure, have favourable effects on vascular and myocardial remodeling and may have direct anti-atherosclerotic actions.[28] Statins reverse dyslipidaemia, stabilize atherosclerotic plaques and help prevent new plaque formation. Additional treatments for secondary prevention post-MI should also be considered, such as omega-3 acid ethyl esters.[29]

Cardiac rehabilitation is a vital component of both the acute stage of care and secondary prevention in post-MI patients. It should begin as soon as possible after hospital admission and continue through discharge, formal rehabilitation and long-term maintenance therapy.[25] Cardiac rehabilitation has been shown to improve prognosis for patients following MI and other manifestations of CHD.[25] When patients are offered comprehensive and tailored help with modifications to their lifestyle involving education, psychological input and exercise training, cardiac rehabilitation can substantially reduce mortality in post-MI patients by as much as 25% over 3 years.[30,31]

Immunisation

The 'Green Book' recommends that patients with chronic heart disease are protected by annual influenza vaccinations and single pneumococcus vaccinations.[32]

Key points

- CHD is the greatest cause of mortality in the UK and in almost all cases of CHD death is due to an MI.
- In 2000, over 270,000 people in the UK had an MI, accounting for one death in five.
- MI is an infarction of the myocardium that results typically from coronary artery occlusion, that may be marked by sudden chest pain, shortness of breath, nausea, sweating and sometimes loss of consciousness, and which can lead to death.
- MI is a clinical presentation of CHD, and is caused by the rupture of an atherosclerotic plaque and the formation of a lumen-occluding thrombus.
- Patients with a suspected MI should be transferred rapidly to a hospital emergency department and a clinical history, physical examination and a 12-lead ECG should be performed as soon as possible.
- Early treatment of MI (prior to and during admission to the emergency department) can keep infarct size to a minimum and prevent complications. To this end, myocardial reperfusion should be started as soon as possible.
- Long-term treatment of all post-MI patients who do not have heart failure should include a β-blocker and an antiplatelet drug, a statin and an ACE inhibitor, except where contra-indicated.
- Additional treatments for secondary prevention post-MI should also be considered, such as omega-3 acid ethyl esters.
- Cardiac rehabilitation should begin as soon as possible after hospital admission and continue through discharge, formal rehabilitation and long-term maintenance therapy.

References

1. The World Health Organization. *The World Health Report 1997. Conquering Suffering, Enriching Humanity.* Geneva: World Health Organization, 1997.
2. British Heart Foundation website. *http://www.bhf.org.uk/*
3. McDonagh MS, Bachmann LM, Golder S *et al*. A rapid and systematic review of the clinical effectiveness and cost-effectiveness of glycoprotein IIb/IIIa antagonists in the medical management of unstable angina. *Health Technol Assess* 2000; **4**: 1–95.
4. Department of Health. *National Service Framework for Older People.* London: Stationery Office, 2001.
5. Scottish Intercollegiate Guidelines Network. Guideline 13: *Management of Patients with Stroke. Part 1.* Edinburgh: SIGN, 1997.
6. Vascular Surgical Society of Great Britain and Ireland. Critical limb ischaemia: management and outcome – report of a national survey. *Eur J Endovasc Surg* 1995; **10**: 108–13.
7. Mehta RH, Eagle KA. Secondary prevention in acute myocardial infarction. *BMJ* 1998; **316**: 838–42.
8. American Heart Association and American Stroke Association. *Heart and Stroke Statistical Update.* Dallas, 2002.
9. Petrie M, McMurray J. *Prescriber* 1998; **9**: 75–88.
10. Loh E, Sutton MS, Wun CC *et al*. Ventricular dysfunction and the risk of stroke after myocardial infarction. *N Eng J Med* 1997; **336**: 251–7.
11. Petersen S, Rayner M. *Coronary Heart Disease Statistics.* British Heart Foundation statistics database 2002. *http://www.dphpc.ox.ac.uk/bhfhprg/stats/2000/2002/pdf/2002Stats.pdf*
12. Reiner Z. Pathophysiology and classification of cardiovascular diseases caused by atherosclerosis. *J Int Fed Clin Chem Lab Med* 2003; **13**: 1–4.
13. Sigurdsson E, Thorgeirsson G, Sigvaldason H, Sigfusson N. Unrecognized myocardial infarction: epidemiology, clinical characteristics, and the prognostic role of angina pectoris: the Reykjavik study. *Ann Intern Med* 1995; **122**: 96–102.
14. Houghton AR, Gray D. *Making Sense of the ECG. A Hands-on Guide.* 2nd Edition. London: Arnold, 2003.
15. Sheridan PJ, Crossman DC. Critical review of unstable angina and non-ST elevation myocardial infarction. *Postgrad Med J* 2002; **78**: 717–26.
16. Libby P. Multiple mechanisms of thrombosis complicating atherosclerotic plaques. *Clin Cardiol* 2000; **23(Suppl 6)**: VI-3–7.
17. Fuster V, Badimon JJ, Chesebro JH. Atherothrombosis: mechanisms and clinical therapeutic approaches. *Vasc Med* 1998; **3**: 231–9.
18. Willeit J, Kiechl S. Biology of arterial atheroma. *Cerebrovasc Dis* 2000; **10(Suppl 5)**: 1–8.
19. Shah PK. New insights into the pathogenesis and prevention of acute coronary syndromes. *Am J Cardiol* 1997; **79**: 17–23.
20. Leys D. Atherothrombosis: a major health burden. *Cerebrovasc Dis* 2001; **11(Suppl 2)**: 1–4.
21. Libby P. Inflammation in atherosclerosis. *Nature* 2002; **420**: 868–74.
22. Pollack CV, Gibler WB. 2000 ACC/AHA guidelines for the management of patients with unstable angina and non-ST-segment elevation myocardial infarction: a practical summary for emergency physicians. *Ann Emerg Med* 2001; **38**: 229–40.
23. National Institute for Clinical Excellence. *Audit of the Management of Post-MI Patients in Primary Care.* 2002. *www.nice.org.uk*
24. Grech ED, Ramsdale DR. ABC of interventional cardiology. Acute coronary syndrome: unstable angina and non-ST segment elevation myocardial infarction. *BMJ* 2003; **326**: 1259–61.
25. National Service Framework for Coronary Heart Disease. March, 2000.
26. Green GB, Bessman E. Emergency department approach to acute myocardial infarction. In: *Cardiovascular Medicine.* 1st Edn. London: Arnold, 2002: 63–83.
27. Grech ED, Ramsdale DR. ABC of interventional cardiology. Acute coronary syndrome: ST segment elevation myocardial infarction. *BMJ* 2003; **326**: 1379–81.
28. Prodigy Guidance – Prior myocardial infarction – prophylactic treatments. August 2003.
29. Din JN, Newby DE, Flapan AD. Omega 3 fatty acids and cardiovascular disease – fishing for a natural treatment. *BMJ* 2004; **328**: 30–5.
30. Oldridge NB, Guyatt GH, Fisher ME, Rimm AA. Cardiac rehabilitation after myocardial infarction: combined experience of randomised clinical trials. *JAMA* 1998; **260**: 945–50.
31. O'Connor GT, Buring GE, Yusuf S *et al*. An overview of randomised trials of rehabilitation with exercise after myocardial infarction. *Circulation* 1989; **80**: 234–44.
32. Immunisation Against Infectious Disease 1996. 'The Green Book'. *http://www.doh.gov.uk/greenbook*

Acknowledgement

Figure 3 is adapted from Libby, 2002.[21]

12. Depression

Dr Richard Clark and Dr Eleanor Bull
CSF Medical Communications Ltd

Summary

Depression is a widespread mental health problem that causes distress, social impairment, increased mortality and has significant societal costs. Characterised by depressed mood and sadness, a loss of interest in activities and decreased energy, depression may range in severity from a normal degree of sadness to severe illness requiring hospitalisation. Mild-to-moderate disorders predominate in a primary-care setting, although these often go unrecognised and many patients go undiagnosed. Patients themselves may be reluctant to seek help in view of the stigma attached to the disease. Primarily, depression results from the dysfunction of serotonergic and noradrenergic pathways within the central nervous system. Current pharmacological treatments aim to correct the neurochemical imbalance that prevails in depression and restore neurotransmitter function through reuptake inhibition, receptor blockade and monoamine oxidase enzyme inhibition. The selective serotonin reuptake inhibitors (SSRIs) have dominated the treatment of depression over the past 10 years. Tricyclic antidepressants and a number of novel therapeutic agents also have proven efficacy, and in most cases, treatment selection is based on the preferences and suitability of the individual patients and the severity of their disease.

Epidemiology

According to the World Health Organization, depressive disorders are amongst the leading causes of disability, both in terms of years lived with disability, and disability-adjusted life years (Figure 1), depression is an extremely prevalent disorder. Worldwide, the annual prevalence of depression is 5.8% for men and 9.5% for women.[1] The lifetime prevalence is 17% in the US, though figures vary between countries, with 10–25% of women and 5–12% of men suffering from major depression at some point during their lifetime.[2–4] In the UK:

- a recent survey estimated that 12% of people in Britain were suffering from depression; one-quarter of these with depression alone and three-quarters with both depression and anxiety (Figure 2)

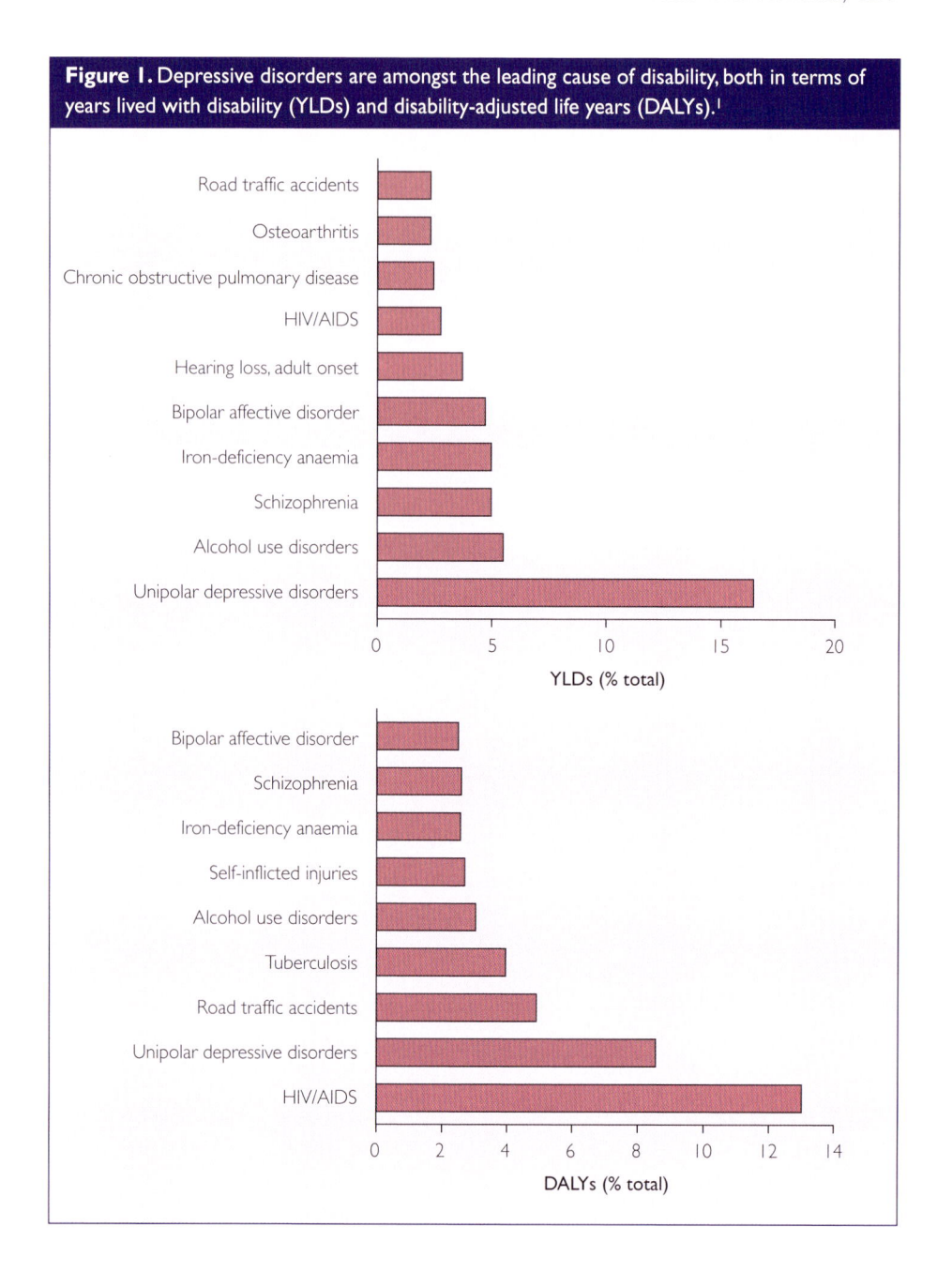

Figure 1. Depressive disorders are amongst the leading cause of disability, both in terms of years lived with disability (YLDs) and disability-adjusted life years (DALYs).[1]

- 5.9% of women and 4.2% of men (approximately 2.9 million people, equivalent to the population of Wales) have depression at any one point in time
- the overwhelming majority of depressed patients are seen by GPs whilst only 3.4% are seen by psychiatrists.[5,6]

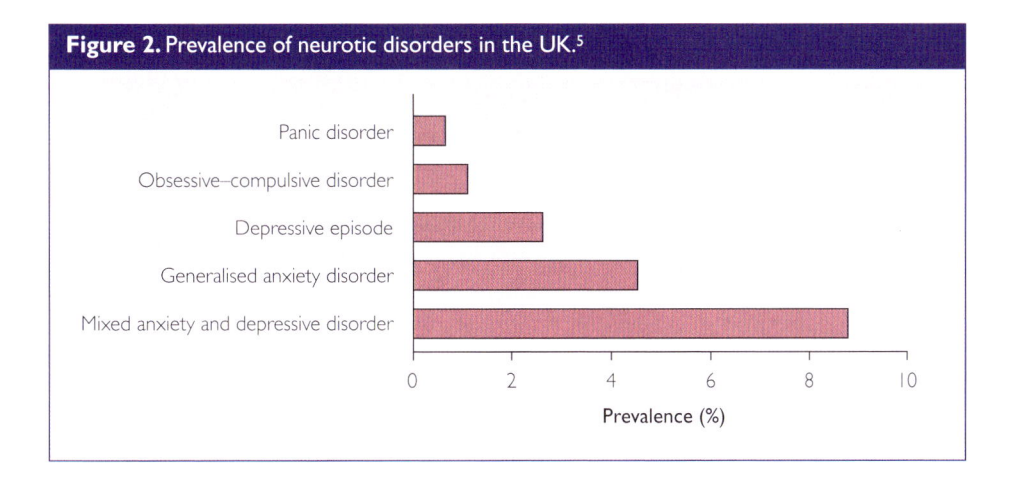

Figure 2. Prevalence of neurotic disorders in the UK.[5]

- Panic disorder
- Obsessive–compulsive disorder
- Depressive episode
- Generalised anxiety disorder
- Mixed anxiety and depressive disorder

Prevalence (%)

Despite the high prevalence of depression, it seems that nearly half of all cases of depression may go unreported, and that when reported, half of these cases may go unrecognised, and even when recognised, are likely to be untreated or mistreated.[7] This is illustrated by a pan-European survey of 78,463 adults who were asked to complete the depressive section of the mini-neuropsychiatric interview (MINI).[8] Of those patients who were depressed, nearly half did not seek any treatment for their condition, over two-thirds had not been prescribed any treatment and only one-quarter had been given antidepressants.

Certain physical conditions such as cancer, stroke, chronic pain, myocardial infarction and Parkinson's disease are often associated with depression, and patients may initially present with somatic symptoms of these diseases.[9,10] Unfortunately, these somatic symptoms may mask depression from the patient and their physician.[10] Alcohol, or other substance abuse, is comorbid with depression in approximately 23% of cases and should also be viewed as a likely indicator of depression.[9] Anxiety and depression are highly comorbid, such that anxiety is often the initial presenting symptom for patients with concomitant depression and anxiety (Figure 3).[9–11] The comorbidity of psychiatric disorders can:
- exacerbate the severity of symptoms
- worsen the overall prognosis
- reduce patients' quality of life
- increase the risk of suicide.[12–14]

Undoubtedly, the overall burden of comorbid depression is substantially greater than that of pure disorders – both in terms of patients' suffering, disability and the course and outcome of their illness, and for the use of healthcare services and the financial burden on the healthcare system.[9]

> Of those patients who were depressed, nearly half did not seek any treatment for their condition, over two-thirds had not been prescribed any treatment and only one-quarter had been given antidepressants.

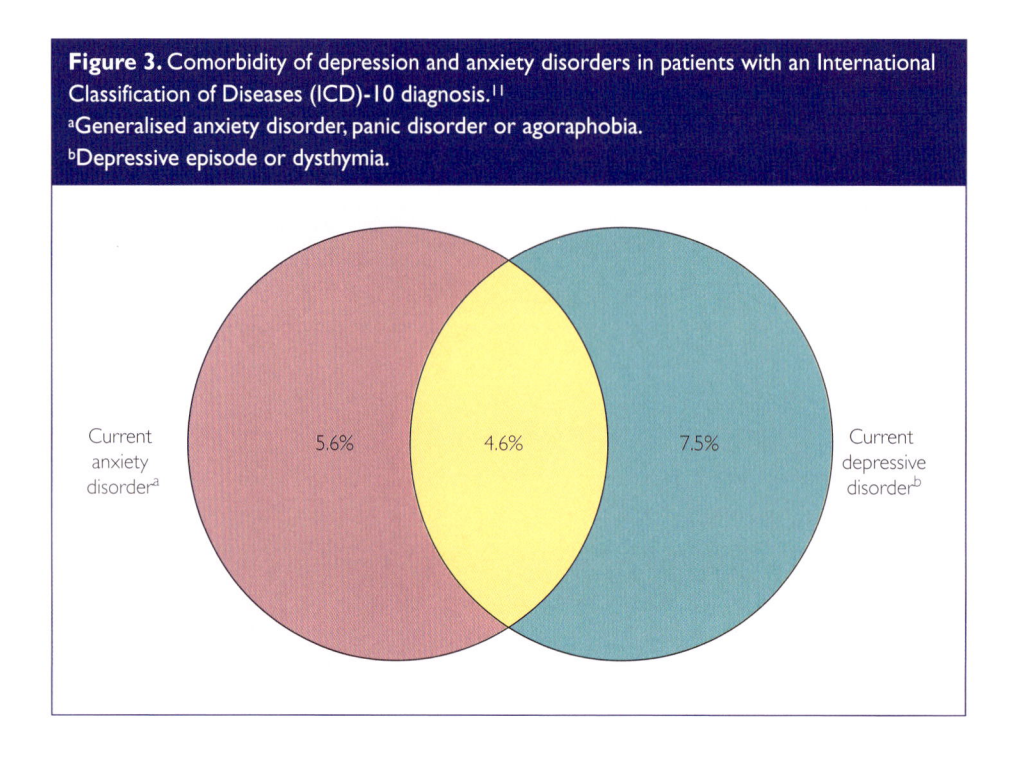

Figure 3. Comorbidity of depression and anxiety disorders in patients with an International Classification of Diseases (ICD)-10 diagnosis.[11]
[a]Generalised anxiety disorder, panic disorder or agoraphobia.
[b]Depressive episode or dysthymia.

Current anxiety disorder[a]: 5.6% | 4.6% | 7.5% : Current depressive disorder[b]

Depression can have significant consequences, and is linked to an increased incidence of suicide, cardiovascular disease, gastrointestinal disorders and physical decline in the elderly.[15–18] Depression has also been linked to cancer and dementia, though usually as a consequence of the former and as a precursor to the latter.[19,20] Certainly, comorbid depression and cancer may affect a patient's prognosis and even their survival.[21]

Although depression can occur at any age, it is often overlooked in young adults, and without prompt and effective intervention their depression can become chronic, with recurrent episodes and/or residual symptoms between episodes.[10,22] Depression is more common in middle age than in the young or elderly. However, depressive symptoms are more likely to be recognised in the elderly, but physicians may be more reluctant to treat this age group for depression.[10] This may be because depression is perceived to be a normal part of the ageing process, or because of a fear of drug interactions in elderly patients with a comorbid physical condition.[10]

Diagnosis

Depression is characterised by affective, cognitive, behavioural and somatic symptoms, some of which – such as hopelessness and low energy – can prevent a patient from actively seeking treatment.[4,23] Even when patients

> Depression is characterised by affective, cognitive, behavioural and somatic symptoms, some of which – such as hopelessness and low energy – can prevent a patient from actively seeking treatment.

present with depression, half of all cases are not diagnosed; thus it is essential to take an informed and rational diagnostic approach.[11] There are two main approaches to the recognition and diagnosis of depression:
- asking patients to complete a depression questionnaire during a routine appointment
- evaluating patients only when clinical presentation triggers the suspicion of depression.[24]

If a patient presents with one or more of the following factors then the likelihood of a depressive disorder is increased markedly:
- chronic medical illness
- chronic pain syndrome
- recent life change or stressor
- fair or poor self-rated health
- unexplained physical symptoms.[25]

Many diagnostic instruments can be used to aid the diagnosis of depression (with or without comorbid anxiety). However, many of these have significant limitations when used in a primary-care setting. They may be time consuming, a wide range of the most common disorders are not covered, their sensitivity or validity have not have been fully explored or few language translations are available.[26] The International Consensus Group on Depression and Anxiety has developed the MINI for both Diagnostic and Statistical Manual of Mental Disorders (DSM)-IV and International Classification of Diseases (ICD)-10 psychiatric disorders in order to overcome these problems. The proposed two-stage process should theoretically detect over 90% of psychiatric conditions encountered by GPs.
- **Screening:** ten questions are used to cover the most prevalent psychiatric disorders (depression, panic disorder, social anxiety disorder, generalised anxiety disorder [GAD] and post-traumatic stress disorder), with the use of additional optional screening questions for the diagnosis of dysthymia, bipolar disorder and obsessive–compulsive disorder.
- **Diagnosis:** diagnostic confirmatory questions are asked for each disorder highlighted by the patient at the screening stage.[26]

The appropriate screening and diagnostic questions for depression are shown in Figure 4.[26]

The International Consensus Group on Depression and Anxiety has also specified that patients with the following diagnoses should be referred to specialist psychiatric care:
- high suicide risk
- severe depression

> **Figure 4.** Screening (recognition) and diagnostic questions for depression.[26]
> [a]Ideally, screening questions for anxiety disorders should also be used due to the high prevalence of comorbid depression and anxiety.
>
> *Screening questions for depression*[a]
> - Have you been consistently depressed or down, most of the day, nearly every day, for the past 2 weeks?
> - In the past 2 weeks, have you been less interested in most things or less able to enjoy the things that you used to enjoy most of the time?
>
> If yes to either question proceed to diagnostic questions for current major depressive episode.
>
> *Diagnostic questions for current major depressive episode*
> Over the past 2 weeks, when you felt depressed or uninterested:
> - Was your appetite decreased or increased nearly every day? Did your weight decrease or increase without trying intentionally? [If yes to either, code as yes.]
> - Did you have trouble sleeping nearly every night?
> - Did you talk or move more slowly than normal, or were you fidgety, restless or having trouble sitting still almost every day?
> - Did you feel tired or without energy almost every day?
> - Did you feel worthless or guilty almost every day?
> - Did you have difficulty concentrating or making decisions almost every day?
> - Did you repeatedly consider hurting yourself, feel suicidal, or wish that you were dead?
>
> If five or more yes answers are given (appetite/weight questions count as one question) then a current major depressive episode can be diagnosed.

- melancholia
- bipolar disorder
- obsessive–compulsive disorder
- substance abuse.[26]

Furthermore, GPs should refer a patient to a psychiatrist if treatment has been initiated in the primary-care setting and the patient's response has been poor, or a patient's clinical prognosis is deteriorating. Referral should also be considered if a patient has a comorbid psychiatric disorder that requires high drug doses or is taking multiple medications or monoamine oxidase inhibitors (MAOIs).[26]

Aetiology and risk factors

Depression is a complex disease and a number of factors may predispose an individual to disease development. There is evidence for genetic and psychosocial determinants, as well as a marked influence of the comorbid disease status of the individual patient.[27]

Genetic predisposition

The inheritance of mood disorders is complex and is unlikely to be determined by dysfunction in a single gene.[28] To date, regions of chromosomes 4, 5, 11, 12, 18 and 21 and the X-chromosome have been implicated in the pathogenesis of depression and a number of candidate genes have been proposed. Genes that code for elements of the serotonergic pathway (e.g. tryptophan hydroxylase, 5-HT transporter, 5-HT$_{2A}$ receptor) are of particular interest and have been associated with suicide and suicidal behaviour.[29]

Psychosocial stressors

There is evidence to suggest that psychosocial stressors in later life, including the death or illness of a relative, marital problems, social isolation and adverse living conditions, play an important role in determining an individual's susceptibility to depression.[30] Furthermore, the impact of these psychosocial risk factors can be enhanced or buffered by personal or environmental factors.[30] Early life experiences may impact on the development of depressive and anxiety disorders, such that children who have been abused either sexually or physically, or who have suffered the death of a parent, are at a higher risk of disease development in later life.[31]

Comorbid disorders or disease

As discussed previously, depression is often comorbid with a number of other diseases including anxiety, stroke, rheumatoid arthritis, dementia, Parkinson's disease, cancer and chronic pain. The relatively high incidence of depression amongst those patients with vascular disease may be partly explained by the 'vascular depression' hypothesis, which proposes that vascular disease may predispose to, precipitate or perpetuate depression.[32] Factors such as hypothalamic–pituitary–adrenal dysregulation, diminished heart rate variability, altered blood platelet function and non-compliance with medial treatments have been proposed as mechanisms underlying the link between depression and cardiovascular disease.[33]

Pathophysiology

Depression is thought to be primarily associated with disturbances in the serotonin, noradrenaline and dopamine neurotransmitter systems, though other mechanisms involving corticotropin-releasing factor and somatostatin may also be involved.[34] The serotonergic and noradrenergic systems are altered most consistently in depressed patients.[35] Thus, antidepressant therapies that target both of these systems might, in theory, be more effective than those affecting a single system.[36] A relative serotonin deficiency has been linked to depression, as suggested by:

- low levels of 5-hydroxyindoleacetic acid (5-HIAA), the major serotonin metabolite, in the cerebrospinal fluid (CSF) of depressed and suicidal patients
- increased density of serotonin receptors in post-mortem brain tissue of depressed and suicidal patients
- decreased density of the serotonin transporter in the brain, detected by functional brain imaging and in post-mortem tissue studies
- efficacy of SSRIs as highly effective antidepressants.[34,35]

Noradrenaline circuit dysfunction has also been linked to depression, as suggested by:

- low levels of noradrenaline metabolites in the urine and CSF of depressed patients
- increased density of noradrenaline receptors in the cortex of depressed patients (post-mortem studies)
- efficacy of noradrenaline reuptake inhibitors as effective antidepressants.[34,35]

Figure 5 illustrates the action of neurotransmitters at nerve synapses, and shows the various stages at which a therapeutic intervention could address an imbalance in specific neurotransmitters.

Clinical management of depression

For patients with depression, the management approach is largely dictated by disease severity. Some drug treatments may prove to be no better than placebo against milder cases of depression, whereas patients with more severe disease tend to respond better to pharmacological intervention.[37] All patients should be assessed on an individual basis and an appropriate management programme tailored to address their needs. Treatment recommendations outlined in a 2001 update of guidelines issued in 1993 by the British Association of Psychopharmacology are presented in Table 1.[38]

Non-pharmacological intervention

Psychotherapy

Counselling, as a non-pharmacological treatment approach, may be preferable or more suitable for some patients, particularly those with milder

Figure 5. The action of neurotransmitters at the synaptic cleft. Most antidepressants are designed to increase the concentration of certain target neurotransmitter(s) at the neuronal synapse. This can be achieved by one or more of the following therapeutic actions: boosting synthesis of the neurotransmitter, blocking its degradation, preventing its reuptake from the synapse into the presynaptic neurone, or mimicking its binding to postsynaptic receptors.

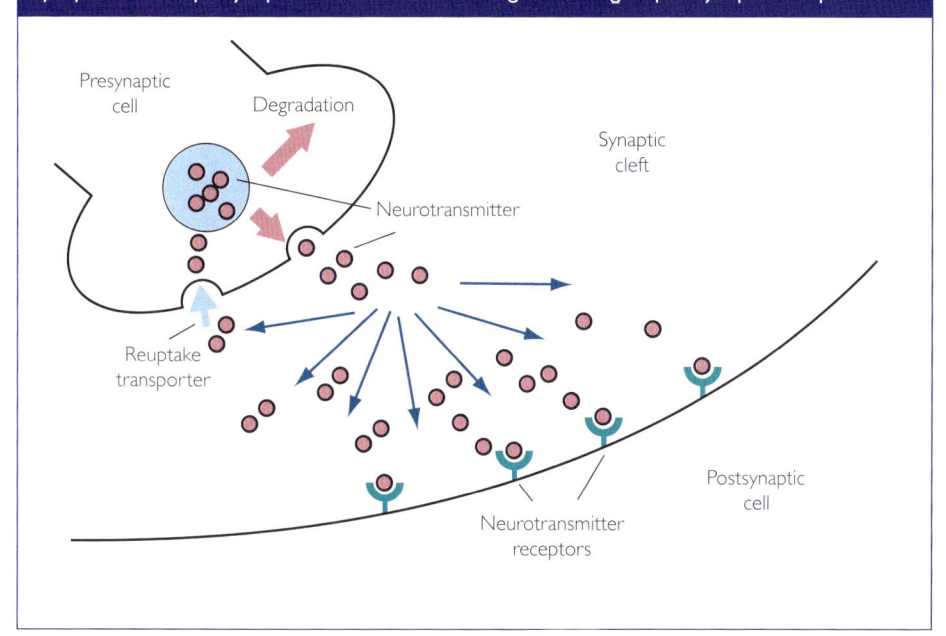

Table 1. Management approaches to depression.[38]

Type of depression	Severity	Recommended treatment approach
Major depression	Mild-to-moderate	• Antidepressant therapy (benefit uncertain for mildest disease severity). • Specific psychological treatments are an effective alternative to antidepressants.
	Severe (hospitalised)	• Antidepressant therapy (used in preference to psychological treatments).
Dysthymia		• Antidepressant therapy (used in preference to psychological treatments).
Milder depression		• Education, support, simple problem solving. • Monitoring for persistence or the development of major depression. • Antidepressants not indicated unless depression persists or there is a history of major depression.

forms of depression.[38] Other patients may benefit from psychotherapy in conjunction with drug treatment.[39] In one study, a generic counselling programme, incorporating six sessions with an experienced councillor, was as effective as antidepressant therapy for the management of mild-to-moderate depressive illness, although there was some evidence that recovery was more rapid with drug treatment.[40] Psychotherapeutic approaches include cognitive behaviour therapy, interpersonal psychotherapy and problem-solving therapy. Of these, no approach emerges as superior to the others, although comparative studies are limited in number.[38]

Electroconvulsive therapy (ECT)

ECT, the stimulation of the brain through electrodes placed on either side of the head, can be effective in the acute treatment of late-life depression.[41] In some patients, ECT may prove more effective than drug treatment, although further investigation of long-term efficacy, morbidity and mortality risks and cost-effectiveness is required.[41,42]

Repetitive transcranial magnetic stimulation (rTMS)

The repeated administration of high-frequency TMS to the cortex may correct some of the cortical abnormalities associated with depression (e.g. altered functioning of fronto-limbic circuits).[43] A novel treatment, rTMS is a non-invasive technique and may serve as a useful alternative to the more invasive ECT in those patients who do not tolerate or respond to drug treatment.[43] Although small in size, the majority of controlled trials of rTMS have demonstrated antidepressant effects compared with a sham condition.[43] However, further evidence derived from large-scale trials is needed before firm conclusions can be drawn as to the benefits of rTMS.[44]

Pharmacological intervention

The majority of patients with depression are managed with drug therapy. Perceptions of antidepressants are largely dependent on the severity of the disease. For milder forms of depression, drugs are generally rated in terms of their tolerability rather than their therapeutic efficacy, whereas patients with severe disease will be more tolerant of side-effects in exchange for symptom relief. Irrespective of the drug selected, approximately 60% of patients with major depression respond to their initial treatment (i.e. a reduction of at least 50% in symptom ratings).[37] The remaining 40% of patients either respond partially or not at all.[37]

> Irrespective of the drug selected, approximately 60% of patients with major depression respond to their initial treatment.

Antidepressants have evolved considerably over the past 50 years (Figure 6).[45] Formerly the cornerstone of treatment, the tricyclic antidepressants have been largely surpassed by the introduction of the SSRIs, which have a more favourable side-effect profile and similar efficacy. Generally, the onset of action of antidepressants is 1–4 weeks, although some agents may take effect more rapidly than others.[37] Following remission of symptoms, treatment should continue at the same dose for at least 4–6 months in order to avoid precipitating adverse events.[46] Patients should be checked regularly for response, compliance, adverse events and suicidal ideation.[37]

Tricyclic antidepressants

The tricyclic antidepressants (e.g. amitriptyline, clomipramine, doxepin, imipramine) act by modulating noradrenergic and serotonergic neurotransmission. The widespread use of some of these agents has been hampered by a considerable side-effect profile and associations with adverse anticholinergic and cardiovascular effects, including arrhythmias and heart block.[45,46] Tricyclic antidepressants are also particularly dangerous in overdose, an inherent risk when medicating patients with depression and

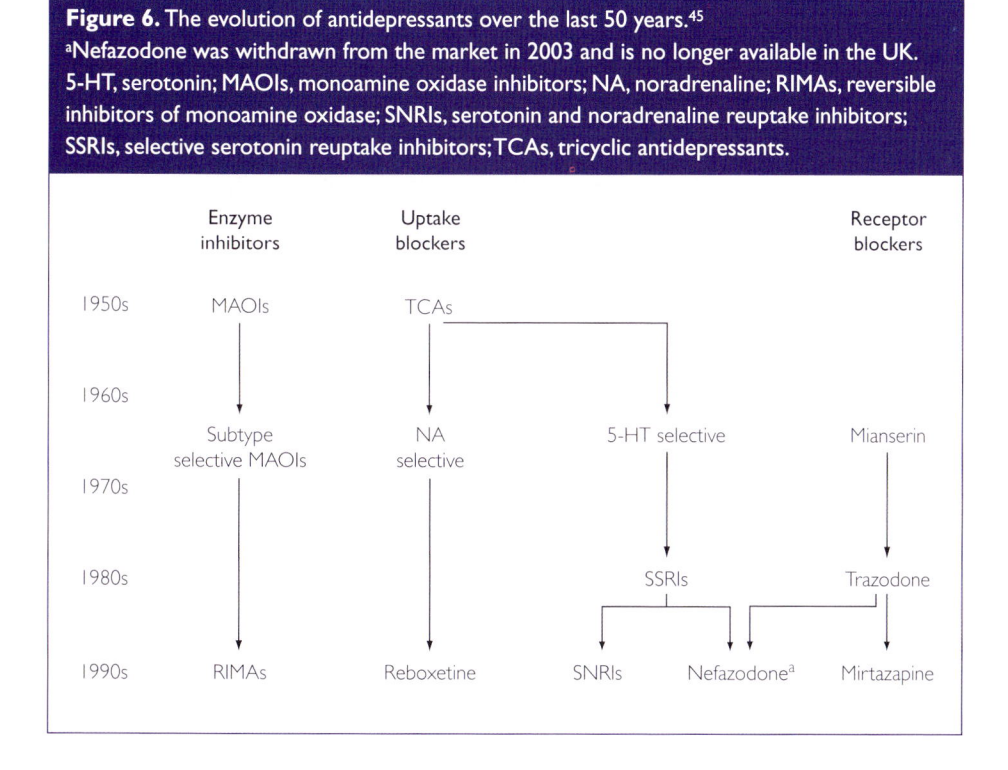

Figure 6. The evolution of antidepressants over the last 50 years.[45]
[a]Nefazodone was withdrawn from the market in 2003 and is no longer available in the UK.
5-HT, serotonin; MAOIs, monoamine oxidase inhibitors; NA, noradrenaline; RIMAs, reversible inhibitors of monoamine oxidase; SNRIs, serotonin and noradrenaline reuptake inhibitors; SSRIs, selective serotonin reuptake inhibitors; TCAs, tricyclic antidepressants.

Decade	Enzyme inhibitors	Uptake blockers			Receptor blockers
1950s	MAOIs	TCAs			
1960s					
1970s	Subtype selective MAOIs	NA selective	5-HT selective		Mianserin
1980s			SSRIs		Trazodone
1990s	RIMAs	Reboxetine	SNRIs	Nefazodone[a]	Mirtazapine

suicidal ideation, and should only be prescribed in limited quantities at a time.[46] Despite these adverse events, the tricyclic antidepressants are highly effective against depression, especially in those patients with severe disease, provided the side-effect profile can be tolerated.

SSRIs

The SSRIs (e.g. citalopram, escitalopram, fluoxetine, paroxetine, sertraline) have dominated the treatment of depression in recent years.[45] By selectively blocking the reuptake of serotonin into the nerve terminal, SSRIs enhance serotonergic neurotransmission and reduce the symptoms of depression with an efficacy comparable with that of the tricyclic agents. However, their efficacy is inferior to that of the tricyclic agents in patients with severe depression. Adverse events associated with SSRIs include nausea, diarrhoea, anxiety, agitation, insomnia, anorexia and sexual dysfunction, although these drugs are less cardiotoxic in overdose than the tricyclic antidepressants.[46]

MAOIs

By inhibiting the monoamine oxidase enzyme, MAOIs (e.g. isocarboxazid, phenelzine, tranylcypromine) prevent the metabolism of serotonin, noradrenaline and dopamine, thus increasing the extracellular concentrations of these neurotransmitters. MAOIs are used less frequently than the SSRIs and tricyclic antidepressants, owing to their potentially dangerous interactions with certain foods (e.g. those containing tyramine) and other drugs.[46]

Other antidepressants

There are a number of antidepressants with unique pharmacological profiles which do not fit into the above classes. These include the noradrenergic and specific serotonergic antidepressant, mirtazapine, and the serotonin and noradrenaline reuptake inhibitor (SNRI), venlafaxine. These agents may be particularly useful in patients who do not respond to SSRIs. Indeed, the available evidence points to a more rapid onset of action for mirtazapine, whilst at certain doses venlafaxine has been shown to exhibit greater efficiency than the SSRIs. Both agents also appear to be useful choices in treating severe depression.

Management of elderly patients

The selection of an antidepressant for the treatment of elderly patients is highly dependent on its tolerability profile. In view of the increased likelihood of comorbid disease and polypharmacy, adverse events and drug–drug interactions are particularly pertinent and may complicate disease management in this patient population.[47] For example, the SSRIs are the preferred treatment option for patients with cardiovascular or cerebrovascular disease, although there is some evidence to suggest that these agents may aggravate the symptoms of Parkinson's disease.[47] Mirtazapine has been shown to be effective in treating elderly depressed patients.

Socioeconomic impact

Depression is prevalent but highly treatable, and yet under-recognition and under-treatment of this disorder has profound socioeconomic consequences.[48] The economic cost of depression is enormous. In the USA, in 1990, depression cost US$44 billion.[49]

- Direct costs (inpatient, outpatient and pharmaceutical costs) were US$12 billion per annum.
- Indirect costs arising from absenteeism from work and reduced productivity whilst at work were US$24 billion per annum.
- Other direct costs arising from depression-related suicides were estimated to cost US$8 billion per annum.

In the UK, the direct cost per year of depression has been estimated at between £220 million and £417 million, with additional indirect annual costs that may exceed £3 billion.[50,51] Cost–benefit analyses indicate that appropriate treatment of depression could provide indirect cost savings that would far outweigh the direct costs associated with such treatments.[52] The number of days of work lost correlates directly with the severity of depression, with those suffering with major depression losing four-times as many working days as those without depression over a 6-month period.[8] Furthermore, the likelihood of depressed subjects being out of paid employment is related to the severity of the depression.[8] Clearly, depression has a major international socioeconomic impact.

Key points

- Depression is widespread, has profound consequences for individuals and society as a whole, and is a leading cause of disability.
- Characterised by hopelessness and a lack of energy, depression affects patients of all ages, although it may be overlooked in young adolescents and the elderly.
- Depressed patients often present with a somatic disorder such as a chronic medical illness, chronic pain or unexplained physical symptoms.
- Depression is primarily associated with disturbances in the serotonin and noradrenaline neurotransmitter systems.
- The management of depression is principally pharmacological, with the SSRIs and tricyclic antidepressant agents representing the cornerstone of drug therapy.
- However, delay in onset of therapeutic action and drug-specific side-effects may affect patient satisfaction and ultimately compliance.
- Depression has profound socioeconomic consequences and cost–benefit analyses indicate that the appropriate treatment of depression could provide indirect cost savings that would far outweigh the direct costs associated with such treatments.

References

1. World Health Organization. *World Health Report 2001. Mental Health: New Understanding, New Hope.* Geneva: WHO, 2001.
2. Lecrubier Y. Prescribing patterns for depression and anxiety worldwide. *J Clin Psychiatry* 2001; **62(Suppl 13)**: 31–6.
3. Kessler RC, McGonagle KA, Zhao S et al. Lifetime and 12-month prevalence of DSM-III-R psychiatric disorders in the United States. Results from the National Comorbidity Survey. *Arch Gen Psychiatry* 1994; **51**: 8–19.
4. American Psychiatric Association. *Diagnostic and Statistical Manual of Mental Disorders.* 4th Edition. Washington, DC: American Psychiatric Association, 1994.
5. Singleton N, Bumpstead R, O'Brien M, Lee A, Meltzer H. *Psychiatric morbidity among adults living in private households (2000).* The Office for National Statistics. London: The Stationery Office, 2001.
6. Ohayon MM, Priest RG, Guilleminault C et al. The prevalence of depressive disorders in the UK. *Biol Psychiatry* 1999; **45**: 300–7.
7. Tylee A. Depression in the community: physician and patient perspective. *J Clin Psychiatry* 1999; **60(Suppl 7)**: 12–16.
8. Lepine JP, Gastpar M, Mendlewicz J, Tylee A. Depression in the community: the first pan-European study DEPRES (Depression Research in European Society). *Int Clin Psychopharmacol* 1997; **12**: 19–29.
9. Wittchen H-U, Lieb R, Wunderlich U, Schuster P. Comorbidity in primary care: presentation and consequences. *J Clin Psychiatry* 1999; **60(Suppl 7)**: 29–36.
10. Ballenger JC, Davidson JR, Lecrubier Y et al. Consensus statement on the primary care management of depression from the International Consensus Group on Depression and Anxiety. *J Clin Psychiatry* 1999; **60(Suppl 7)**: 54–61.
11. Sartorius N, Ustun TB, Lecrubier Y, Wittchen HU. Depression comorbid with anxiety: results from the WHO study on psychological disorders in primary health care. *Br J Psychiatry* 1996; **30(Suppl)**: 38–43.
12. Rouillon F. Anxiety with depression: a treatment need. *Eur Neuropsychopharmacol* 1999; **9**: S87–92.
13. Clayton PJ. The comorbidity factor: establishing the primary diagnosis in patients with mixed symptoms of anxiety and depression. *J Clin Psychiatry* 1990; **51(Suppl 11)**: 35–9.
14. Zajecka JM, Ross JS. Management of comorbid anxiety and depression. *J Clin Psychiatry* 1995; **56(Suppl 2)**: 10–13.
15. Inskip HM, Harris EC, Barraclough B. Lifetime risk of suicide for affective disorder, alcoholism and schizophrenia. *Br J Psychiatry* 1998; **172**: 35–7.
16. Nemeroff CB, Musselman DL, Evans DL. Depression and cardiac disease. *Depress Anxiety* 1998; **8(Suppl 1)**: 71–9.
17. Ballenger JC, Davidson JRT, Lecrubier Y et al. Consensus statement on depression, anxiety and functional gastrointestinal disorders. *J Clin Psychiatry* 2001; **62(Suppl 8)**: 48–51.
18. Penninx BW, Guralnik JM, Ferrucci L, Simonsick EM, Deeg DJ, Wallace RB. Depressive symptoms and physical decline in community-dwelling older persons. *JAMA* 1998; **279**: 1720–6.
19. Penninx BW, Guralnik JM, Pahor M et al. Chronically depressed mood and cancer risk in older persons. *J Natl Cancer Inst* 1998; **90**: 1888–93.
20. Jorm AF. Is depression a risk factor for dementia or cognitive decline? A review. *Gerontology* 2000; **46**: 219–27.
21. Ballenger JC, Davidson JR, Lecrubier Y, Nutt DJ, Jones RD, Berard RM. International Consensus Group on Depression and Anxiety. Consensus statement on depression, anxiety, and oncology. *J Clin Psychiatry* 2001; **62(Suppl 8)**: 64–7.
22. Wunderlich U, Bronisch T, Wittchen H-U. Comorbidity patterns in adolescents and young adults with suicide attempts. *Eur Arch Psychiatry Clin Neurosci* 1998; **248**: 87–95.
23. World Health Organization. *International Statistical Classification of Diseases and Related Health Problems, tenth revision (ICD-10).* Geneva: WHO, 1992.
24. Williams JW, Nöel PH, Cordes JA, Ramirez G, Pignone M. Is this patient clinically depressed? *JAMA* 2002; **287**: 1160–70.
25. Kroenke K, Spitzer RL, Williams JB et al. Physical symptoms in primary care: predictors of psychiatric disorders and functional impairment. *Arch Fam Med* 1994; **3**: 774–9.
26. Ballenger JC, Davidson JRT, Lecrubier Y, Nutt DJ (International Consensus Group on Depression and Anxiety). A proposed algorithm for improved recognition and treatment of the depression/anxiety spectrum in primary care. *Primary Care Companion J Clin Psychiatry* 2001; **3**: 44–52.
27. Riso L, Miyatake R, Thase M. The search for determinants of chronic depression: a review of six factors. *J Affect Disord* 2002; **70**: 103–15.
28. Souery D, Rivelli S, Mendlewicz J. Molecular genetic and family studies in affective disorders: state of the art. *J Affect Disord* 2001; **62**: 45–55.
29. Du L, Faludi G, Palkovits M, Bakish D, Hrdina P. Serotonergic genes and suicidality. *Crisis* 2001; **22**: 54–60.
30. Bruce M. Psychosocial risk factors for depressive disorders in late life. *Biol Psychiatry* 2002; **52**: 175–84.
31. Nemeroff C. Neurobiological consequences of childhood trauma. *J Clin Psychiatry* 2004; **65**: 18–28.
32. Thomas A, Kalaria R, O'Brien J. Depression and vascular disease: what is the relationship? *J Affect Disord* 2004; **79**: 81–5.
33. Grippo A, Johnson A. Biological mechanisms in the relationship between depression and heart disease. *Neurosci Biobehav Rev* 2002; **26**: 941–62.
34. Nemeroff CB. The neurobiology of depression. *Sci Am* 1998; **278**: 42–9.
35. Garlow SJ, Musselman DL, Nemeroff CB. The neurochemistry of mood disorders: clinical studies. In: Charney DS, Nestler EJ, Bunney BS, eds. *Neurobiology of Mental Illness.* New York and Oxford: Oxford University Press, 1999.
36. Nelson JC. Synergistic benefits of serotonin and noradrenaline reuptake inhibition. *Depress Anxiety* 1998; **7(Suppl 1)**: 5–6.
37. Spigset O, Martensson B. Fortnightly review: drug treatment of depression. *BMJ* 1999; **318**: 1188–91.
38. Anderson I, Nutt D, Deakin J. Evidence-based guidelines for treating depressive disorders with antidepressants: a revision of the 1993 British Association for Psychopharmacology guidelines.British Association for Psychopharmacology. *J Psychopharmacol.* 2000; **14**: 3–20

39 Persons J, Thase M, Crits-Christoph P. The role of psychotherapy in the treatment of depression: review of two practice guidelines. *Arch Gen Psychiatry* 1996; **53**: 283–90.
40 Chilvers C, Dewey M, Fielding K *et al.* Antidepressant drugs and generic counselling for treatment of major depression in primary care: randomised trial with patient preference arms. *BMJ* 2001; **322**: 1–5.
41 van der Wurff F, Stek M, Hoogendijk W, Beekman A. The efficacy and safety of ECT in depressed older adults: a literature review. *Int J Geriatr Psychiatry* 2003; **18**: 894–904.
42 UK ECT Review Group. Efficacy and safety of electroconvulsive therapy in depressive disorders: a systematic review and meta-analysis. *Lancet* 2003; **361**: 799–808.
43 Padberg F, Moller H. Repetitive transcranial magnetic stimulation: does it have potential in the treatment of depression? *CNS Drugs* 2003; **17**: 383–403.
44 Martin J, Barbanoj M, Schlaepfer T et al. Repetitive transcranial magnetic stimulation for the treatment of depression. Systematic review and meta-analysis. *Br J Psychiatry* 2003; **182**: 480–91.
45 Artigas F, Nutt DJ, Shelton R. Mechanism of action of antidepressants. *Psychopharmacol Bull* 2002; **36 Suppl 2**: 123–32.
46 *British National Formulary (BNF) 47*. London: the British Medical Association and the Royal Pharmaceutical Society of Great Britain, September 2004.
47 Baldwin R, Anderson D, Black S *et al*. Guideline for the management of late-life depression in primary care. *Int J Geriatr Psychiatry* 2003; **18**: 829–38.
48 Davidson JR, Meltzer-Brody SE. The underrecognition and undertreatment of depression: what is the breadth and depth of the problem? *J Clin Psychiatry* 1999; **60(Suppl 7)**: 4–9.
49 Greenberg PE, Stiglin LE, Finkelstein SN, Berndt ER. The economic burden of depression in 1990. *J Clin Psychiatry* 1993; **54**: 405–18.
50 Jonsson B, Bebbington PE. What price depression? The cost of depression and the cost-effectiveness of pharmacological treatment. *Br J Psychiatry* 1994; **164**: 665–73.
51 Kind P, Sorensen J. The costs of depression. *Int Clin Psychopharmacol* 1993; **7**: 191–5.
52 Simon GE, Barber C, Birnbaum HG *et al*. Depression and work productivity: the comparative costs of treatment versus nontreatment. *J Occup Environ Med* 2001;**43**: 2–9.

Acknowledgements

Figure 3 is adapted from Sartorius *et al*., 1996.[11]
Figure 4 is adapted from Ballenger *et al*., 2001.[26]
Figure 6 is adapted from Artigas *et al*., 2002.[45]

13. Diabetes

Dr Richard Clark
CSF Medical Communications Ltd

Summary

The term diabetes mellitus describes a metabolic disorder of multiple aetiology characterised by chronic hyperglycaemia with disturbances of carbohydrate, fat and protein metabolism resulting from defects in insulin secretion, insulin action, or both. Symptoms such as polyuria and polydipsia are indicative of diabetes, but abnormal hyperglycaemia (fasting plasma glucose [FPG] >7.0 mmol/L or random plasma glucose >11.1 mmol/L) are required to confirm a diagnosis.

Epidemiology and impact of diabetes

The global prevalence of diabetes is increasing dramatically, with the number of people with diabetes predicted to rise from about 118 million in 1995, to 220 million in 2010 and 300 million in 2025.[1,2] Most cases are type 2 diabetes, which has the highest prevalence in developed countries as it is strongly associated with obesity and a sedentary lifestyle.[3] In the UK:

- there are approximately 1.4 million people with diabetes (about 2% of the population), and an estimated further 1 million undiagnosed cases[4,5]
- approximately 85–90% of diabetics have type 2 diabetes[1,6]
- the prevalence of diabetes increases with age (Figure 1)[6,7]
- 1 in 20 people over the age of 65 and 1 in 5 people over the age of 85 have type 2 diabetes[6]
- there is a slightly higher prevalence of type 2 diabetes amongst men than women (Figure 1).[7]

There are ethnic variations in the prevalence of diabetes. In the UK, diabetes is six times more common in people of South-Asian descent and up to three times more common in those of African and Afro-Caribbean descent, compared with the Caucasian population.[6] It is noteworthy that in Indo-Asians the prevalence of type 2 diabetes can be as high as 12% in the UK, and that the condition generally presents at an earlier age.[8,9]

The long-term effects of type 2 diabetes can include progressive development of the specific microvascular complications of retinopathy

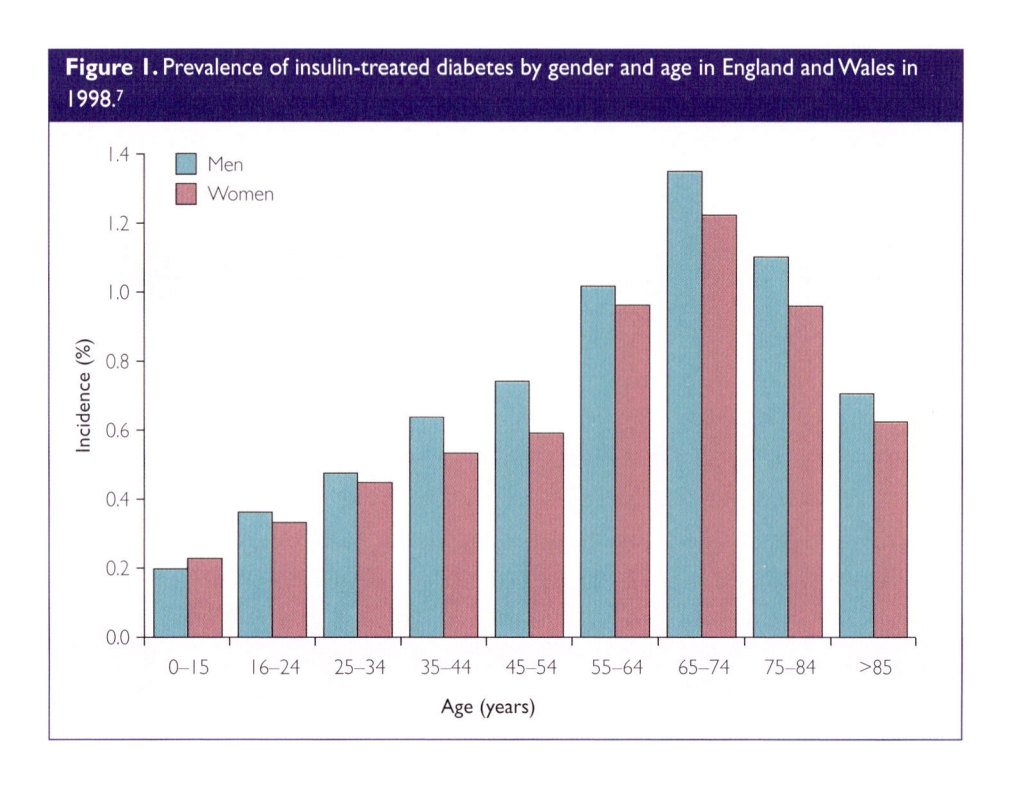

Figure 1. Prevalence of insulin-treated diabetes by gender and age in England and Wales in 1998.[7]

> Mortality rates from coronary heart disease (CHD) and stroke are up to five- and three-times higher in people with diabetes than the general population, and in the UK, type 2 diabetes reduces life expectancy by up to 10 years.

with potential blindness, nephropathy that may lead to renal failure, and/or neuropathy with risk of foot ulcers, limb amputation, Charcot joints, and features of autonomic dysfunction, including sexual dysfunction.[10] Rates of macrovascular diseases, such as myocardial infarction (MI), stroke and peripheral vascular disease are much higher for patients with type 2 diabetes than the normal population, and account for greater than 70% of deaths in this group.[11] Mortality rates from coronary heart disease (CHD) and stroke are up to five and three times higher in people with diabetes than the general population.[6] In the UK, type 2 diabetes reduces life expectancy by up to 10 years.[6] Severe and chronic complications, notably retinopathy, nephropathy, cardiovascular disease (CVD) and stroke, associated with type 2 diabetes have a profound impact on individuals and the health services, consuming 5% of total NHS resources and up to 10% of hospital in patient resources.[6] The mortality rate for all types of diabetes mellitus are considered for the UK for the last 30 or so years in Figure 2.[12] More men than women have diabetes as a cause of death, and despite increases in the incidence of diabetes, mortality rates in the UK seem reasonably stable during this time frame (Figure 2).[12] Furthermore, the indirect contribution of diabetes to mortality rates has an even more profound impact.

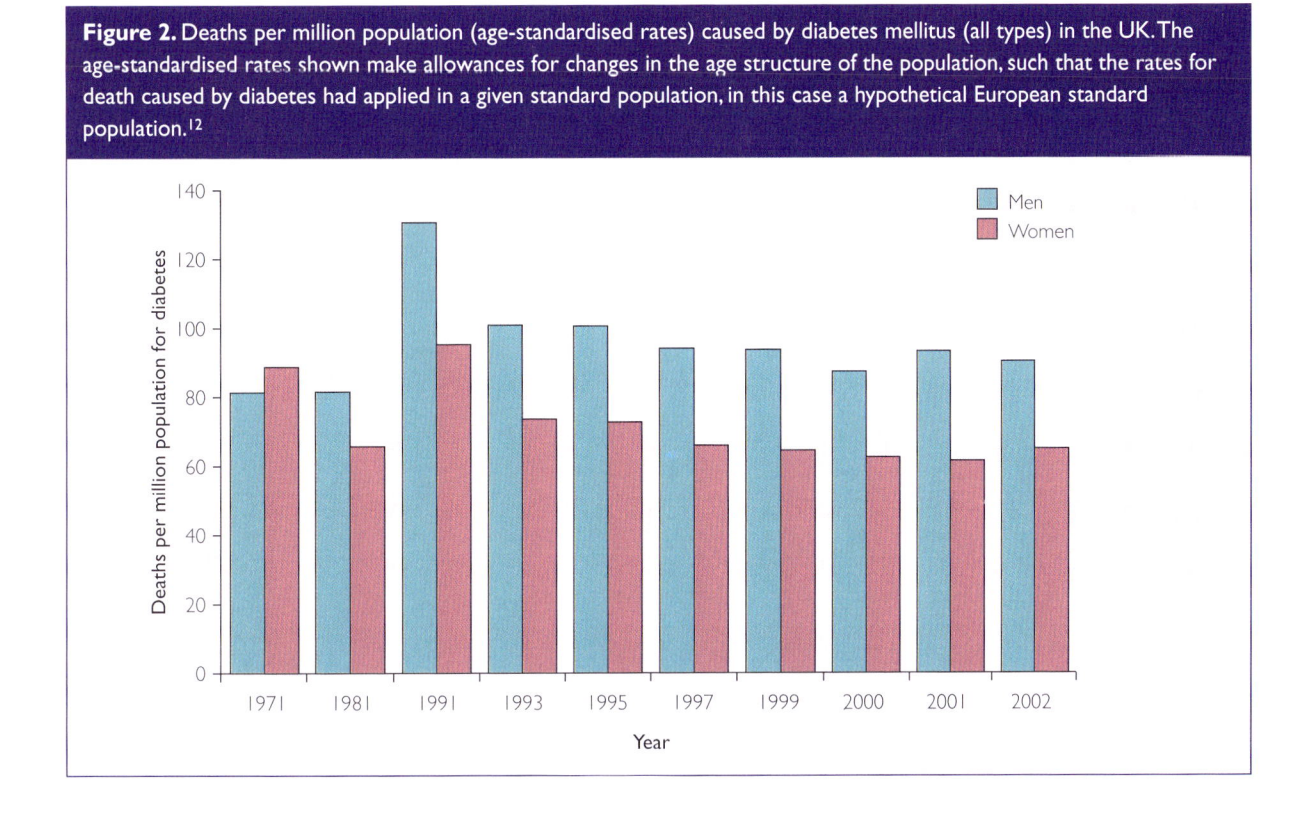

Figure 2. Deaths per million population (age-standardised rates) caused by diabetes mellitus (all types) in the UK. The age-standardised rates shown make allowances for changes in the age structure of the population, such that the rates for death caused by diabetes had applied in a given standard population, in this case a hypothetical European standard population.[12]

Classification, diagnosis and disease progression

There are two main types of diabetes: type 1 and type 2, previously known as insulin-dependent and non-insulin dependent diabetes, respectively. Type 1 diabetes develops if the body is unable to produce insulin, and requires insulin injections for treatment.[4] Type 2 diabetes encompasses people who have relative, rather than absolute, insulin deficiency. They exhibit various degrees of resistance to the action of insulin, and their diabetes may go undiagnosed for many years as hyperglycaemia may not be severe enough to provoke obvious symptoms of diabetes.[10] Initially, and often throughout their lifetime, these individuals do not need insulin treatment to survive.[10] The most recent World Health Organization (WHO) recommendations also recognise:
- gestational diabetes
- impaired glucose tolerance (IGT)
- impaired fasting glycaemia (IFG).[10]

> Type 2 diabetes may go undiagnosed for many years as hyperglycaemia may not be severe enough to provoke obvious symptoms of diabetes.

Gestational diabetes is carbohydrate intolerance resulting in hyperglycaemia with onset or first recognition in pregnancy.[10] People with

IGT and IFG have impaired glucose regulation, but these states should be differentiated from diabetes. IGT and IFG are metabolic states intermediate between normal glucose homeostasis and diabetes (Figure 3).[10] IGT and IFG are not clinical entities in their own right, but rather risk categories for CVD and future diabetes, respectively.[13] IGT is a stage in the natural history of disordered carbohydrate metabolism (FPG <7.0 mmol/L and oral glucose tolerance test 2-hour value ≥7.8 mmol/L, but <11.1 mmol/L), and patients with IGT often progress to diabetes and cardiovascular disease.[10,13] IFG occurs in individuals who have fasting glucose values above the normal range but below those diagnostic of diabetes (FPG ≥6.1 mmol/L, but <7.0 mmol/L).[10]

The WHO and UK guidelines advise that plasma glucose levels indicative of diabetes mellitus are as follows:
- random venous plasma glucose greater than or equal to 11.1 mmol/L

Figure 3. Disorders of glycaemia showing aetiological types and clinical stages.[10]
IFG, impaired fasting glucose; IGT, impaired glucose tolerance.
[a]In rare cases patients in these categories may require insulin for survival (e.g. presenting during pregnancy).

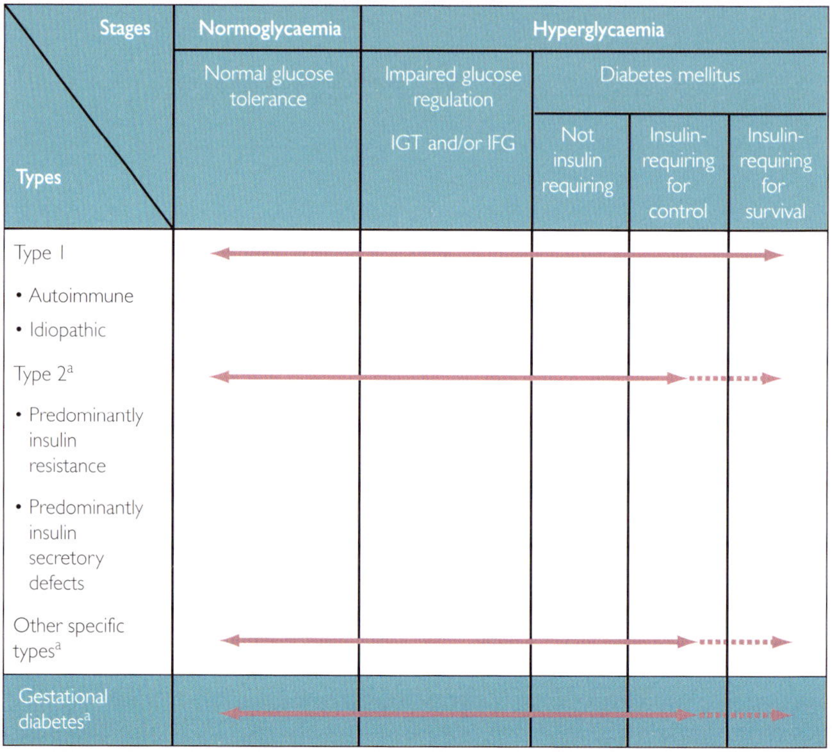

Types \ Stages	Normoglycaemia	Hyperglycaemia			
	Normal glucose tolerance	Impaired glucose regulation	Diabetes mellitus		
		IGT and/or IFG	Not insulin requiring	Insulin-requiring for control	Insulin-requiring for survival
Type 1 • Autoimmune • Idiopathic	←――――――――――――――――→				
Type 2[a] • Predominantly insulin resistance • Predominantly insulin secretory defects	←―――――――――――――・・・・・→				
Other specific types[a]	←―――――――――――――・・・・・→				
Gestational diabetes[a]	←・・・・――――――・・・・→				

- FPG greater than or equal to 7.0 mmol/L
- plasma glucose greater than or equal to 11.1 mmol/L at 2 hours after a 75 g oral glucose load (oral glucose tolerance test [OGTT]).[5,10,13]

For individuals without symptoms of diabetes (e.g. thirst, polyuria, polydipsia, and unexplained weight loss) at least one additional plasma glucose measurement with a value in the diabetic range above is essential to diagnose diabetes. This may be from a fasting (casual sample) or from an OGTT.[5,10,13]

The 'gold standard' test for diabetes is the OGTT, but this may not always be feasible, whereas FPG levels are more convenient than OGTT and more sensitive than random plasma glucose levels, and so is often the measurement of choice.[5]

Plasma glucose levels are the preferred measure for the diagnosis of diabetes.[14] However, HbA_{1C} (glycated haemoglobin) can be useful in the clinical diagnosis of type 2 diabetes, provided that confirmatory venous plasma glucose estimations are obtained, results are reviewed for presence of abnormal haemoglobin and erythrocyte turnover is not abnormal.[14]

- HbA_{1c} greater than 7.5% is approximately equivalent to FPG levels of greater than or equal to 7.0 mmol/L.
- HbA_{1c} greater than 6.5% is approximately equivalent to FPG levels of greater than 6.0 mmol/L.[14]

Risk factors

The following are risk factors for the development of type 2 diabetes:
- increasing age
- obesity and/or increased percentage of fat in the abdominal region
- lack of physical activity
- history of gestational diabetes
- IGT or IFG (see classification and diagnosis section)
- hypertension
- familial predisposition.[5]

Some risk factors are modifiable, such as obesity and lack of exercise, by a change in lifestyle. However, there is a strong genetic component for type 2 diabetes. The concordance rate for monozygotic twins is fairly high (approximately 70%), but as it is below unity this implies an environmental component to its aetiology.[15] This is also suggested by the fact that the risk to dizygotic twins is slightly higher than to ordinary siblings.[15]

The oral glucose tolerance test (OGTT) is the 'gold standard' test for diabetes, but fasting plasma glucose (FPG) is often the measurement of choice.

Pathophysiology

The primary defect in those with type 1 diabetes is the failure of production of insulin, due to the autoimmune destruction of pancreatic β-cells.[16] In contrast, the pathophysiology of type 2 diabetes stems from insulin resistance and insulin secretion defects, usually in combination.[11] Initially, hepatic and skeletal muscle tissues lose sensitivity to the action of insulin (insulin resistance), but the β-cells are able to increase insulin secretion to compensate.[17] Obesity is an important contributor to insulin resistance and this state is associated with hyperinsulinaemia.[18] The overt hyperglycaemia that characterises type 2 diabetes occurs when insulin secretion can no longer overcome the individual's level of insulin resistance.[18] A deterioration of β-cell function and further increases in insulin resistance exacerbate the disease. As the disease worsens, a loss in β-cell mass may occur due to glucotoxicity.[19] Furthermore, as insulin-mediated glucose uptake occurs mainly in the postprandial state, the metabolic consequences of type 2 diabetes are closely linked with postprandial metabolism.[18]

Prevention and treatment

The management of diabetes should address:
- increased insulin resistance
- impaired insulin secretion
- complications
- comorbid disorders.

Clearly, a combination of lifestyle modification and pharmacological intervention(s) are required to meet these challenges.

Lifestyle modifications

It is now clear that type 2 diabetes and CHD are linked. Diabetes is a risk factor for CHD, and CHD accounts for much of the serious morbidity and premature mortality associated with type 2 diabetes.[20] The type of lifestyle modification that reduces the risk of CHD will also be effective in the prevention of type 2 diabetes. The following dietary modifications are recommended:
- weight normalisation
- reduce the intake of saturated fat as much as possible
- increase the intake of vegetables (including legumes and pulses), fruit and wholegrain cereals
- increase the intake of fish, particularly oily fish, as these contain high levels of omega-3 polyunsaturated fatty acids (eicosapentaenoic and docosahexaenoic acids).[20]

Type 2 diabetes results from an interaction between genetic predisposition and lifestyle factors, including diet, physical activity and obesity.[3] The effect of lifestyle interventions on patients 'at risk' of developing diabetes (i.e. those with IGT) has been extensively investigated, as exemplified by a recent trial in 522 middle-aged overweight people with IGT.[21] The progression to diabetes was reduced by 58% over 4 years by interventions to reduce total and saturated fat intake, increase exercise and raise dietary fibre intake.[21] This confirmed results obtained in other studies – that diet and exercise reduce the incidence of type 2 diabetes in patients with IGT.[22,23]

As IGT or IFG precedes type 2 diabetes, it may provide an opportunity for targeted intervention, but reversing the overall trend for increased obesity in the general population should remain the primary objective.[3,6,20] Interestingly, physical activity of moderate intensity and duration can substantially reduce the risk of type 2 diabetes, as shown by an 8-year study in over 70,000 nurses without diabetes, as equivalent energy expenditure walking or engaged in vigorous activity resulted in comparable magnitudes of risk reduction.[24]

> Diet and exercise reduce the incidence of type 2 diabetes in patients with IGT.

Pharmacological therapies

Prevention

Although lifestyle modifications can reduce the progression from IGT to diabetes by over 50% it may not always be possible to maintain these changes. Benefits have been found in large cohorts of patients with IGT for a range of antidiabetic agents (e.g. acarbose, metformin and troglitazone).[3] These trials produced a 25–56% reduction in progression to the diabetic state.[3]

Treatment of hypertension, dyslipidaemia and nephropathy

The treatment of hyperglycaemia – by any means – is the primary objective of the management of type 2 diabetes, and thus this will be the focus of this section. However, it is important to consider the complications of diabetes. The recent UK Prospective Diabetes Study (UKPDS) confirmed the relationship between hyperglycaemia and microvascular complications, such as nephropathy, neuropathy and retinopathy.[25] By tight control of glycaemia these microvascular diseases were prevented. There also seems to be a relationship between risk factors for macrovascular disease and diabetes, and up to 70% of adults with type 2 diabetes have raised blood pressure and more than 70% have raised cholesterol levels.[6]

> Treatment of patients with diabetes for dyslipidaemia and hypertension, in particular, is sensible.

It is reasonable to be aware of these potential comorbidities and to treat them. Treatment of patients with diabetes for dyslipidaemia and hypertension, in particular, is sensible. The use of statins to treat dyslipidaemia and thus help prevent atherosclerosis should be considered. Statins are the preferred lipid-lowering therapy for the majority of patients and may be particularly effective in risk reduction amongst diabetics, even if LDL-C levels are comparatively low (<3.2 mmol/L).[26,27,28] The DAIS (Diabetes Atherosclerosis Intervention Study) found that the fibrate, fenofibrate, was effective in reducing the progression of atherosclerosis in diabetics.[29] The risk of cardiovascular events in hypertensive diabetics has been demonstrated to be significantly reduced in diabetics by intensive blood pressure lowering.[30] In addition, angiotensin converting enzyme (ACE) inhibition may reduce cardiovascular risk by directly affecting endothelial dysfunction, atherosclerosis and thrombus formation.[31]

The progression of diabetic nephropathy is associated with an incremental risk of cardiovascular disease and microalbuminuria is the leading predictor of CHD in patients with type 2 diabetes, ahead of smoking, diastolic blood pressure and serum cholesterol.[26] Results from several trials have suggested that angiotensin (AT) II receptor antagonists and ACE-inhibitors may be effective in protecting against the progression of nephropathy resulting from type 2 diabetes by mechanisms that may be independent of their blood-pressure lowering effects.[32,33]

Antidiabetic agents

The management of diabetic patients should focus on good glycaemic control compatible with a good quality of life and the reduction of microvascular risks, in addition to attention to major risk factors for macrovascular disease, such as hypertension and dyslipidaemia (Figure 4). The following agents are used in glycaemic control in type 2 diabetics.

Sulphonylureas: these agents have been in use for many years and stimulate insulin secretion. Though this class is very effective in controlling glycaemia in many patients they are associated with hypoglycaemia, which can be a particular problem in those whose glucose levels are under tight control, the elderly, people who perform intermittent intense exercise or commonly miss or delay meals.[11] Sulphonylureas can also sometimes cause hypoinsulinaemia in some instances, which further accentuates the adverse metabolic situation already present in the majority of people with type 2 diabetes.[16]

Biguanides: metformin is the only currently available biguanide. It is now preferred as first-line therapy over sulphonylureas in most patients as it is less likely to cause hyperinsulinaemia.[16] Metformin can achieve tight

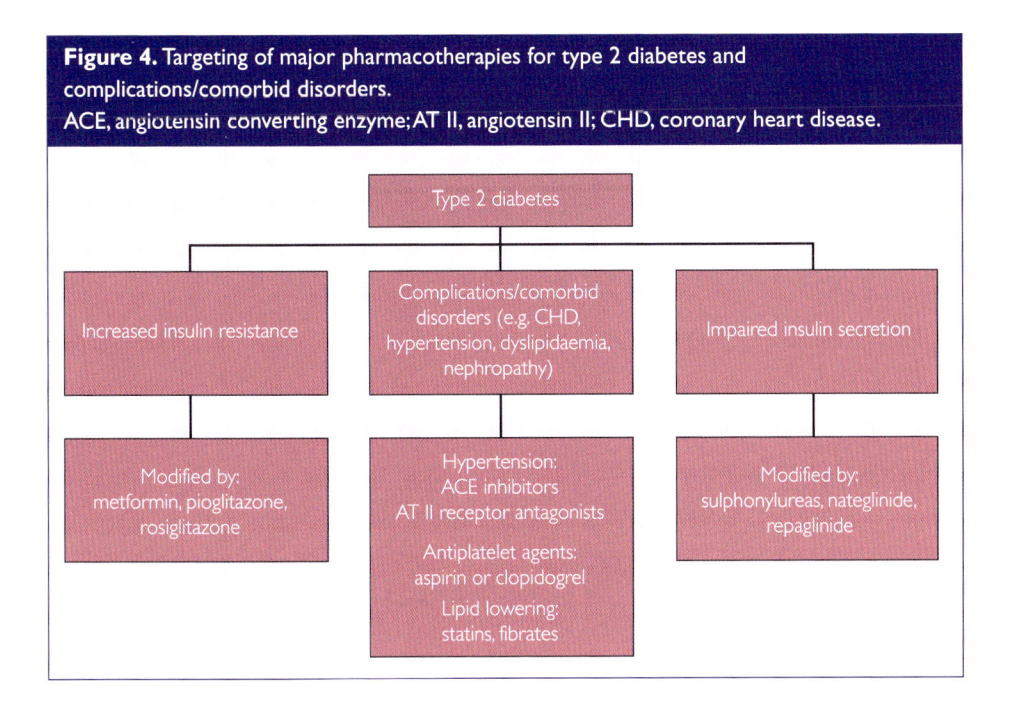

Figure 4. Targeting of major pharmacotherapies for type 2 diabetes and complications/comorbid disorders.
ACE, angiotensin converting enzyme; AT II, angiotensin II; CHD, coronary heart disease.

```
                          Type 2 diabetes
          ┌──────────────────┼──────────────────┐
   Increased insulin    Complications/comorbid    Impaired insulin
      resistance        disorders (e.g. CHD,         secretion
                        hypertension, dyslipidaemia,
                        nephropathy)
          │                   │                        │
     Modified by:        Hypertension:            Modified by:
      metformin,         ACE inhibitors          sulphonylureas,
     pioglitazone,       AT II receptor antagonists  nateglinide,
     rosiglitazone                                 repaglinide
                         Antiplatelet agents:
                         aspirin or clopidogrel
                         Lipid lowering:
                         statins, fibrates
```

glycaemic control associated with minimal weight gain (often weight loss), and reduce morbidity and mortality associated with diabetes in overweight patients.[34] Thus, metformin is often the preferred antidiabetic in obese patients. It affects glucose levels by inhibiting hepatic gluconeogenesis, increasing peripheral glucose uptake and decreasing intestinal adsorption of glucose.[16] Metformin is often used as combination therapy along with a sulphonylurea as these two types of agent have different and complementary mechanisms of action.

Early-phase insulin secretion agents: these agents (nateglinide, repaglinide) act directly on pancreatic β-cells to stimulate insulin secretion that is rapid, of short duration and is dependent on ambient glucose.[35] As such, these agents are particularly suitable for reducing postprandial hyperglycaemia and allow for more flexibility in lifestyle such that meals can be skipped without risking hypoglycaemia.[35] Their mode of action is complementary to agents that target insulin resistance (e.g. metformin or thiazolidinediones).

Thiazolidinediones: (e.g. pioglitazone, rosiglitazone) are commonly called 'glitazones' and enhance insulin-mediated glucose uptake (i.e. reducing insulin resistance) in skeletal muscle, hepatic and adipose tissue.[11,16] They enhance insulin action by increasing the number of glucose transporters in insulin-resistant tissues, thereby improving insulin-stimulated glucose transport.[17] However, this class of agents is associated with a slight risk of liver damage, so liver function should be tested before and at intervals after starting therapy. They may also cause hypoglycaemia if meals are missed.[5] However, a recent consensus statement from the American Heart Association and American Diabetic Association has expressed warnings concerning the use of thiazolidinediones in patients with heart failure.[36]

α-*glucosidase inhibitor:* acarbose is the only currently available member of this class. These act by delaying carbohydrate absorption, attenuating postprandial peak glucose levels.[11] However, they are associated with diarrhoea, flatulence and bloating and require slow dose titration.[11] Thus, acarbose is used only in patients unable to tolerate other oral treatments.[5]

Combination therapy

There is no overall accepted standard approach to the pharmacological management of type 2 diabetes, but metformin is widely recommended as first-line therapy, particularly in obese patients. Combining antidiabetic agents can take advantage of synergistic modes of action to enable better glycaemic control. The combination of metformin and a sulphonylurea is commonly used, though more recently other options such as metformin plus either a thiazolidinedione or an early-phase insulin secretion agent have become available. Furthermore, combination therapy can postpone the use of insulin, but as the disease progresses it is often required, either alone or in combination, to restore glycaemic control.[37]

Key points

- The global prevalence of diabetes is increasing dramatically, with the number of people with diabetes predicted to rise to 220 million in 2010.
- Type 2 diabetes is far more common than type 1 diabetes and has the highest prevalence in developed countries as it is strongly associated with obesity and a sedentary lifestyle.
- Type 2 diabetes is associated with microvascular and macrovascular complications, the latter being strongly associated with premature mortality amongst diabetic patients.
- Some risk factors for type 2 diabetes such as obesity and lack of exercise are modifiable by a change in lifestyle, but there is also a strong genetic component for type 2 diabetes.
- The pathophysiology of type 2 diabetes stems from insulin resistance and insulin secretion defects, usually in combination.
- Patients with type 2 diabetes should receive treatment for concurrent disorders such as dyslipidaemia and hypertension.
- A range of antidiabetic agents is available to ensure adequate glycaemic control, and these are often used in combination with one another.

References

1. Amos AF, McCarty DJ, Zimmet P. The rising global burden of diabetes and its complications: estimates and projections to the year 2010. *Diabet Med* 1997; **14(Suppl 5)**: S1–85.
2. King H, Aubert RE, Herman WH. Global burden of diabetes, 1995–2025: prevalence, numerical estimates, and projections. *Diabetes Care* 1998; **21**: 1414–31.
3. Simpson RW, Shaw JE, Zimmet PZ. The prevention of type 2 diabetes—lifestyle change or pharmacotherapy? A challenge for the 21st century. *Diabetes Res Clin Pract* 2003; **59**: 165–80.
4. Diabetes UK website. *http://www.diabetes.org.uk*
5. Prodigy guidance. Diabetes type 2 – blood glucose management. September 2002.
6. National Service Framework for Diabetes: Standards (2001). *http://www.doh.gov.uk/nsf/diabetes/*
7. Office for National Statistics. *Key Health Statistics from General Practice 1998*. Series MB6 No. 2. London: National Statistics.
8. Mather HM, Keen H. The Southall Diabetes Survey: prevalence of known diabetes in Asians and Europeans. *Br Med J (Clin Res Ed)* 1985; **291**: 1081–4.
9. Allawi J, Rao PV, Gilbert R *et al*. Microalbuminuria in non-insulin-dependent diabetes: its prevalence in Indian compared with Europid patients. *Br Med J (Clin Res Ed)* 1988; **296**: 462–4.
10. World Health Organization. *Definition, diagnosis and classification of diabetes mellitus and its complications*. Geneva: World Health Organization, 1999.
11. Ahmann AJ, Riddle MC. Current oral agents for type 2 diabetes. Many options, but which to choose when? *Postgrad Med* 2002; **111**: 32–46.
12. Office for National Statistics. *Health Statistics Quarterly*. No. 20, Winter 2003. London: National Statistics.
13. Scottish Intercollegiate Guidelines Network (SIGN) guideline. *Management of diabetes*. September 2001.
14. European Diabetes Policy Group. A desktop guide to Type 2 diabetes mellitus. *Diabet Med* 1999; **16**: 716–30.
15. Kyvik KO, Green A, Beck-Nielsen H. Concordance rates of insulin dependent diabetes mellitus: a population based study of young Danish twins. *BMJ* 1995; **311**: 913–7.
16. Takiya L, Chawla S. Therapeutic options for the management of type 2 diabetes mellitus. *Am J Manag Care* 2002; **8**: 1009–23.
17. Rosak C. The pathophysiologic basis of efficacy and clinical experience with the new oral antidiabetic agents. *J Diabetes Complications* 2002; **16**: 123–32.
18. Dornhorst A. Insulinotropic meglitinide analogues. *Lancet* 2001; **358**: 1709–16.
19. Federici M, Hribal M, Perego L *et al*. High glucose causes apoptosis in cultured human pancreatic islets of Langerhans: a potential role for regulation of specific Bcl family genes toward an apoptotic cell death program. *Diabetes* 2001; **50**: 1290–301.
20. Mann JI. Diet and risk of coronary heart disease and type 2 diabetes. *Lancet* 2002; **360**: 783–9.
21. Tuomilehto J, Lindstrom J, Eriksson JG *et al*. Prevention of type 2 diabetes mellitus by changes in lifestyle among subjects with impaired glucose tolerance. *N Engl J Med* 2001; **344**: 1343–50.
22. Knowler WC, Barrett-Connor E, Fowler SE *et al*. Reduction in the incidence of type 2 diabetes with lifestyle intervention or metformin. *N Engl J Med* 2002; **346**: 393–403.
23. Pan XR, Li GW, Hu YH *et al*. Effects of diet and exercise in preventing NIDDM in people with impaired glucose tolerance. The Da Qing IGT and Diabetes Study. *Diabetes Care* 1997; **20**: 537–44.
24. Hu FB, Sigal RJ, Rich-Edwards JW *et al*. Walking compared with vigorous physical activity and risk of type 2 diabetes in women: a prospective study. *JAMA* 1999; **282**: 1433–9.
25. Stratton IM, Adler AI, Neil HA *et al*. Association of glycaemia with macrovascular and microvascular complications of type 2 diabetes (UKPDS 35): prospective observational study. *BMJ* 2000; **321**: 405–12.
26. Betteridge D, Morrell J. *Clinician's Guide to Lipids and Coronary Heart Disease*. 2nd edn. London: Arnold, 2003.
27. Sacks FM, Tonkin AM, Craven T *et al*. Coronary heart disease in patients with low LDL-cholesterol: benefit of pravastatin in diabetics and enhanced role for HDL-cholesterol and triglycerides as risk factors. *Circulation* 2002; **105**: 1424–8.
28. MRC/BHF Heart Protection Study of cholesterol-lowering therapy and of antioxidant vitamin supplementation in a wide range of patients at increased risk of coronary heart disease death: early safety and efficacy experience. *Eur Heart J* 1999; **20**: 725–41.
29. Effect of fenofibrate on progression of coronary-artery disease in type 2 diabetes: the Diabetes Atherosclerosis Intervention Study, a randomised study. *Lancet* 2001; **357**: 905–10.
30. Tight blood pressure control and risk of macrovascular and microvascular complications in type 2 diabetes: UKPDS 38. UK Prospective Diabetes Study Group. *BMJ* 1998; **317**: 703–13.
31. Heinig RE. What should the role of ACE inhibitors be in the treatment of diabetes? Lessons from HOPE and MICRO-HOPE. *Diabetes Obes Metab* 2002; **4(Suppl 1)**: S19–25.
32. Parving HH, Lehnert H, Brochner-Mortensen J *et al*. The effect of irbesartan on the development of diabetic nephropathy in patients with type 2 diabetes. *N Engl J Med* 2001; **345**: 870–8.
33. Overlack A, Adamczak M, Bachmann W *et al*. ACE-inhibition with perindopril in essential hypertensive patients with concomitant diseases. The Perindopril Therapeutic Safety Collaborative Research Group. *Am J Med* 1994; **97**: 126–34.
34. Effect of intensive blood-glucose control with metformin on complications in overweight patients with type 2 diabetes (UKPDS 34). UK Prospective Diabetes Study (UKPDS) Group. *Lancet* 1998; **352**: 854–65.
35. Standl E, Fuchtenbusch M. The role of oral antidiabetic agents: why and when to use an early-phase insulin secretion agent in type 2 diabetes mellitus. *Diabetologia* 2003; **46(Suppl 1)**: M30–6.
36. Nesto R, Bell D, Bonow R *et al*. Thiazolidinedione use, fluid retention and congestive heart failure. A consensus statement from the American Heart Association and American Diabetes Association. *Circulation* 2003; **108**: 2941–8.
37. Van Gaal LF, De Leeuw IH. Rationale and options for combination therapy in the treatment of Type 2 diabetes. *Diabetologia* 2003; **46(Suppl 1)**: M44–50.

Acknowledgement

Figures 1 and 3 are adapted from the World Health Organization, 1999.[10]

14. Erectile dysfunction

Dr Scott Chambers
CSF Medical Communications Ltd

Summary

Erectile dysfunction (ED) is defined as the consistent inability to achieve or maintain an erection sufficient for satisfactory sexual performance. It is highly prevalent, affecting more than half the male population. Moreover, its prevalence is on the increase, and is expected to double over the next 20 years.

ED has a variety of aetiologies and risk factors, and is classified principally according to whether it derives from organic and/or psychogenic sources. ED has a strong age-dependent and progressive course. The age-related increase in its prevalence is consistent with the chronic nature of the disorder and its association with a number of other serious and life-threatening conditions, including cardiovascular disease and diabetes. Indeed, each of these conditions share common risk factors, and thus, it has been widely postulated that ED represents an early warning sign for coronary heart disease (CHD). ED also has a significant and profoundly negative impact on quality of life, impacting upon the individual, their partner and social inter-relationships.

Whilst for many years the treatment of ED has not been optimal, the availability of oral therapy, in particular the phosphodiesterase type 5 (PDE5) inhibitors, in the late 1990s, has greatly increased the awareness of the disorder, and has led to a significant improvement in the management of this serious condition.

Epidemiology of ED

ED, or the consistent inability to achieve or maintain an erection sufficient for satisfactory sexual performance, is a highly prevalent condition, with over 50% of men over 40 years of age affected by it at some point in their lives.[1,2] In 1995, an estimated 150 million men worldwide had experienced ED of some degree. By 2025 its prevalence has been predicted to more than double to 320 million, principally due to the twin drivers of ageing populations in the western world and population growth in developing nations (Figure 1).[3,4] The prevalence of ED has been shown to increase with

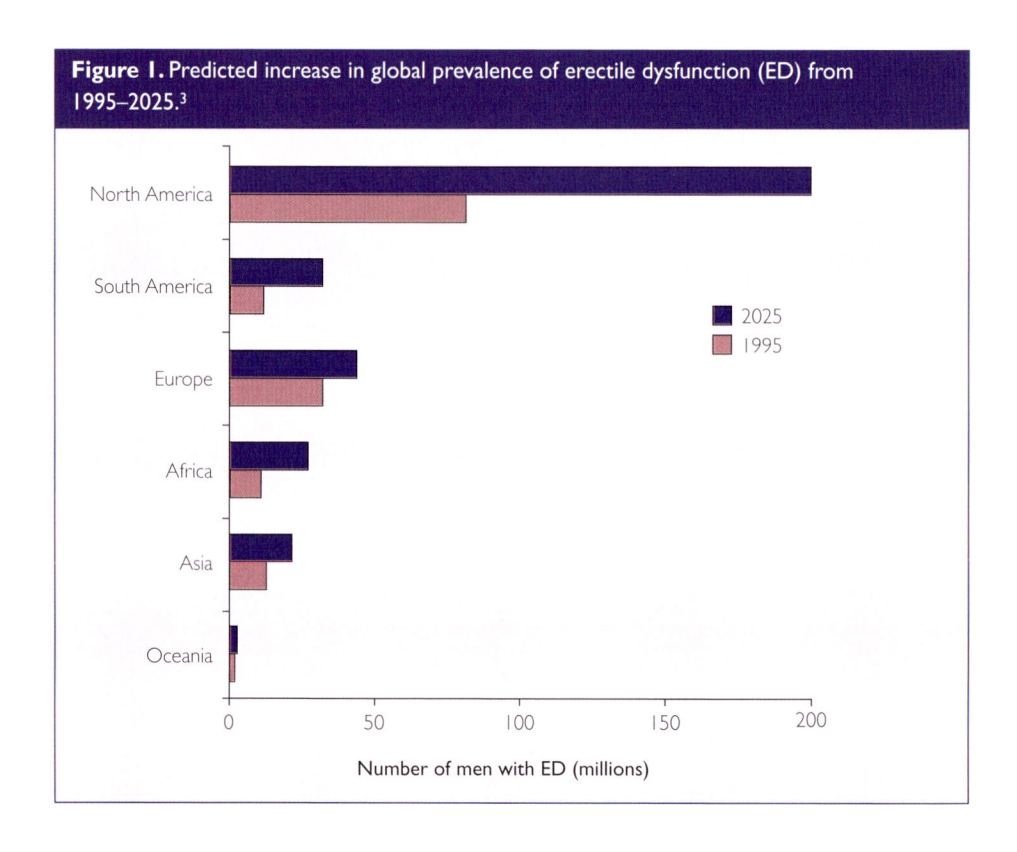

Figure 1. Predicted increase in global prevalence of erectile dysfunction (ED) from 1995–2025.[3]

advancing age, whilst older men are remaining sexually active as they move into their later years, factors that further increase the pool of potential ED patients.[5]

The majority of ED-related epidemiological data is from US sources, whilst UK-based data are relatively scarce with no major population-based studies reported. However, calculations suggest that ED affects approximately 2.3 million, or 1 in 10 of the male population.[6] These figures may represent an underestimate, given that many men are stigmatised by their condition and feel discouraged from seeking and continuing treatment. This is exemplified by a number of studies showing that more than 75% of patients do not receive any treatment for their condition.[4] However, the introduction of PDE5 inhibitors in the late 1990s has fostered a greater awareness of the condition amongst both patients and physicians, and has increased the numbers seeking and receiving treatment. Consequently, these factors have brought the management of ED into the domain of the primary care physician.[7]

A cross-sectional study of patients attending a central London genitourinary clinic reported that 19% of attendees had ED (median age 30 years, range 16–78).[8] A survey of over 2000 men aged 55–70 presenting at 11 community clinics in Wales, reported that 13.2% of patients had complete ED.[9] In addition, this survey demonstrated a clear age-related increase in the burden of the condition: ED was found in 6.9% of men aged 55–60 years, 12.5% in those aged 61–65 years and 22.2% of those 66–70 years. When the authors of this study extrapolated their findings to the entire UK population, approximately 500,000 men were predicted to be affected.[9] However, this is likely to represent an underestimate of the total ED patient population in the UK as these data relate specifically to complete ED and thus exclude those with less severe forms of the condition. In the 1990s, the number of reported diagnoses of ED in the UK increased, mainly due to an expansion in the awareness of the condition and the availability of non-invasive therapy, principally the first PDE5 inhibitor, sildenafil.[10]

The US-based Massachusetts Male Aging Study (MMAS) has provided some of the most illuminating data relating to the prevalence of ED in men aged between 40 and 70 years, and has estimated the number of men affected in the US at up to 30 million.[11] The MMAS was a cross-sectional, random sample survey that reported a mean probability of any form of ED of 52% in the entire patient cohort (minimal ED 17.2%, moderate ED 25.2% or complete ED 9.6%). Again, a clear age-dependent increase in the burden of ED was reported in the MMAS such that by the age of 70 years, 67% of men were affected. The severity of the condition also showed an age-dependent relationship: three-times more patients aged 70 years or older (15%) had complete ED compared with men aged 40 years (5%).[11] A follow-up study of the MMAS estimated that the annual incidence of new cases of ED was about 24 cases per 1000 men.[12]

It should be noted that the prevalence of moderate-to-severe ED in the MMAS (~35%) is somewhat higher than findings from other surveys (5–20%).[13] This may be a reflection of differences in methodology and definitions of severity employed in the different studies, but may also reflect real differences between populations.[13]

The age-related increase in the burden of ED reported in these epidemiological surveys is typical of chronic disease and consistent with an increased occurrence of cardiovascular disease, diabetes and other risk factors in older men with ED.[11,14] Vascular disease of various types is associated with ED, including myocardial infarction, coronary artery diseases, cerebrovascular disease, peripheral vascular disease, hypertension and atherosclerosis.[15] Conversely, the incidence of ED increases in men with diabetes, hypertension, cardiovascular disease or depression. For example, in the MMAS, men with diabetes had an overall prevalence of ED of 35%.[11]

The age-related increase in the burden of ED is typical of chronic disease and consistent with an increased occurrence of cardiovascular disease, diabetes and other risk factors.

ED represents a huge burden on public health, and impacts on society, the individual, and the patient's partner and family.[14] ED has a significant and profoundly negative impact on patients' quality of life,[16] and can lead to an increase in emotional stress, which may further damage patient–partner relationships.[14] Subsequent withdrawal from the social support of intimate relationships may also have a detrimental effect on patients' physical and mental well-being, particularly amongst the elderly.[1] ED often results in anxiety and depression,[17] and can impact upon a patient's self-esteem and self-image, which can perpetuate the psychogenic element of ED even further.

Risk factors and aetiology

The aetiology of ED is multifactorial and arises from disturbances in vascular, neurological, hormonal, anatomical and iatrogenic (organic) factors and/or psychological (psychogenic) factors (Table 1).[7] Furthermore, ED can be subdivided into mild (minimal), moderate or severe (complete) according to the extent of the dysfunction.

Over the past 20 years, there has been a radical shift in our understanding of the aetiology of ED as we gain greater insight into molecular, neurological and physiological aspects of erection.[18] Two main concepts have emerged from this shift in our understanding. First, ED is no longer considered as an inevitable part of ageing. Second, the majority of ED has an organic origin, contrasting with the previously accepted view that the majority of cases were due to psychological disturbances.[18,19] Despite this, psychological disturbances are still responsible for a significant proportion of ED, with about 20–30% of patients having psychogenic ED. A further sizeable proportion of patients suffer ED of both organic and psychological origin (mixed ED). Psychological issues also contribute to the severity of organic ED.

Of the organic causative factors, disruptions to the vascular system account for some 70% of cases (Figure 2).[20] Indeed, because of the association between vascular disease and ED, it is now accepted that ED represents an 'early warning sign' for cardiovascular disease, and may be apparent prior to the presentation of any other clinical symptoms. For example, ED is four-times more likely to be present in men with diabetes, hypertension or CHD than in those without these diseases.[21]

Commonly prescribed drugs used to treat many of the comorbidities associated with ED are another important trigger of ED (Table 2).[2] Thiazide diuretics are the most common cause of ED amongst prescribed drugs, and increase ED in part by reducing systemic blood pressure which is important in maintaining penile rigidity. Other factors unrelated to blood

Table 1. The aetiology of erectile dysfunction.[2]

Aetiology of ED	Common comorbidity
Organic	
Vasculogenic	Atherosclerosis
	Hypertension
	Diabetes mellitus
	Peripheral vascular disease
	Trauma
	Peyronie's disease
Neurogenic	Stroke or Alzheimer's dementia
	Spinal cord injury
	Radical pelvic surgery
	Diabetic neuropathy
	Pelvic injury
	Multiple sclerosis
Hormonal	Hypogonadism
	Hyperprolactinaemia
Iatrogenic	Antihypertensive and antidepressant drugs
	Antiandrogens
Lifestyle	Alcohol and drug abuse
	Cigarette smoking
Psychogenic	Performance anxiety
	Relationship problems
	Stress
	Depression

pressure reduction may also contribute to ED caused by thiazide diuretics. Indeed, given that hypertension is more common in patients with ED, the group that receive antihypertensive medications would be expected to be more likely to have erectile difficulties.

Psychogenic ED may result from performance anxiety, psychiatric disorders (e.g. depression and schizophrenia), relationship issues, confusion over sexual orientation and lack of sexual arousal.[2] There is also a strong association between depression and ED, which, paradoxically, can be further exasperated by the treatment with certain antidepressants.[17]

Neurogenic ED can be caused by Parkinson's disease, Alzheimer's dementia, stroke, spinal cord injury, multiple sclerosis and cerebral trauma. These disorders cause ED by decreasing overall libido or by preventing the initiating neurological signal that promotes erection.[2]

Figure 2. The aetiology of organic ED.[20]

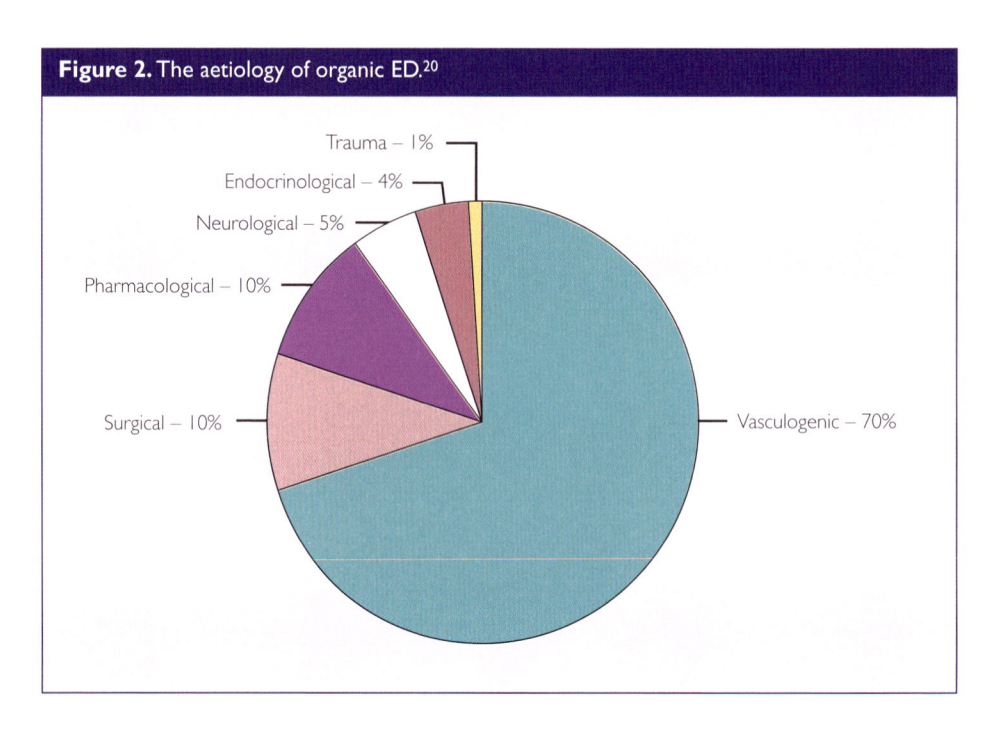

- Trauma – 1%
- Endocrinological – 4%
- Neurological – 5%
- Pharmacological – 10%
- Surgical – 10%
- Vasculogenic – 70%

Table 2. Pharmacological agents associated with erectile dysfunction.[2]

Drug class	Example
Antihypertensives	β-blockers, thiazide diuretics, potassium sparing diuretics
Antidepressants	Selective serotonin reuptake inhibitors, serotonin and noradrenaline reuptake inhibitors (e.g. venlafaxine), tricyclic antidepressants, monoamine oxidase inhibitors
Antipsychotics	Phenothiazines, carbamazepine, risperidone
Hormonal agents	Cyproterone acetate, luteinising hormone releasing hormone analogues, oestrogens
Lipid regulators	Gemfibrozil, clofibrate
Anticonvulsants	Phenytoin, carbamazepine
Parkinson's treatments	Levodopa
Dyspepsia drugs	H_2 receptor antagonists
Miscellaneous	Allopurinol, indometacin, disulfiram, phenothiazine antihistamines, phenothiazine antiemetics

Physiology of erection

To understand the natural history of ED, it is necessary to review the anatomy of the penis and the normal physiological processes that result in an erection (Figure 3). The penis comprises three separate 'cylinders' or corpora, which include the corpus spongiosum that houses the urethra, and

Figure 3. Anatomy of the penis.

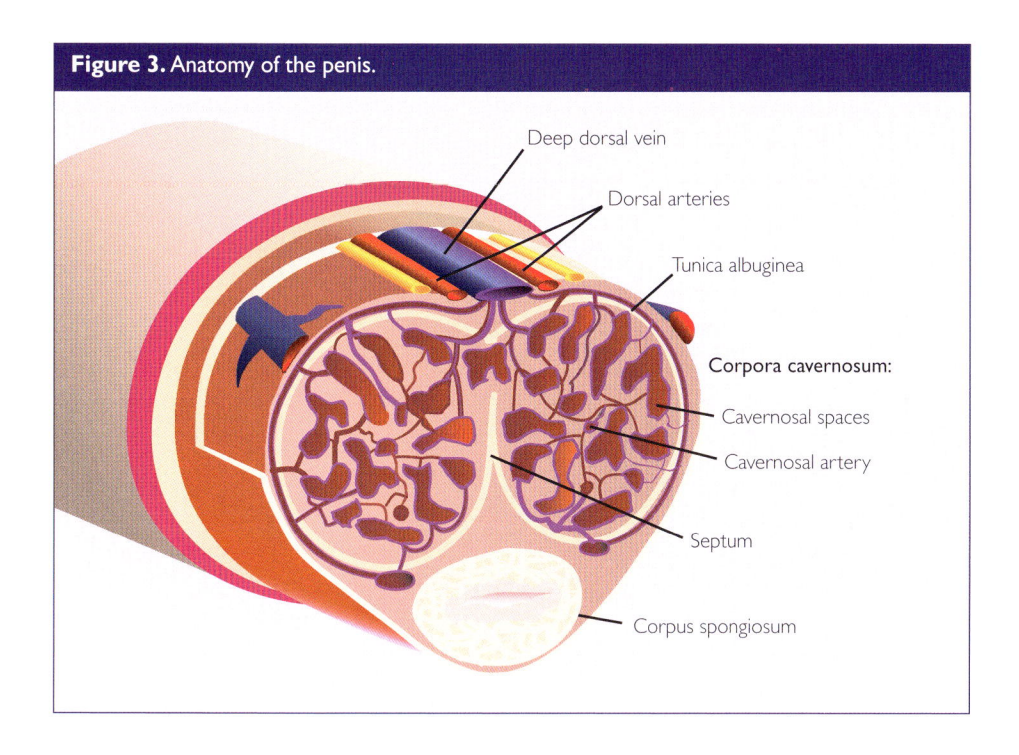

- Deep dorsal vein
- Dorsal arteries
- Tunica albuginea
- Corpora cavernosum:
  - Cavernosal spaces
  - Cavernosal artery
- Septum
- Corpus spongiosum

the corpora cavernosa. These are surrounded by a thick fibro-elastic sheath called the tunica albuginea. Within the penis are multiple sinusoidal spaces surrounded by trabeculae of smooth muscle which form the functional erectile tissue. Briefly, in haemodynamic terms, erection depends upon an increased blood flow in the paired cavernosal arteries (branches of the main penile artery) and subsequent filling of the sinusoidal spaces from helicine arteries (branches of the cavernosal arteries).[22] Increases in arterial pressure lead to expansion of the trabecular walls and the tunica albuginea, resulting in compression of the draining venules and reduced outflow of blood, a process known as veno-occlusion. The combination of these effects leads to engorgement of the penis with blood and thus an erection. Restoration to a flaccid state, or detumescence, occurs essentially by a reversal of these processes. Thus, the smooth muscle of the helicine arteries contracts, reducing arterial inflow, followed by the collapse of lacunar spaces and increased venous outflow, restoring the penis to its resting flaccid state.

Erection occurs as a result of a complex interplay of neural, neurochemical, hormonal and vascular mechanisms.[23,24] Disruptions to any one of these mechanisms can potentially lead to ED. In the absence of sexual stimulation, the penis is maintained in a normal flaccid state by α-adrenergically mediated contraction of cavernosal and vascular smooth muscle, thereby limiting blood flow into the penis. In response to sensory

> Erection depends upon an increased blood flow in the paired cavernosal arteries and subsequent filling of the sinusoidal spaces from helicine arteries.

stimuli, neurochemical signals are generated and transmitted from the paraventricular nucleus in the hypothalamus to an erection centre in the spinal cord. These signals induce the release of the principal chemical mediator of erection, nitric oxide (NO), from non-adrenergic, non-cholinergic (NANC) nerve terminals in the corpora cavernosa and endothelial cells of the arterioles in the penis. NO acts by promoting smooth muscle relaxation within localised arteries and in the cavernosal tissue.[25] It achieves this by activating guanylate cyclase, an enzyme which regulates the conversion of guanosine triphosphate (GTP) to cyclic guanosine monophosphate (cGMP; Figure 4). cGMP is a key second messenger involved in intracellular signal transduction and acts via protein activation mechanisms to reduce intracellular Ca^{2+} concentrations. Thus, calcium uptake into the smooth muscle of the vasculature and corpora cavernosa is reduced, leading to smooth muscle relaxation, increased blood flow and ultimately erection, via the haemodynamic mechanisms discussed above.[23,24] Subsequent hydrolysis of cGMP by the enzyme PDE5, restores the penis to its flaccid state by restoring the contractile tone of the smooth muscle (Figure 4).

Normal erectile function is a delicate balance between vasoconstriction and vasodilation of the smooth muscle in the corpora cavernosa. As discussed in the previous section, vascular disease accounts for the majority of organic cases of ED and disrupts this delicate balance. Vasculogenic ED may arise either as a consequence of poor arterial blood flow or poor

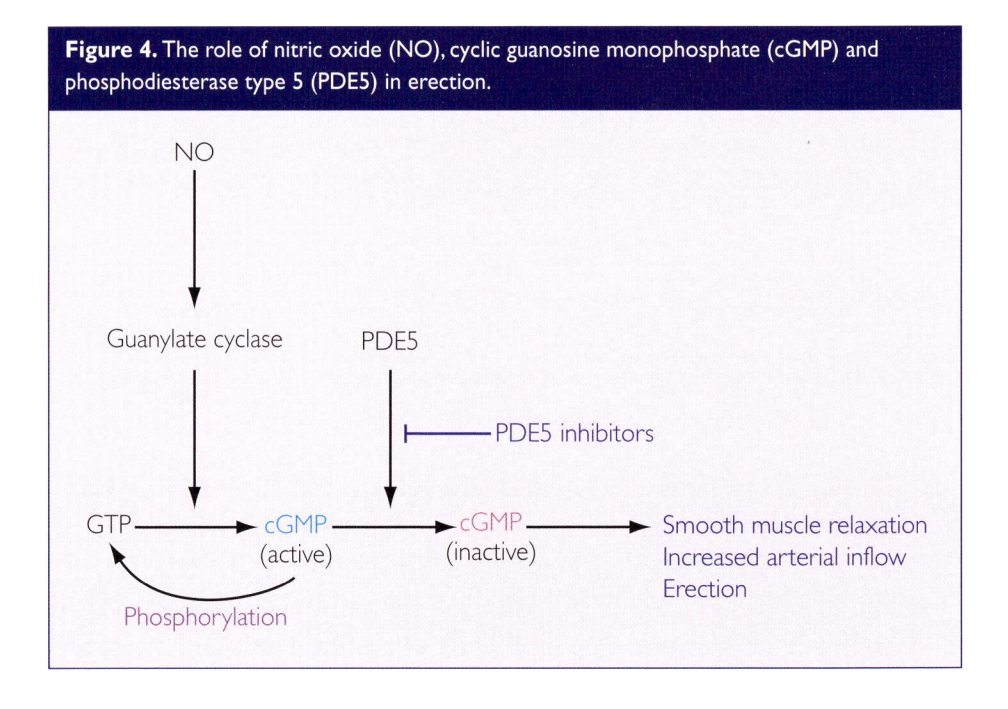

> Normal erectile function is a delicate balance between vasoconstriction and vasodilation of the smooth muscle in the corpora cavernosa.

Figure 4. The role of nitric oxide (NO), cyclic guanosine monophosphate (cGMP) and phosphodiesterase type 5 (PDE5) in erection.

cavernosal trapping of penile blood. A combination of veno-occlusive dysfunction and arterial insufficiency limits the ability of corporal smooth muscle to relax, reduces dilatation in the sinusoids and thereby reduces arterial blood flow into the penis.

Diagnosis

The Erectile Dysfunction Alliance published guidelines for the management of ED in the UK in 2000.[26] These guidelines emphasise the importance of ED as a marker for other common major diseases, such as cardiovascular disease and diabetes, and the need to provide adequate "attention, consideration, proper investigation and appropriate treatment."[26]

According to these guidelines, a critical first step in effective diagnosis of ED is a thorough history (medical, sexual and psychosocial) and physical examination (Figure 5). Such assessments should evaluate the nature of the sexual problem, in order to differentiate ED from other problems with sexual function such as premature ejaculation or loss of libido.[26] Thus, men with ED normally present with unimpaired ejaculatory function and normal libido.[27] In addition, an assessment of the nature of ED can allow the physician to accurately differentiate between psychogenic and organic ED, thereby enabling an appropriate management strategy to be determined. For example, psychogenic ED occurs suddenly and in specific situations and is accompanied by normal nocturnal and early morning erections. In contrast, organic ED is normally persistent, and is associated with loss of early morning erections.[27]

Other risk factors that should be noted when taking a medical history include:
- medical risk factors (e.g. diabetes, hypertension, hypercholesterolaemia, cardiovascular disease, spinal cord injury, peripheral vascular disease, pelvic injury/surgery, depression, trauma)
- lifestyle risk factors (e.g. smoking, alcohol and drug misuse, obesity)
- iatrogenic risk factors (e.g. thiazide diuretics, β-blockers, antidepressants).

The physical examination should focus on the genitourinary, vascular and neurological systems. Important assessments include blood pressure, heart rate and femoral pulses. Assessment of secondary sexual characteristics will indicate the adequacy of androgen concentrations, and thus whether androgen replacement is necessary. An examination of the genitalia should include checking testicular size and consistency and the presence of penile plaques and deformities to exclude disorders such as Peyronie's disease. A digital rectal examination will assist in evaluating whether the prostate is enlarged, and is particularly useful in older patients aged over 50 years.

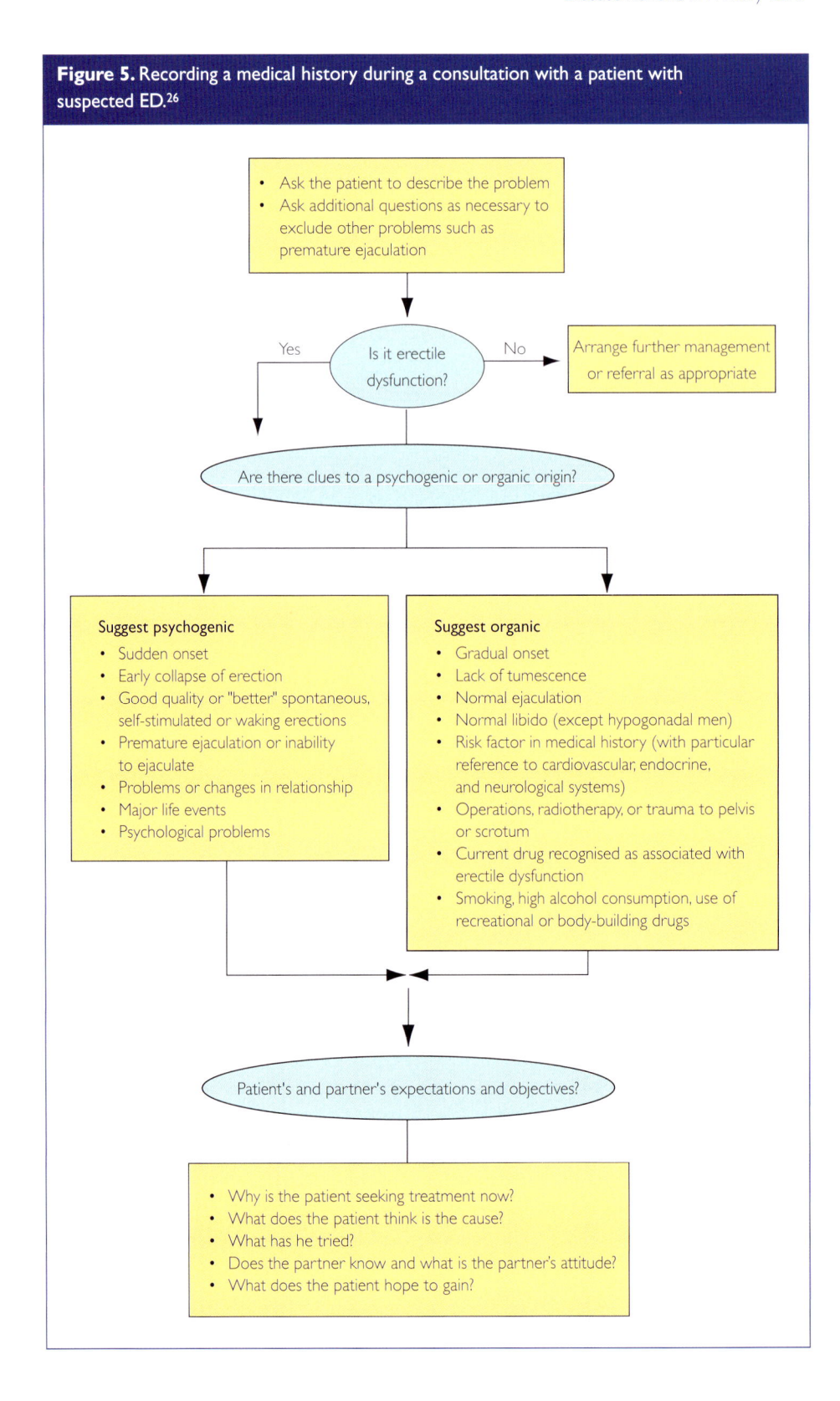

Figure 5. Recording a medical history during a consultation with a patient with suspected ED.[26]

- Ask the patient to describe the problem
- Ask additional questions as necessary to exclude other problems such as premature ejaculation

↓

Is it erectile dysfunction?

- No → Arrange further management or referral as appropriate
- Yes ↓

Are there clues to a psychogenic or organic origin?

Suggest psychogenic
- Sudden onset
- Early collapse of erection
- Good quality or "better" spontaneous, self-stimulated or waking erections
- Premature ejaculation or inability to ejaculate
- Problems or changes in relationship
- Major life events
- Psychological problems

Suggest organic
- Gradual onset
- Lack of tumescence
- Normal ejaculation
- Normal libido (except hypogonadal men)
- Risk factor in medical history (with particular reference to cardiovascular, endocrine, and neurological systems)
- Operations, radiotherapy, or trauma to pelvis or scrotum
- Current drug recognised as associated with erectile dysfunction
- Smoking, high alcohol consumption, use of recreational or body-building drugs

↓

Patient's and partner's expectations and objectives?

- Why is the patient seeking treatment now?
- What does the patient think is the cause?
- What has he tried?
- Does the partner know and what is the partner's attitude?
- What does the patient hope to gain?

A number of laboratory investigations may provide further insight into the aetiology and severity of the ED, and will also serve to assist in identifying other comorbid conditions. The determination of which laboratory investigations to perform very much depends on the information garnered during the initial medical history assessment. Investigations that may be of value include:
- fasting blood glucose or glycosylated haemoglobin (HbA_{1C})
- serum testosterone, prolactin, luteinising hormone
- thyroid, liver and renal function tests
- full blood count
- fasting lipid profile
- prostate specific antigen (PSA) testing, with appropriate counselling.

Other more specialised tests are available to diagnose ED, including imaging studies, angiography and evaluation of vascular function within the penis. However, these require specialised equipment and, therefore, usually demand referral to a urology specialist.[2]

A number of validated questionnaires have been developed which may assist in the diagnosis and allow an assessment of the severity of ED and also its response to appropriate treatment. In addition, they may promote dialogue between the patient and their physician, which is an important factor in patient management.

Such tools include the International Index of Erectile Function (IIEF), which is a sensitive, specific and standardised 15-item questionnaire that assesses five domains of male sexual function ranked by the patient on a five-point Likert scale.[28] Normal erectile function is defined as an IIEF score of 26 or greater, and thus a score below this threshold is an indication of poorer sexual and erectile function. The IIEF has been well validated across different cultural backgrounds and translated into more than ten different languages. The five domains of male sexual function assessed by the IIEF are:
- erectile function
- intercourse satisfaction
- overall satisfaction
- orgasmic function
- sexual desire.

The six questions which comprise the erectile function domain of the IIEF are shown in Table 3.

Table 3. The erectile function domain of the International Index of Erectile Function (IIEF) questionnaire.[28]

Question	Response options
Erection frequency Q1. How often were you able to get an erection during sexual activity? **Erection firmness** Q2. When you had erections with sexual stimulation, how often were your erections hard enough for penetration?	0= No sexual activity 1= Almost never/never 2= A few times (much less than half the time) 3= Sometimes (about half the time) 4= Most times (much more than half the time) 5= Almost always/always
Frequency of penetration Q3. When you attempted sexual intercourse, how often were you able to penetrate (enter) your partner? **Erection maintenance** Q4. During sexual intercourse, how often were you able to maintain your erection after you had penetrated (entered) your partner?	0= Did not attempt intercourse 1= Almost never/never 2= A few times (much less than half the time) 3= Sometimes (about half the time) 4= Most times (much more than half the time) 5= Almost always/always
Successful completion Q5. During sexual intercourse, how difficult was it to maintain your erection to completion of intercourse?	0= Did not attempt intercourse 1= Extremely difficult 2= Very difficult 3= Difficult 4= Slightly difficult 5= Not difficult
Confidence Q6. How do you rate your confidence that you could get and keep an erection?	1= Very low 2= Low 3= Moderate 4= High 5= Very high

Treatment

Over the past 30 years, significant advances have been made in the management of ED, from psychosexual therapy and penile prostheses in the 1970s, revascularisation, vacuum constriction devices and intracavernosal injection therapy in the 1980s, to transurethral and oral drug therapy in the 1990s.[2]

Despite the availability of these different treatment options, lifestyle changes represent an important first step in patient management, as poor

lifestyle choices can make a significant contribution to the condition, and can be modified with appropriate support. Whilst effective lifestyle modification can benefit the global health of an individual, the actual evidence relating to its long-term benefit in ED is limited. However, suggested lifestyle changes that can be implemented which may aid patient outcome include:
- smoking cessation
- reduction in alcohol intake
- stress management
- exercise and weight reduction
- adoption of a healthy diet
- avoidance of recreational drugs.

Effective communication and education is also a critical factor in improving patient management, and should involve both the patient and their partner wherever possible, particularly when determining a treatment strategy (Figure 6).[26] Without such an approach the patient may continue on a downward spiral with possible deterioration in their symptoms.

First-line therapy

The ultimate aim of any therapy for ED is to normalise the sexual response and free the patient from the pressure of performing sexually within a designated time frame. Many couples prefer non-invasive, easily administered treatments that are reversible and offer convenience, without impacting upon the natural spontaneity of the sexual experience. Thus, oral therapy is considered by the World Health Organization[29] and other country-specific guidelines[30–32] to be a first-line approach in the treatment of ED.

There are two main classes of oral pharmacological agents currently licensed for the management of ED in the UK: the dopamine agonist, apomorphine, which acts centrally, and the PDE5 inhibitors, which affect the local regulation of erectile function by potentiating the effects of NO. Both classes of agent have been shown to significantly enhance erectile function in clinical trials, thereby increasing the likelihood of successful sexual intercourse, independently of the aetiology or the severity of ED.

PDE5 inhibitors

Inhibitors of PDE5 were originally developed for the treatment of angina, due to their predicted vasodilatory effects on the coronary vasculature.[23] However, the first PDE5 inhibitor to be developed commercially, sildenafil,

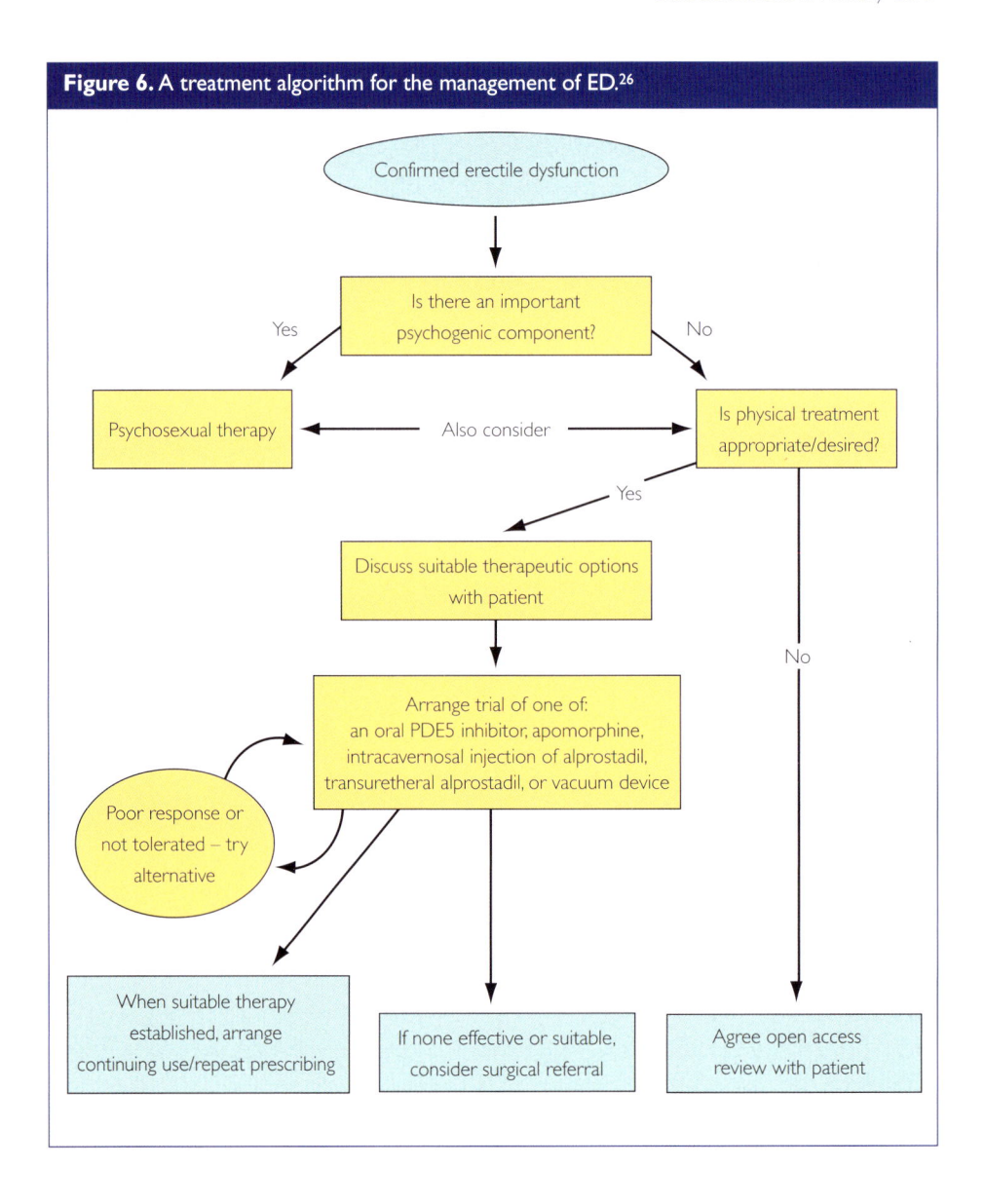

Figure 6. A treatment algorithm for the management of ED.[26]

> PDE5 inhibitors potently and selectively inhibit the breakdown of cGMP by PDE5, thereby potentiating the pro-erectile responses to NO.

was shown in clinical trials to have no effect on angina. Intriguingly, pro-erectile responses were reported by a significant number of patients, leading to its commercial development as a treatment for ED.[23]

PDE5 inhibitors potently and selectively inhibit the breakdown of cGMP by PDE5, thereby potentiating the pro-erectile responses to NO (Figure 4). As sexual arousal is necessary to stimulate the production of NO, these agents do not provide benefit in its absence. Three PDE5 inhibitors are currently licensed for use in the UK – sildenafil, tadalafil and vardenafil – and whilst clinical studies have shown that all agents offer broadly similar levels of efficacy in terms of erectile response, there are a number of differences in their pharmacodynamics and pharmacokinetics which may translate to different efficacy and safety profiles. PDE5 inhibitors are effective across a broad spectrum of patients with ED of varying severity and aetiology.

All agents in this class produce small reductions in blood pressure and are thus contraindicated in patients who are receiving organic nitrates due to the augmentation of hypotensive effects when both agents are co-administered. Likewise, concomitant administration of α-blockers, such as doxazosin, with PDE5 inhibitors has been shown to lead to symptomatic hypotension in some patients. Therefore, co-administration of PDE5 inhibitors and α-blockers should be performed with caution. PDE5 inhibitors are generally well tolerated and have similar side-effect profiles, with reported adverse events including headaches, flushing, dyspepsia and nasal congestion.

Apomorphine

Apomorphine is administered sublingually and can generate an erection within 20 minutes.[33] It acts centrally by selectively stimulating dopamine D_1 and D_2 receptors, which activate specific pro-erectile neural events within the paraventricular nucleus of the hypothalamus. Stimulation of NO and oxytocin by these processes results in relaxation of the smooth muscle in the corpora cavernosum, engorgement of the sinusoids and erection. As apomorphine is an emetic, the most common side-effects associated with its use are nausea and vomiting.[33] Apomorphine does not appear to be as effective as PDE5 inhibition in terms of erectile response.

Other oral agents

A number of other oral agents have been investigated for the treatment of ED including phentolamine (an α-adrenergic receptor blocker) and yohimbine (an $α_1/α_2$-adrenoreceptor antagonist). Phentolamine acts by shifting the balance away from α-adrenergically mediated contraction of corporal cavernosum and thus flaccidity, towards parasympathetic mechanisms, thereby activating NO synthase.[33] Yohimbine is thought to act centrally on adrenergic receptors in the brain associated with libido and penile erection. However, its use in treating ED is viewed with some suspicion. Neither phentolamine nor yohimbine are currently licensed for use in the UK for treating ED.

Psychosexual therapy

Psychosexual therapy may offer some benefit to those patients who have ED of a clear psychogenic origin or in those who refuse medical and surgical

> Psychosexual therapy may offer some benefit to those patients who have ED of a clear psychogenic origin or in those who refuse medical and surgical intervention.

intervention. It may also be useful in combination with pharmacological treatment in those with ED of mixed aetiology.[22] Its primary objective is to decrease performance anxiety by increasing the range of sexual activities not requiring an erection of sufficient rigidity for penetration, thereby increasing a couple's intimacy and their ability to openly communicate about sex.[27] Psychosexual therapy requires close co-operation of the patient and their sexual partner, and therefore its success is dependent on the motivation of both parties. Promising results are possible in the short-term, although longer-term responses have been variable.[26] In addition, psychosexual therapy can be time consuming and may only be available to limited sections of the patient population.[26]

Second-line therapy

Vasoactive drugs which can be administered both intracavernosally by injection or intraurethrally are available for those patients who do not respond to oral drug therapy or for those who cannot tolerate such agents. Indeed, intraurethral and intracavernosal therapy are now used almost exclusively in those patients who fail to respond to oral therapy.[34]

Intracavernosal alprostadil (prostaglandin E1)

Alprostadil is a synthetic prostaglandin E1 and is currently the most widely used agent given by either intracavernosal injection or by intraurethral application. It possesses vasoactive properties which generate an erection by inhibiting the prevailing α_1 adrenergic activity that promotes the smooth muscle contraction that maintains the penis in a flaccid state.

Intracavernosal injection therapy with alprostadil is effective in 60–90% of patients with ED, and is associated with a rapid onset of erection (5–15 minutes) producing erections firm enough for penetration that last 30–60 minutes.[35] However, patient comfort and education are essential elements in the success of this treatment, whilst the involvement of the patient's partner may be necessary in those with limited manual dexterity.[30] Side-effects of intracavernosal injection therapy include priapism, penile pain and fibrosis.

Intraurethral alprostadil

Recently, a semi-solid pellet formulation of alprostadil has become available and is administered transurethrally via a polypropylene applicator with a hollow stem.[35] There is a high degree of patient satisfaction with this method due to its perceived lack of invasiveness, although its clinical success is somewhat lower than that achieved with intracavernosal injection of alprostadil.[30,35] In some cases, the use of a constrictive band at the base of the penis may provide more rigid erections.

Hormone treatment

Only a small proportion of cases of ED are caused by hormone abnormalities. The most frequent hormone abnormality is a reduced level of testosterone caused by hypogonadism which can be restored by appropriate testosterone replacement. However, testosterone replacement therapy should only be reserved for patients with confirmed hypogonadism.[2]

Vacuum devices

Vacuum erection devices are a non-invasive treatment option that comprise an external cylinder which is fitted to the penis, allowing air to be pumped out, thereby promoting blood flow into the penis and subsequent erection.[26] The erection is maintained by fitting a constriction band around the base of the penis. These devices are useful in patients in whom oral therapy has failed or is unacceptable and in those who are averse to needles and other invasive therapies. However, they can be cumbersome and thus detract from the natural spontaneity of the sexual experience.

Third-line therapy

Penile prosthesis and surgery

There are two main types of penile prostheses which are inserted into the penis during surgery, and used to generate an erect state. Semi-rigid, malleable rods maintain the penis in a state of permanent rigidity, but also allow the penis to be bent out of the way when the patient is not sexually active. The inflatable implant is more sophisticated and involves insertion of a hydraulic device which causes stiffening of the penis when a pump, implanted in the scrotum, is activated. Such prostheses should only be considered in those in whom other approaches have failed or who are unwilling or unable to continue with medical treatment or external devices, because permanent damage to the erectile tissue may arise after surgery.[26] Indeed, since effective oral treatments for ED have become available, these techniques play a minimal role in patient management.

> Since effective oral treatments for ED have become available, these techniques play a minimal role in patient management.

Key points

- ED is a highly prevalent, progressive condition that is associated with a profound and negative impact on quality of life.

- ED is significantly more prevalent in older patients, although it is not an inevitable consequence of ageing. Its greater prevalence in the elderly is consistent with a greater prevalence of cardiovascular disease, diabetes and other risk factors, which are all associated with an increase in ED.

- Due to its association with many types of vascular disease and diabetes, ED is now thought to be an early warning sign for these comorbid conditions.

- Currently, ED is not effectively treated with a significant proportion of patients not seeking treatment due to the stigma associated with the condition. However, the availability of oral treatments, particularly the PDE5 inhibitors, has greatly increased awareness of the condition.

- The principal neurochemical mediator of erection is NO, and this signalling pathway serves as a useful therapeutic target in order to treat ED.

- Effective diagnosis of ED may also provide an opportunity to detect serious underlying clinical comorbidities including diabetes, CHD, hypertension and depression.

- Diagnosis should involve a targeted patient history, physical examination and appropriate laboratory investigations.

- Oral treatments, such as the PDE5 inhibitors and apomorphine, are widely considered to be the first-line agents in the treatment of ED. However, lifestyle modification also plays a critical role, as does doctor–patient communication and education.

References

1. NIH Consensus Conference. Impotence. NIH Consensus Development Panel on Impotence. *JAMA* 1993; **270**: 83–90.
2. Lue TF. Erectile dysfunction. *N Engl J Med* 2000; **342**: 1802–13.
3. Ayta IA, McKinlay JB, Krane RJ. The likely worldwide increase in erectile dysfunction between 1995 and 2025 and some possible policy consequences. *BJU Int* 1999; **84**: 50–6.
4. Giuliano F. Introduction: Advances in the treatment of erectile dysfunction. *Euro Urol Suppl* 2002; **1**: 1–3.
5. Braun M, Wassmer G, Klotz T *et al.* Epidemiology of erectile dysfunction: results of the Cologne Male Survey. *Int J Impot Res* 2000; **12**: 305–11.
6. Holmes S. Tadalafil: a new treatment for erectile dysfunction. *BJU Int* 2003; **91**: 466–8.
7. Shabsigh R. Recent developments in male sexual dysfunction. *Curr Psychiatry Rep* 2000; **2**: 196–200.
8. Goldmeier D, Keane FE, Carter P *et al.* Prevalence of sexual dysfunction in heterosexual patients attending a central London genitourinary medicine clinic. *Int J STD AIDS* 1997; **8**: 303–6.
9. Green JS, Holden ST, Ingram P *et al.* An investigation of erectile dysfunction in Gwent, Wales. *BJU Int* 2001; **88**: 551–3.
10. Kaye JA, Jick H. Incidence of erectile dysfunction and characteristics of patients before and after the introduction of sildenafil in the United Kingdom: cross sectional study with comparison patients. *BMJ* 2003; **326**: 424–5.
11. Feldman HA, Goldstein I, Hatzichristou DG, Krane RJ, McKinlay JB. Impotence and its medical and psychosocial correlates: results of the Massachusetts Male Aging Study. *J Urol* 1994; **151**: 54–61.
12. Johannes CB, Araujo AB, Feldman HA *et al.* Incidence of erectile dysfunction in men 40 to 69 years old: longitudinal results from the Massachusetts male aging study. *J Urol* 2000; **163**: 460–3.
13. Kubin M, Wagner G, Fugl-Meyer AR. Epidemiology of erectile dysfunction. *Int J Impot Res* 2003; **15**: 63–71.
14. Porst H. Restoring a normal sexual response: The ultimate goal of erectile dysfunction therapy. *Eur Urol Suppl* 2002; **1**: 19–24.
15. Kirby M. Management of erectile dysfunction in men with cardiovascular disease. *Br J Cardiol* 2003; **10**: 305–7.
16. Fugl-Meyer AR, Lodnert G, Branholm IB, Fugl-Meyer KS. On life satisfaction in male erectile dysfunction. *Int J Impot Res* 1997; **9**: 141–8.
17. Nurnberg HG, Seidman SN, Gelenberg AJ *et al.* Depression, antidepressant therapies, and erectile dysfunction: clinical trials of sildenafil citrate (Viagra) in treated and untreated patients with depression. *Urology* 2002; **60**: 58–66.
18. Melman A, Gingell JC. The epidemiology and pathophysiology of erectile dysfunction. *J Urol* 1999; **161**: 5–11.
19. Kaiser FE. Erectile dysfunction in the aging man. *Med Clin North Am* 1999; **83**: 1267–78.
20. Brock GB. Issues in the assessment and treatment of erectile dysfunction: individualising and optimizing therapy for "the silent majority". *Rete Reviews* 2002; **1**: 1–70.
21. Kim S, Narayanan S, Song JC. Tadalafil. *Formulary* 2002; **37**: 289.
22. Wagner G, Saenz de Tejada I. Update on male erectile dysfunction. *BMJ* 1998; **316**: 678–82.
23. Rosen RC, McKenna KE. PDE-5 inhibition and sexual response: pharmacological mechanisms and clinical outcomes. *Annu Rev Sex Res* 2002; **13**: 36–88.
24. Moreland RB, Hsieh G, Nakane M, Brioni JD. The biochemical and neurologic basis for the treatment of male erectile dysfunction. *J Pharmacol Exp Ther* 2001; **296**: 225–34.
25. Rajfer J, Aronson WJ, Bush PA, Dorey FJ, Ignarro LJ. Nitric oxide as a mediator of relaxation of the corpus cavernosum in response to nonadrenergic, noncholinergic neurotransmission. *N Engl J Med* 1992; **326**: 90–4.
26. Ralph D, McNicholas T. UK management guidelines for erectile dysfunction. *BMJ* 2000; **321**: 499–503.
27. Kirby RS. Impotence: diagnosis and management of male erectile dysfunction. *BMJ* 1994; **308**: 957–61.
28. Rosen RC, Riley A, Wagner G *et al.* The international index of erectile function (IIEF): a multidimensional scale for assessment of erectile dysfunction. *Urology* 1997; **49**: 822–30.
29. Jardin A, Wagner G, Khoury S *et al.* Recommendations of the First International Consultation on Erectile Dysfunction, co-sponsored by the World Health Organization (WHO). Plymouth: Health Publications Ltd, 2000.
30. Wespes E, Amar E, Hatzichristou D *et al.* Guidelines on erectile dysfunction. *Eur Urol* 2002; **41**: 1–5.
31. The Process of Care Consensus Panel. The process of care model for evaluation and treatment of erectile dysfunction. *Int J Impot Res* 1999; **11**: 59–70.
32. Erectile dysfunction practice guidelines. *Can J Urol* 2002; **9**: 1583–7.
33. Vitezic D, Pelcic JM. Erectile dysfunction: oral pharmacotherapy options. *Int J Clin Pharmacol Ther* 2002; **40**: 393–403.
34. Montorsi F, Salonia A, Deho F *et al.* Pharmacological management of erectile dysfunction. *BJU Int* 2003; **91**: 446–54.
35. Cohan P, Korenman SG. Erectile dysfunction. *J Clin Endocrinol Metab* 2001; **86**: 2391–4.

Acknowledgements

Figures 5 and 6 are adapted from Ralph and McNicholas, 2000.[26]

Notes

Notes